1991
YEAR BOOK OF
SURGERY®

The 1991 Year Book® Series

Year Book of Anesthesia®: Drs. Miller, Kirby, Ostheimer, Roizen, and Stoelting

Year Book of Cardiology®: Drs. Schlant, Collins, Engle, Frye, Kaplan, and O'Rourke

Year Book of Critical Care Medicine®: Drs. Rogers and Parrillo

Year Book of Dentistry®: Drs. Meskin, Currier, Kennedy, Leinfelder, Matukas, and Rovin

Year Book of Dermatology®: Drs. Sober and Fitzpatrick

Year Book of Diagnostic Radiology®: Drs. Hendee, Keats, Kirkpatrick, Miller, Osborn, Reed, and Thompson

Year Book of Digestive Diseases®: Drs. Greenberger and Moody

Year Book of Drug Therapy®: Drs. Lasagna and Weintraub

Year Book of Emergency Medicine®: Drs. Wagner, Burdick, Davidson, Roberts, and Spivey

Year Book of Endocrinology®: Drs. Bagdade, Braverman, Halter, Horton, Kannan, Molitch, Morley, Odell, Rogol, Ryan, and Sherwin

Year Book of Family Practice®: Drs. Berg, Bowman, Dietrich, Green, and Scherger

Year Book of Geriatrics and Gerontology®: Drs. Beck, Abrass, Burton, Cummings, Makinodan, and Small

Year Book of Hand Surgery®: Drs. Dobyns, Chase, and Amadio

Year Book of Health Care Management: Drs. Heyssel, King, and Steinberg, Ms. Avakian, and Messrs. Berman, Brock, Kues, and Rosenberg

Year Book of Hematology®: Drs. Spivak, Bell, Ness, Quesenberry, and Wiernik

Year Book of Infectious Diseases®: Drs. Wolff, Barza, Keusch, Klempner, and Snydman

Year Book of Infertility: Drs. Mishell, Paulsen, and Lobo

Year Book of Medicine®: Drs. Rogers, Des Prez, Cline, Braunwald, Greenberger, Utiger, Epstein, and Malawista

Year Book of Neonatal and Perinatal Medicine: Drs. Klaus and Fanaroff

Year Book of Neurology and Neurosurgery®: Drs. Currier and Crowell

Year Book of Nuclear Medicine®: Drs. Hoffer, Gore, Gottschalk, Sostman, Zaret, and Zubal

Year Book of Obstetrics and Gynecology®: Drs. Mishell, Kirschbaum, and Morrow

1991

The Year Book of SURGERY®

Editor

Seymour I. Schwartz, M.D.
Professor and Chair, Department of Surgery, University of Rochester, School of Medicine and Dentistry

Associate Editors

Olga Jonasson, M.D.
Robert M. Zollinger Professor and Chair, Department of Surgery, The Ohio State University, Columbus

Martin C. Robson, M.D.
Chief of Division of Plastic Surgery, University of Texas Medical Branch, Galveston

G. Tom Shires, M.D.
Professor and Chairman, Department of Surgery, New York Hospital—Cornell Medical Center

Frank C. Spencer, M.D.
George David Stewart Professor of Surgery; Chairman, Department of Surgery, New York University; Director, Department of Surgery, New York University Medical Center and Bellevue Hospital

James C. Thompson, M.D.
John Woods Harris Professor and Chairman, Department of Surgery; Chief of Surgery, University Hospitals, The University of Texas Medical Branch, Galveston

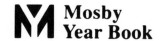

Mosby Year Book

St. Louis   Baltimore   Boston   Chicago   London   Philadelphia   Sydney   Toronto

Editor-in-Chief, Year Book Publishing: Nancy Gorham
Sponsoring Editor: Carla L. White
Manager, Medical Information Services: Edith M. Podrazik
Senior Medical Information Specialist: Terri Strorigl
Senior Medical Writer: David A. Cramer, M.D.
Assistant Director, Manuscript Services: Frances M. Perveiler
Associate Managing Editor, Year Book Editing Services: Elizabeth Fitch
Production Coordinator: Max F. Perez
Proofroom Manager: Barbara M. Kelly

Editorial Office:
Mosby–Year Book, Inc.
200 North LaSalle St.
Chicago IL 60601

International Standard Serial Number: 0090-3671
International Standard Book Number: 0-8151-7790-9

Table of Contents

The material covered in this volume represents literature reviewed up to November 1990.

Journals Represented

Mosby–Year Book subscribes to and surveys nearly 850 U.S. and foreign medical and allied health journals. From these journals, the Editors select the articles to be abstracted. Journals represented in this YEAR BOOK are listed below.

Acta Chirurgica Scandinavica
American Journal of Clinical Pathology
American Journal of Epidemiology
American Journal of Pathology
American Journal of Physiology
American Journal of Surgery
American Surgeon
Anesthesiology
Annals of Emergency Medicine
Annals of Internal Medicine
Annals of Plastic Surgery
Annals of Surgery
Annals of Thoracic Surgery
Annals of the Royal College of Surgeons of England
Archives of Otolaryngology–Head and Neck Surgery
Archives of Pathology and Laboratory Medicine
Archives of Surgery
Blood
British Journal of Haematology
British Journal of Plastic Surgery
British Journal of Surgery
British Medical Journal
Burns
Canadian Journal of Cardiology
Cancer
Cancer Research
Circulation
Circulatory Shock
Clinical Imaging
Contemporary Orthopedics
Digestive Diseases and Sciences
European Journal of Plastic Surgery
European Journal of Vascular Surgery
Gastroenterology
Head and Neck
Heart and Vessels
Infections in Surgery
International Journal of Radiation, Oncology, Biology, and Physics
Journal of Burn Care and Rehabilitation
Journal of Cardiac Surgery
Journal of Cardiovascular Surgery
Journal of Clinical Endocrinology and Metabolism
Journal of Computer Assisted Tomography
Journal of Cranio-Maxillo-Facial Surgery
Journal of Experimental Medicine
Journal of Heart Transplantation
Journal of Immunology
Journal of Investigative Dermatology

Journal of Laboratory and Clinical Medicine
Journal of Paediatrics & Child Health
Journal of Parenteral and Enteral Nutrition
Journal of Pathology
Journal of Pediatric Surgery
Journal of Surgical Research
Journal of Thoracic and Cardiovascular Surgery
Journal of Trauma
Journal of Vascular Surgery
Journal of the American College of Cardiology
Journal of the American Medical Association
Journal of the Royal College of Surgeons of Edinburgh
Laboratory Investigation
Lancet
Laryngoscope
Mayo Clinic Proceedings
Nephrology, Dialysis, Transplantation
New England Journal of Medicine
Plastic and Reconstructive Surgery
Respiratory Medicine
Scandinavian Journal of Plastic and Reconstructive Surgery and Hand Surgery
Scandinavian Journal of Thoracic and Cardiovascular Surgery
Science
Southern Medical Journal
Surgery
Surgery, Gynecology and Obstetrics
Surgical Research Communications
Transplantation
Ultrasound in Medicine and Biology
World Journal of Surgery

STANDARD ABBREVIATIONS

The following terms are abbreviated in this edition: acquired immunodeficiency syndrome (AIDS), central nervous system (CNS), cerebrospinal fluid (CSF), computed tomography (CT), electrocardiography (ECG), human immunodeficiency virus (HIV).

Annual Overview

General Considerations

A strong case is made for performing elective surgery without transfusion if at all possible. It has been emphasized that the chronically anemic patient has already compensated by increasing stroke volume, and it is not appropriate to "prophylactically" transfuse a patient unless there is an anticipated major blood loss. As prediction of myocardial infarction assumes a greater importance in an aging population, dipyridamole thallium imaging has been shown to be superior to exercise testing and clinical variables for predicting cardiac events related to surgery. A long-term study of the effects of partial ileal bypass has demonstrated significant reductions in plasma cholesterol that persist for prolonged periods of time. The rise in high-density lipoprotein cholesterol associated with this approach is relatively low, and it is known that the rise significantly correlates with myocardial infarction.

Seymour I. Schwartz, M.D.

Shock

Studies during the past year on the mechanisms and management of shock continue to comprise a significant amount of research effort. At the present time, such studies are focusing primarily on mediators as a major source of mortality related to hemorrhagic shock. The role of resuscitation, on the other hand, is focusing increasingly on better access, more rapid transportation, and the composition of fluids required for resuscitation. Insofar as resuscitation is concerned, there is a continuing effort to develop the use of an intraosseous infusion device, particularly for children and for small-volume initial fluid resuscitation in adults. A self-tapping unit was devised that seems to work well in this regard. This device was developed, however, largely in an attempt to increase the use of small-volume infusion in the prehospital setting with hypertonic saline. The continuing studies on hypertonic saline indicate once again that the increased blood pressure and powerful peripheral vasodilatation brought about by hypertonic saline does, at least in the experimental setting, increase blood pressure and increase early mortality. The utility of a volume of hypertonic saline that is approximately only half the volume of isotonic fluid usually administered is really seriously in doubt.

The benefit of hypothermia in hemorrhagic shock continues to be evaluated. Studies this year indicate that modest hypothermia, that is more than 33° C, may well be a protective mechanism in hemorrhagic shock, whereas severe hypothermia below 33° C may be deleterious. One has to be concerned about any hypothermia at all, however, in view of the fact that only mild hypothermia, which may be physiologically protective, is damaging to platelet function, which may lead to serious bleeding in the injured patient who has sustained shock.

A tremendous number of articles have appeared in the past year in relation to the mediator tumor necrosis factor (TNF) and its relationship to bacterial translocation. Many studies now indicate that translocated bacteria from the intestine, spurred on by hemorrhagic shock or sepsis at a different and remote site, may well be a major factor in the development of multiple organ failure and adult respiratory distress syndrome (ARDS) following injury. Labeled *Escherichia coli* organisms indicate early translocation in hemorrhagic shock. Among the many factors that influence removal of the gut barrier to translocation appears to be reduced intestinal blood flow. Others certainly include the immunocompromised state; in addition, the presence of malnutrition or some specific drug therapy may alter the flora of the intestine and enable bacterial translocation to occur.

The exact relationship of bacterial translocation to TNF elaboration is yet to be worked out, but it certainly appears that TNF elaboration is one of the stress hormones responsive to shock and trauma; it may be the most important one, however, because it has been shown clearly that TNF can cause ARDS. Other specific studies (e.g., acid aspiration injury) also indicate clearly that TNF is the mediator even in this direct pulmonary injury. Studies continue to show that the monocyte is a major source for the elaboration of TNF; therefore, even though TNF is a paracrine substance with monocytes being the organ of production, it is clear that this mediator can be formed in any organ.

There are continuing attempts to identify early the immunosuppression that occurs in response to injury. It appears that the macrophage is a major source of the immunologic changes, and immunotherapy is being tried with varying degrees of success.

Trauma

Good clinical research related to better management of specific injuries continues in abundance. More outcome data are appearing with regard to mode of transportation of the injured. Studies this year indicate that if an intensive care unit setting is available with the necessary personnel, whether in a helicopter or in an even longer-range fixed wing aircraft, the results are far superior to those associated with any other mode of transportation. Combining such data with previously documented studies showing that patients have a better outcome when treated in a trauma center, the benefits of intensive care while moving patients to trauma centers become very significant.

Several studies this year evaluated the use of the acute physiology and chronic health evaluation (APACHE) system for predicting the outcome from injuries or intensive care of severely ill patients and indicated that this system does not predict either multiple organ failure or death in any meaningful way. As a consequence, its usefulness is probably not sustained. This system would not predict the need for operation or other therapeutic approach, or the number of days required in intensive care. Any predictive value simply could not be demonstrated in these studies.

Articles continue to appear annually examining the use of presumptive antibiotics in the traumatized patient. The word presumptive is used because the antibiotics are not present at the time of injury, but are given, rather on the presumption that the injury will certainly cause bacterial contamination. Studies indicate that short-term presumptive antibiotics are still a logical form of therapy, but at least in one study there was an indication that the short-term antibiotic should be given in high doses.

Another study indicates that, although patients over the age of 65 have a decreased incidence of trauma, their morbidity and mortality rates are higher. This should serve to increase the focus on the active, immediate, and aggressive care of the injured elderly patient.

Diagnostic peritoneal lavage continues to stand the test of time. Several studies again this year show that it is a highly sensitive diagnostic test that is low in cost, rapid, accurate, safe, avoids disruptions in patient care with other forms of evaluation or views, and is particularly useful in evaluating patients with blunt abdominal trauma. Other articles continue to indicate that the presence of red blood cells in significant numbers is probably the only valid correlate to come from the diagnostic peritoneal lavage fluid.

Controversy continues to swirl about the management of penetrating neck injuries. As more data are accumulated, it still appears that if the platysma muscle is violated, particularly in zone II, operative exploration remains the safest method of management.

Other recent articles indicate that the degree of splenic damage demonstrated after injury by computerized axial tomography (CAT) scan is not a good predictor of which patients can safely be observed and which need operative intervention. It appears more and more than this decision must be an operative one, and if much blood is required, these patients should probably be operated on earlier. A further limitation of CAT scanning becomes more apparent when intestinal injuries are present. More and more series indicate that intestinal injury, even with free perforation, is not well diagnosed by CAT scanning.

The problem with deep vein thrombosis in the traumatized patient continues to be assessed. Current studies indicate that the incidence rises with increasing age. However, because most such prospective studies with venography show the presence of clots, the incidence of pulmonary embolism is quite low and prophylactic anticoagulation should probably be limited, therefore, to a few groups who are at high risk for significant deep venous thrombosis.

There are continuing articles this year on the utility of the atrial caval shunt when dealing with retrohepatic venous injuries. When trauma centers have such shunts immediately available in the operating room, more and more survivors are being reported. Similarly, the use of a closed suction drainage device, such as the Jackson-Pratt device, appears to result in a lower incidence of subsequent infection than use of an open sump drainage.

Although the management of severe intra-abdominal trauma has tended to be more and more conservative, there are still times when heroic efforts (e.g., doing an atrial caval shunt or pancreaticoduodenectomy) are the only way to salvage patients with severe combined or multiple intra-abdominal injuries.

Fluid Electrolytes and Nutrition

For the third year in a row there continue to be examinations of appropriate amino acid concentratios and compositions in total parenteral nutrition. The selective addition of branched chain amino acids in this kind of support offers no benefit over the standard amino acid mixtures.

Specific studies on energy expenditure in patients with sepsis and trauma continue to reveal the variety of responses that are not always hypermetabolic. In fact, several groups of patients have been studied in whom there is hypometabolism in the face of sepsis or trauma. As a consequence, it would appear that reliance on formulas for determining the need for excessive caloric replacement needs to be reexamined. Probably, direct measurement of resting energy expenditure will be needed to optimize therapy and minimize complications.

Interest continues on the value of human growth hormone in improving nutrition in patients receiving total parenteral nutrition. Better and longer-term studies on the protein-sparing effect of growth hormone, resulting probably from oxidation of fat in preference to protein, are badly needed.

Wound Healing

The past year was the year for recombinant technology to come to the forefront of wound healing. This technology has allowed various peptide growth factors to be manufactured in large amounts. At least 32 such growth factors have now been isolated. Animal models of impaired healing allow "windows" to be opened, permitting observations to be made. Growth factors such as bFGF, PDGF, TGF_B, and EGF can be used singly, or in combination, to effect improvement in some process of healing. From the various studies reported, it is clear that wound healing must be divided into processes such as angiogenesis, inflammation, fibroplasia, extracellular matrix definition, contraction, and epithelialization. This will allow the surgeon to be much more sophisticated in attempts at wound modulation.

As the various humoral substances are being elucidated, so are the cellular factors in wound healing. Lymphocytes are being investigated, and various subsets reportedly have different roles both in normal healing and in proliferative scar formation, as reported by Linares.

Because of the increase in knowledge of wound healing, the possibility is rapidly approaching that clinicians will be able to modulate wound repair. Clinical trials of some of the recombinant products have not yet been published, but the past year did see the report of an autologous platelet-derived formula rich in growth factors. Clinical trials with these new wound healing agents will be difficult to control; however, we will read of many in the coming year. Just as normal healing will be modified, scar formation may also be affected. Therefore, a new look at keloid and hypertrophic scar formation is included.

The problem of fetal wound repair remains perplexing, but a single paper appears to yield many answers. However, species are different, and contradictory findings may be forthcoming. Also, the time of gestation for wound healing events differs. At present, the usefulness of fetal wound healing information is questionable, except to the specialist in fetal surgery.

Infection

One of the most interesting papers to emerge this past year was one on methicillin-resistant *Staphylococcus aureus* (MRSA). The authors from the United States Army Institute for Surgical Research showed that, although methicillin resistance is a convenient marker, MRSA should not enjoy such notoriety. It is exquisitely sensitive to vancomycin and should not require the expensive efforts presently attributed to its management.

An organism that remains a problem is *Candida*. Because drugs used to treat candidemia are often toxic, an early accurate diagnosis would be useful. The use of the polymerase chain reaction may be more accurate and more rapid than standard fungal cultures.

Novel ways to deliver antibiotics were also reported this year. Among the most promising was a paper on liposomes. The slow release of antibiotics from liposomes appeared to be life-saving in a rodent model of peritonitis. Another delivery system, reported by Russell, is transference of a muscle flap into an infected fibrotic abscess cavity. This allowed high levels of systemically administered antibiotics to be delivered into a relatively avascular space. Clinically, the use of vascularized muscle to eradicate infection continues to be reported. One-stage débridement and flap closure of the infected mediastinum proved to be more efficacious than staged procedures.

Warnings have appeared about certain age-old practices. Occlusive dressings were shown to entrap bacteria and increase infection rates. These dressings are safe only over clean wounds; when placed over contaminated wounds they function to close over an abscess. A nice study was reported pointing out the potential dangers of bone wax. In addition to infection, these include pulmonary emboli, inflammatory cysts, fibrosis, inhibition of osteogenesis, and, potentially, nonunion.

A refreshing article in this day of worrying about infectious postoperative complications is a report of more than 700 operations on morbidly obese patients, with a very low infection rate resulting. The author gives helpful hints on keeping infections at a minimum and outlines subtle changes to be aware of for early diagnosis.

Burns

The American Burn Association updated the guidelines this year to describe the resources needed to operate a burn center to achieve optimal patient care. Although standards are not popular, the United States delivers the best burn care in the world, and these standards should be required reading for all who care for thermally injured patients.

The pathophysiology of burn injury continues to be of interest. Lipid peroxidation products and cytokines are produced as a result of thermal trauma. These remain longer than originally thought and their exact role is not clear. Many of the oxidants are hamrful, as are cytokines, e.g., TNF. Exactly how to deal with these harmful metabolites awaits further research.

Metabolism after burns and trauma is the concern of many investigators. From resuscitation and wound closure to nutrition, postburn hypermetabolism is a problem. A new resuscitation regimen has been suggested using hypertonic saline dextran instead of isotonic fluid alone. Stable isotope technology is a noninvasive method that may allow comparisons of various resuscitative techniques. Possibly, this technology will allow a study of blood turnover to determine accurate losses from the thermal injury vs. loss from therapeutic maneuvers. Lack of the ability to measure operative blood loss meticulously has made comparison of operative techniques difficult. An attempt made to measure such loss suggested that early massive burn wound excision resulted in less blood loss than when excision was performed later on in the burn course.

An interesting paper was presented by McCauley dealing with burn alopecia. The group described a large series and classified the alopecia for treatment purposes. This paper reported the largest series of patients with burn alopecia corrected by tissue expansion and outlines the benefits of that experience.

Bacterial translocation was thought by many to be a complication of burns only in the experimental animal. During the year, Deitch reported conclusive evidence that this phenomenon can occur after uncomplicated thermal injury in man. Unfortunately, the methodology of this report required the patients to be fasting, and early enteral feeding may be one of the best ways to prevent bacterial translocation. Therefore, although the paper appears to answer the question definitively, the answer may still be yes, maybe.

Transplantation

Clinical transplantation received great recognition in October 1990 when Joseph E. Murray and E. Donnell Thomas won the 1990 Nobel Prize in Medicine for their pioneering clinical procedures in kidney and bone marrow transplantation, respectively. Organ transplantation, first performed successfully in the 1950s, is now the treatment of choice for many otherwise fatal conditions; it is one of the most common surgical procedures performed in many large medical centers.

In fact, organ transplantation has become so desirable that major problems of access to transplantation face many patients, given that the supply of donor organs remains sharply limited. More than 20,000 patients are on waiting lists for organs, including 18,000 potential kidney recipients and 1,000 to 2,000 potential liver and heart recipients. Loosening of indications for liver transplantation to include patients with alcoholic liver disease has been especially controversial, as has the use of living related donors for liver and pancreatic transplantation.

The social and political issues of organ donation and distribution remain at the forefront of problems for the transplantation community. With reauthorization of the National Organ Transplant Act and renewal of the contract for the Organ Procurement and Transplantation Network with the United Network for Organ Sharing, more emphasis will be placed on implementation of uniform standards for organ distribution, and we hope, for improved organ donation. In this regard, the efforts of Callender and others in improving the participation of minority populations in organ donation is especially noteworthy. The present emphasis on organ distribution based on HLA phenotype when a good match is available places some ethnic minorities at a disadvantage because their HLA phenotypes differ from the largely Caucasian donor pool. Also, socioeconomic factors have had an adverse impact on rates of organ transplantation for economically disadvantaged patients.

Matching donors with recipients on the basis of HLA and phenotype remains controversial, especially because the success rates of all allograft procedures is now high, at least for the first two years. The polymorphism of the HLA system is so great that "perfect matches" are unrealistic; there is a report of rejection of a bone marrow transplant related to a single amino acid difference in an HLA-DR antigen, and micropolymorphisms are present in many defined HLA phenotypes. Nonetheless, as discussed in the chapter on Transplantation, when strict criteria for definition of a good match are used, there continues to be a clear graft survival advantage not outweighed by modern immunosuppressive therapy.

There have been a number of advances in immunosuppression. Monoclonal antibodies to the T cell receptor anti-CD4 interfere with T cell triggering and initiation of the immune response. Antibodies to the interleukin-2 receptor selectively destroy activated lymphocytes. These agents are now in trials either in primate systems or clinically. New immunosuppressive agents with actions similar or related to the actions of cyclosporine have also received clinical trials, and the reports about FK506 from Pittsburgh are encouraging. Late failures of allografts are largely caused by rejection and, unfortunately, many of these are because of the patient's noncompliance with the immunosuppressive regimen. Of considerable concern is the increasing incidence of viral-related lymphomas, seen especially in recipients of extrarenal organs in whom immunosuppression is likely to be intense. Thus, although today's immunosuppression is vastly superior to that of even a decade ago, the current regimens are far from ideal; immunosuppression must be continued indefinitely, often at prohibitive cost, and global immunosuppression removes important host surveillance mechanisms. The report of Barker's group is of special interest in this context. By inoculating pancreatic islet cells into the thymus while simultaneously administering antilymphocyte serum to the recipient to deplete the peripheral circulation of T cells and accelerate stem cell traffic into the thymus, a state of tolerance appears to have been induced. Other experimental approaches to selective immunosuppression are under active investigation.

Transplantation of the small bowel remains experimental, with no reports as yet of long-term success in humans. Experience in large animal models continues to be encouraging, and discussion now revolves around the indications for small bowel transplantation, especially in children, given the reasonably good maintenance achieved with parenteral nutrition. Transplantation of the pancreas also remains controversial. As stated in an editorial in the *Lancet* (335:1371–1372, 1990): "Before advocating early pancreas transplantation it is necessary to show that the gains in terms of prevention of severe complications of diabetes justify the risks of surgery and lifelong immunosuppression." Islet transplantation in an immunoprotected form, or even gene therapy, for instance, insertion of the insulin gene into fibroblasts, may be a better alternative. At present, however, the morbidity and mortality of pancreas transplantation continue to fall, and patients with successful pancreas transplants achieve a much improved quality of life, even though the complications of the disease are unaffected.

Tumor Immunology

Advances in molecular biology and molecular genetics have provided many new insights into carcinogenesis, growth, and spread of tumors. Control of cells by growth factors, the importance of cell-to-cell contact, and the mechanisms of cell interaction and adhesion have been of special interest because the receptors for the factors involved may prove to be targets for directed therapy. The role of macrophages and cytokines such as TNF and the interleukins, in cytolysis and immune surveillance are of increasing interest. Monoclonal antibodies to the receptors or to the factors themselves, or molecular analogues, can be used as immunotoxins to carry isotopes or endotoxins to the specific cells of interest. Genetic engineering techniques have been applied to modify monoclonal antibodies to reduce immune elimination by replacing much of the mouse sequences with human groups.

The promise of genetic engineering, replacing key elements of mutant oncogenes, for instance, came closer to reality with the seminal report of gene transfer into humans by Rosenberg and his colleagues at the National Cancer Institute. Using the model of immunotherapy of melanoma with expanded clones of tumor-infiltrating lymphocytes (TIL), the genome of the TIL was modified by introduction of a genetic marker, resistance to an antibiotic, by a harmless retrovirus. Other genes could be introduced instead of the inert marker, for instance, the genes for cytokines or adhesion molecules that could improve the TIL cytotoxic effect. The demonstration that this technique is safe for humans opens the door to many possibilities of gene therapy for a variety of diseases.

Another promising and ingenious approach to cancer therapy has been the use of monoclonal antibodies conjugated with toxins or with iron to sweep bone marrow of metastatic cancer cells before reinfusion into patients who have been treated with lethal chemotherapy. Also, bone marrow stem cell colony-stimulating factors can improve the proportion of hematopoietic stem cells in the infusate and in the patient. Surprisingly good results are reported by a number of groups, and large clinical trials are beginning. Breast cancer and lung cancer are especially appropriate for these approaches.

Immunotherapy of cancer long has been a frustration. With these new approaches made possible by the advances in molecular biology and genetics, some real progress in the understanding and treatment of cancer has been recorded during this past year.

Skin

Noninvasive techniques to sample skin in various normal and pathologic conditions may soon be available. Ultrasonic measurements made with a laser acoustic microscope combined with nuclear magnetic resonance spectroscopy allow such "sampling" to occur and may provide the answer to many questions in the near future.

Substitutes for skin continue to be sought. Questions still abound concerning cultured epithelial grafts. It appears that a dermal substitute will be required. Even with an adequate dermal substitute, the epithelial layer must stick to the dermis and proliferate. The matrix peptide RGD was suggested as a means to solve this problem.

Until a successful skin substitute is found, flaps and tissue expansion are still reported. Manders and his group reported that immediate tissue expansion is not as good as originally thought and probably is no better than wide undermining. Multiple free tissue transfers performed simultaneously appear to be cost effective and may perform the need for closure of very large defects. When such large defects are closed by conventional flaps, tissue necrosis is a frequent complication. This year, electrical nerve stimulation (ENS) was suggested as a way to prevent ischemic necrosis. The paper was not totally convincing, but it was enticing enough to hold hope for the future, if substantiated by controlled trials.

Two interesting papers on malignant melanoma were chosen for review. A study of all the various classifications of melanoma revealed that a combination of tumor thickness and depth of invasion had the best prognostic ability. It is hoped that this paper will end the search for more classifications. Another definitive paper appeared this year demonstrating that "wide" margins are unnecessary to control malignant melanoma. This is so important to realize if the patient is going to be offered flap reconstruction after ablation. Because all recent papers are in agreement, we hope that practicing surgeons will soon act as though they agree with the data.

Breast

The efficacy of perioperative antibiotic prophylaxis for patients undergoing excision of a breast mass, mastectomy, or herniorrhaphy was assessed, and it was concluded that perioperative antibiotic prophylaxis with Cephonacid was useful as a method of reducing postoperative wound infection. It has been shown that the nipple discharges associated in greater degree with malignancy are those that are either clear and watery or serosanguinous. A case is made for the routine excision of fibroadenomas of the breast. Only 1 of 10 cases of cystosarcoma phalloides represents a malignant lesion. The issue of axillary dissection as a routine approach for these patients remains controversial.

A study of the natural history of in situ breast carcinoma indicates that the ductal in situ and lobular carcinomas have similar courses, and that lymph node dissection is unnecessary. A study of patients who underwent breast biopsy for calcifications in nonpalpable lesions indicates that the Wolfe pattern on mammography had no relationship to the incidence of malignancy. There was a marked correlation between malignancy and more than 15 calcifications, or calcifications that appeared in a linear or branching pattern.

Assessing the outcome of surgery for nonpalpable mammographic abnormalities, it has been demonstrated that if the specimen radiograph does not show the mammographic abnormality within the pieces of tissues excised and there is no palpable nodule, it may be best to conclude the biopsy because the missed lesions are usually benign. Levels I and II axillary dissection without clearance of the axillary vein is sufficient in the staging of early-stage breast cancer and reduces morbidity. Although the standard for patients undergoing conservative breast surgery is the addition of radiation, data from a series of patients suggests that postoperative radiotherapy may not be required in every patient treated by segmental mastectomy. The issue of systemic therapy in patients with node negative breast cancer remains controversial with some groups suggesting that all women with node-negative breast cancer, whether positive or negative for estrogen receptor, should receive systemic therapy. This form of breast cancer remains a disease with an extremely poor prognosis. The data suggest that patients receiving chemotherapy before local therapy or mastectomy have a significantly improved 5-year survival.

Head and Neck

Prevention of head and neck cancer will eventually prove more useful than treatment. Prevention of second primary tumors was the subject of a study using isotretinoin. Its use suggested a decrease in the appearance of a second primary tumor. If these data hold up in a larger study population, it will be a significant advance.

Treatment papers were prevalent. Postoperative radiotherapy, reported from Memorial Sloan-Kettering Cancer Center, was effective in stages III and IV salivary gland tumors. Modified neck dissections again were demonstrated to be efficacious in patients with clinically N_0 necks. Stages T_{1-3}, N_0, M_0 supraglottic laryngeal tumors respond well to radiotherapy alone, allowing voice preservation. Another interesting paper on tumor therapy discussed intraoperative radiotherapy. Most disturbing about this modality was the number of local recurrences that the authors report "outside the margin of the port." The figures presented are not convincing that the complex logistics of patient transfer are justified.

Two practical papers are presented that may be of use to the head and neck surgeon. The first deals with accurate measurement of blood loss and the use of autologous blood transfusions. In this day of fear of bloodborne diseases, critically analyzing a surgeon's blood loss for specific procedures is to be applauded. Another of this year's papers described an attempt to evaluate functional reconstruction. Certainly, total rehabilitation of the head and neck cancer patient includes reconstruction. That reconstruction must be functional, and standards for function are needed. This paper suggests that the same rigid standards devised for cleft palate patients be applied to postoperative speech patterns for the head and neck cancer patient.

The Thorax

With bronchogenic carcinoma, early diagnosis remains one of the most significant factors influencing prognosis. The paper by Read well describes the favorable results with T_1, N_0 lesions less than 2 cm in size. About 78% of 244 patients treated over a period of 19 years had 5-year freedom from a cancer-related death.

With pulmonary metastases, Marincola reported interesting experiences with more than 140 patients treated at Stanford. A sternotomy incision was preferred because bilateral metastases were often first recognized at this time. A 5-year survival rate approaching 50% was obtained with most neoplasms, with the striking exception of melanoma or breast cancer.

The paper by Estrera, describing nine patients with systemic air embolism from a penetrating lung injury, should be studied in detail. Almost surely, this occurs more commonly than is recognized; the diagnosis was made at operation by observing air in the coronary arteries. The critical features that combined to produce this grave complication include a penetrating injury near the hilum that simultaneously injures a large bronchus and pulmonary vein. Prompt clamping of the hilar structures supplying the injured lung segment is the keystone of emergency therapy.

Two significant papers deal with empyema. The report by Forty of experiences with 52 late cases, 47 of which were treated by decortication, well documents its efficacy. These patients were referred, often after 3 weeks of ineffective tube drainage. One wonders if the more frequent use of limited thoracotomy, as described in the 1989 YEAR BOOK in a report by Van Way, might make the late use of decortication needed less often.

The paper by Pairolero discusses experiences with 45 patients with postpneumonectomy empyema, 28 of whom had an associated bronchopleural fistula. Early muscle transposition was clearly of great value in initial treatment. These 45 cases were almost surely referred to the Mayo Clinic from a wide area. I am reminded, however, of the unusual report from England by Sarsam reviewed in this section in 1990. This group reported a series of 332 pneumonectomies over a period of 10 years; in none of these patients did a bronchopleural fistula develop, raising again the question of how often bronchopleural fistulas can be prevented with appropriate technique.

The impressive report by Grillo, summarizing experiences with tracheal tumors, must represent the most extensive experience in the world. It was quite impressive that more than 50% of the patients required a carinal resection; nonetheless, mortality was less than 5%, with a 5-year survival of nearly 80% of patients with more favorable histologic types.

The report by Wright, describing experiences with 48 patients treated for a primary mediastinal nonseminomatous germ cell tumor, dramatically documents the importance of early use of chemotherapy, such as cisplatin. Twenty-two of 28 patients treated with this method had an excellent response, with a 57% 5-year survival, but 20 other patients treated late, referred after initial unsuccessful therapy elsewhere, had dismal results.

Regarding pediatric pulmonary problems, the report from Pittsburgh describes experiences with 105 children hospitalized for thoracic trauma, 97% being blunt injuries. There was a striking difference from the type of pathology seen after similar injuries in the adult. Traumatic aortic injury, cardiac contusion, or rupture of the diaphragm were uncommon. Thoracotomy was needed in only 5% of the group.

Finally, the interesting report by Adzick documents a zealous approach with the unsolved problem of high mortality with congenital diaphragmatic hernia. This report describes 38 cases diagnosed in utero and treated promptly, including use of an extracorporeal membrane oxygenator. Unfortunately, the overall survival was poor, well documenting that a high percentage of these unfortunate infants, thus far, seem to have an incurable problem.

Congenital Heart Disease

The long-term prognosis following a Fontan operation, in which pulmonary blood flow is determined by systemic venous pressure rather than by the contractile force of the right ventricle, is unknown. An important report by Fontan analyzed, mathematically, the long-term results among 334 patients in whom classic risk factors were small. These studies identified a significant decline in function that began about 6 years after operation and gradually progressed. Predicted survival was 86% 5 years after operation but only 73% at 15 years.

The harmful effect of transannular patching during operative correction of tetralogy of Fallot has been long debated. The important report by Kirklin found, among 814 patients, very little difference in long-term function and survival in the first 20 years after operation. These data relate to the significance of the report by Clarke, who described experiences with 122 cryopreserved allograft valves, using a pulmonary allograft conduit in 55 of the group. The present data indicate that there is little need to perform the complex allograft operation as a primary repair as long as significant distal stenoses in the pulmonary arterial tree are not present.

Whether or not subclavian flap angioplasty is the best operation for coarctation in infants is considered in the report from Holland by van Son. Among a group of 70 infants operated on during a period of more than 14 years, 5 years after operation results with the subclavian flap procedure were considerably inferior to those obtained with resection and end-to-end anastomosis. A more radical resection of the abnormal ductus tissue in the aorta at the site of coarctation, followed by an extensive anastomosis that extends onto the undersurface of the aortic arch, may prove to give the best long-term results. Finally, the Mayo Clinic report by Cohen evaluated results in what is probably the largest group of patients with repair of coarctation—646 patients with a mean long-term follow-up for as long as 20 years. The data clearly showed that patients operated on before 9 years of age had better results, which suggests that irreversible injury may develop insidiously in the first few years of life unless repair is performed.

Valvular Heart Disease

Valve allografts are being used with increasing frequency, especially in children. Documentation of good results for as long as 20 years, combined with the increased availability of such valves, has encouraged their wider usage. The report by Mark O'Brien from Australia, a leading investigator of allograft valves for more than 20 years, is of particular interest. His different techniques of implantation are described in detail.

With allograft valves, there is uncertainty about whether or not preservation of donor cells is ideal. This question is examined in the short case report by Gonzalez-Lavin, who carefully studied the origin of cells in a cryopreserved aortic homograft explanted 10 months after operation.

Long-term results with porcine prostheses are described by Jamieson, a major investigator of this subject, as their total experience includes nearly 3,000 patients. The supra-annular prosthesis has been used in 1,700 patients since 1981. As with other reports, however, excellent function is present at 5 years in the majority of patients, but subsequent increasing frequency of degeneration results in only 77% functioning well 10 years after operation.

The timing of valve replacement was analyzed in the detailed report by Lindblom, who performed an extensive long-term follow-up of 2,800 patients over a period of 15 years. The cogent argument is made that earlier operation should be seriously considered with present techniques as the frequency of valve-related deaths is now only about 5% within 10 years after operation.

MITRAL VALVE OPERATIONS

DeLoche described results in 206 patients operated on by Carpentier's group more than 10 years earlier. Only 13% had been reoperated on. There was a striking freedom from thromboembolism (94%), as well as endocarditis (97%).

Hennein clearly demonstrated better cardiac function after mitral valve replacement when some chordae were preserved. Among 69 patients studied, the 14 with preservation of some chordae had much better cardiac function than the 55 who did not. Interestingly enough, preservation of only posterior chordae was as effective as more extensive chordae preservation.

Replacing chordae tendineae with polytetrafluoroethylene (PTFE) sutures was studied in 22 patients by David, using a 5–0 Gore-Tex suture. The results in this short-term report were encouraging, as no major failures have thus far been recognized.

The report by Panos from Toronto is an impressive one. Experiences with 19 patients operated on acutely for severe mitral regurgitation and shock after myocardial infarction are described. Only two deaths occurred, a remarkably low mortality considering the fact that for years the reported operative mortality for this serious problem has ranged between 30% and 70%. The author's use of continuous blood cardioplegia may be a significant fact. It has long been a puzzle why correction of a severe mechanical defect, such as rupture of the mitral valve apparatus after myocardial infarction, was still associated with such a high operative mortality. If the physiologic problem from the massive mitral insufficiency were corrected, the high mortality must represent either the stress of operation or inadequate myocardial preservation.

Aortic Valve Operations

Galloway described excellent results from my institution after aortic valve replacement in patients older than 70 years. The operative mortality was near 5%; the 5-year survival from late cardiac death was 81%. These data refute the frequently heard assertion that the high mortality and morbidity following aortic valve replacement in this group of patients justifies the use of palliative balloon valvuloplasty, which produces far less satisfactory results.

The influence of the stent on the durability of a porcine prosthesis was investigated by David. Short-term results in 25 patients were excellent, inserting a stentless porcine valve with the same technique as that used for an aortic allograft. Carpentier cautioned that this technique had been evaluated more than 20 years earlier, but it remains unknown whether the theoretical improved durability would outweigh the technical hazards of implantation.

Finally, the report by Stelzer from London described experiences in 17 patients with a hypoplastic aortic annulus who were treated with a pulmonary allograft conduit. For the unusual patient with severe hypoplasia of the aortic outflow tract, this may be the ideal technique.

Endocarditis

The impressive report by Dreyfus clearly documented that valve repair, as opposed to valve replacement, is relatively safe when treating acute endocarditis. Among a group of 40 patients, there was only one operative death; one patient required reoperation, and no recurrent endocarditis developed, an impressive fact. Similar excellent results were described briefly in a workshop by Turley. He stated that in a period of 8 years, 19 patients with tricuspid endocarditis were treated by repair, which was successful in 14; endocarditis recurred in 2.

Reul, reporting from Houston, analyzed the long-term results between bioprosthetic valves and metallic valves when performing valve replacement for acute endocarditis. The early mortality rate was similar, but 5 years after operation the metallic prostheses performed much better (95% free of reoperation), compared to the bioprostheses (75% free of reoperation).

Coronary Heart Disease

Goldman reported results from the extensive cooperative study in the Veterans Administration of antiplatelet therapy after bypass. The value of aspirin was strongly reaffirmed, expecially in vessels smaller than 2 mm; the thrombosis rate was 20% with aspirin but 32% without.

There is a paucity of long-term data following bilateral mammary grafts. Galbut described the experiences of the Miami group with more than 1,000 patients over a period of several years. The results are most impressive: 80% survival at 10 years; a frequency of nonfatal infarction of 1% per patient year; and rare reoperation—.3% per year. A unique characteristic of their data is that the mammary artery was used as an isolated artery, independent of fascia, vein, or lymphatics. Possibly, this small pedicle contributed to the very low rate of sternal infection, 1.5%.

Kitamura described astonishingly good results with bilateral internal mammary grafts in eight children with Kawasaki disease. The average age at operation was 8 years. One hundred percent patency of both mammary arteries was obtained in all patients.

The major question of the importance vs. the expense of keeping an operating room "ready" while an angioplasty is performed was analyzed in the report by Cameron. Urgent bypass is needed in only about 5% of patients undergoing angioplasty. In a questionnaire survey, a wide variation in patterns was found. Using the next operating room available in a center with a busy operating suite is one popular approach. Another, not widely used, is timing the performance of the potentially hazardous angioplasty with the availability of an operating room.

Emory University, in the report by Talley, analyzed the influence on long-term results of failed angioplasty followed by revascularization. Among a group of 430 patients seen in a period of 5 years, 25% had a perioperative infarction, but excellent long-term results were obtained whether or not an infarction occurred. It should be emphasized, however, that a high percentage of the patients operated on originally had single-vessel disease, so the applicability of these data to patients with severe triple-vessel disease is unknown.

The report by Floten, describing data from Starzl's group in Oregon, reaffirmed the safety of bypass between 1 and 30 days after an infarction. Experiences with 832 patients treated in a period of 13 years are described. Five- and 10-year long-term results were surprisingly similar between those who had a recent infarction and those who had one in the past.

Experiences with coronary revascularization in patients who survived a prehospital cardiac arrest were described in the report by Kelly from the Massachusetts General Hospital. Eighty percent of the 50 patients had inducible arrhythmias beforehand. Revascularization decreased the frequency to about 50%, clearly leaving a large percentage who may require treatment with an implantable defibrillator.

The extensive report by Loop from Cleveland of 2,509 reoperations for myocardial revascularization must be the largest in the world. There was an encouraging decrease in operative mortality to 2.9% in the most recent group, as well as a decrease in frequency of infarction from 8% to 4%. Vein graft atherosclerosis was the leading indication for reoperation.

Miscellaneous Cardiac Conditions and the Great Vessels

CARDIOPULMONARY BYPASS TECHNIQUES

The question of the importance of low oncotic pressure during cardiopulmonary bypass was investigated in the report by Marelli, evaluating the use of 50 g of albumin in the perfusate. No clinical differences could be found in patients whether or not albumin was added. As albumin is expensive, this is also an important economic consideration.

The ideal level of anticoagulation during bypass was discussed in two different reports, one by Metz and the other by Gravlee. An activated coagulation time (ACT) near 400 seconds seemed the best. Surprisingly enough, the report by Gravlee found more bleeding with higher levels of ACT, suggesting that larger doses of heparin are not always innocuous.

Data are gradually accumulating to indicate that there is a significant difference between the response of neonatal and adult myocardium to cardioplegia. The report by Yang and Hearse described laboratory studies evaluating the biochemical reasons for this difference, pointing out that the key biochemical mechanisms for energy production are quite different between the immature and the adult myocardium.

The value and safety of closure of the pericardial cavity with bovine pericardium after bypass remain uncertain. The report by Eng describes seerious problems with adhesions in four patients who required reoperation within 3–8 years after the initial operation, at which time bovine pericardium was used. For these reasons the routine use of bovine pericardium has been abandoned.

The report by Bashein studied the long-discussed question of the best method of carbon dioxide management during hypothermic cardiopulmonary bypass. In one group the PCO_2 was kept near 40 mm as measured at room temperature, whereas in the other group the PCO_2 was corrected to the degree of hypothermia. There were no hemodynamic or neurologic differences.

COMPLICATIONS OF CARDIOPULMONARY BYPASS

A neurologic injury remains the most serious complication of cardiopulmonary bypass. The frequency, although small, increases steadily in patients older than 60 years of age. Various physiologic studies in the past few years have not yet identified any failure of cerebral autoregulation in older patients, so the basic cause usually remains unknown. The report by Arom analyzed computerized electroencephalographic monitoring as an index of cerebral blood flow. The report should be viewed as a preliminary one, with its importance to be determined by future studies, but the authors detected changes in the intensity of electrical signals recorded that could be altered by changes in perfusion technique. Unfortunately, specific details were not given.

Blauth, in England, has reported several studies about microemboli viewed in the retina during cardiopulmonary bypass. In the most recent report, retinal emboli were visible in all of 30 patients perfused with the bubble oxygenator. These were estimated to be about 20 μ in diameter. The clinical significance remains uncertain.

The short report by Sugimoto analyzed the physiologic mechanism underlying the effectiveness of treating late pericardial tamponade with a pericardial window. The clinically quite interesting conclusion is that fusion of the epicardium to the pericardium is the basic mechanism, rather than maintaining an open "window." This concept emphasizes that maintenance of tube drainage of the pericardial cavity is more important than the extent of the pericardial window created.

A short report from Sweden studied focal dysfunction after cricothyroidotomy in 19 patients. Complex physiologic studies of voice function were done. Ten of the 19, nearly 50%, were judged to have some changes from a normal voice. Because no dysfunction of the cricothyroid muscle could be found, the possibility was suggested that the abnormalities resulted from formation of scar tissue. The voice changes were minimal in all but 3 patients.

A comparable study of changes following conventional tracheostomy was not done. I studied this report in some detail, because cricothyroidotomy has been widely employed at NYU for more than a decade and has been found particularly useful as an alternative to long-term intubation after cardiopulmonary bypass. Permanent changes in voice function have not been recognized, but detailed physiologic studies have not been done.

Two reports discussed the frequency and importance of impaired function of the diaphragm following open-heart surgery. The report by Bogers found diaphragmatic elevation in 7% of 370 operations, but normal function returned within a year in 90% of them. The report by Graham is of unusual value, assessing long-term results following unilateral diaphragmatic plication in 17 patients. It is impressive that the changes produced by plication remained satisfactory in 6 patients studied more than 5 years after operation.

Infection of the sternotomy incision, although infrequent, remains a serious cause of morbidity and mortality after open-heart operations. Loop described sternal wound complications in 1.1% of 6,500 patients operated on in a period of 20 years. Infection was particularly increased in diabetic patients in whom bilateral mammary grafts were used. Similar findings have been reported by others. These indicate that bilateral mammary grafts should be approached with considerable caution in the diabetic patient.

There is a puzzling discrepancy among different reports about the frequency of sternal infection after placement of bilateral mammary grafts with resulting sternal ischemia. The strong possibility exists, but is not proven, that this may be related to the size of the mammary pedicle created, as well as to the extensive use of the cautery, both of which would injure collateral circulation.

The interesting report by Fine suggested that delayed sternotomy pain could be related to hypersensitivity to nickle in a few patients. The authors state that sternotomy wires usually contain about 8% nickle. Among the general population there is a hypersensitivity to nickle in about 10% of females, about 2% of males. Removal of the wires in the unusual case described in this report produced prompt relief.

CARDIAC TRAUMA AND TUMORS

The report by Baxter emphsizes again that many patients with blunt chest trauma are "overtreated" because of the fear of problems from myocardial contusion. Data on 290 patients indicated that significant contusion could be detected regularly within 12 hours. In the 1990 overview, similar conclusions were described in other reports, reemphasizing that serious problems from myocardial contusion can be either detected or excluded within 24 hours after injury.

The unusual but vexing problem of intracardiac missiles was reviewed by Symbas, summarizing available information in the English literature as well as their personal experience with 24 patients. This report is a valuable reference source in helping to decide which missiles should be removed and which should be left alone.

The report by Rosenberg described experiences with 30 patients with blunt vascular injuries to the brachiocephalic branches of the aortic arch. The diagnosis was established by angiography, for the clinical picture was identical to the more common traumatic rupture of the aorta. Although 27 of the 30 patients survived, none with paralysis from brachial injury had a return of neurologic function.

The unusual but troublesome question about the possible recurrence of an intracardiac myxoma was studied by Bartolotti in a 20-year follow-up of 54 patients. During this time the tumor was routinely excised with a small amount of adjacent tissue at the stalk. There have been no instances of tumor recurrence.

AORTIC DISEASE

The monumental report from Stanley Crawford describes experiences with 717 patients with aneurysmal disease in the ascending and transverse aortic arch treated over a period of 9 years, with a 30-day survival of 91%. The manuscript contains a wealth of technical information. It is quite interesting that since 1986, the technique of using a 10-mm dacron graft for attaching the coronary ostia to the aortic prosthesis, rather than the classic method of side-to-side anastomosis between the coronary ostia and an aortic opening, has been performed in 94 patients.

In the report by Oz, the cumulative experience by Lemole and his group with a sutureless ring graft for replacement of the aorta was described in 49 patients with disease in the ascending and transverse aorta. The results were not much better than those achieved with conventional techniques, but it was of particular interest that the tape ligating the spool of the prosthesis in position did not erode and cause hemorrhage, nor did the prosthesis migrate because of insufficient fixation.

MISCELLANY

Kuppermann analyzes the sobering problem of the cost of the implantable defibrillator. Data obtained by the Health Care Financing Administration on 138 patients found the initial hospitalization cost for defibrillator implantation to approach $50,000. A detailed economic analysis of the cost:benefit ratio, as compared to recurrent hospitalization for treatment of arrhythmias, however, found a significant cost saving of between $5,000 and $15,000 per life-year saved. Although it is beyond my competence to analyze these findings in detail, such economic considerations are especially important in this time of rising medical costs. If the defibrillators are to be widely used, however, some appropriate method of insurance reimbursement is necessary.

Arteries and Veins

The results in a series of patients who underwent carotid endarterectomy and were followed for 2–6 years demonstrate the durability of the procedure. Carotid endarterectomy contralateral to an occluded artery may be carried out with acceptable risk and low stroke-free and survival rates comparable to those seen in other patients undergoing carotid endarterectomy. Reevaluation of the issue of celiac artery decompression demonstrates that the operation should not be undertaken in patients with vague upper abdominal complaints and compression observed on angiography, because favorable results associated with the procedure cannot be demonstrated uniformly. In a study of patients with abdominal aortic aneurysms who were followed with nonoperative management, the individual rates of expansion proved to be variable and unpredictable. Patients with small aneurysms can be safely followed if their pulse pressure is controlled and elective repair is then performed when the aneurysm reaches 5–6 cm based on sequential ultrasonographic measurements.

The argument persists with regard to the relative advantage of transperitoneal vs. retroperitoneal approach for aortic reconstruction; one prospective randomized control could show no advantage for either technique. The incidence of 13.3% was reported for the development of false aneurysm after prosthetic reconstructions for aortic-iliac obstructive disease, leading to the advocacy of the use of a long-term follow-up scheduled with periodic angiography and ultrasonography for these patients.

Popliteal artery entrapment should be considered in the young adult with claudication and is seen with greater frequency in an increasingly active population. A treadmill test, followed by biplane arteriography, established a diagnosis in all of the patients. This supports the concept of prophylactic revision of an infrainguinal bypass graft in a patient with no symptoms if the ankle/brachial index is reduced and the duplex scan result is abnormal. Duplex examination of femorodistal graft is an effective screening tool for detecting stenoses, which occur in about 20% of the grafts. In approximately 25% of femoral distal grafts, graft-related stenosis develops, and graft surveillance is worthwhile but only for the first year of operation, according to one report.

Although the in situ vein graft is increasing in popularity, one report indicates a preference for the use of the reversed vein bypass for lower extremity revascularization based on the excellent results achieved. An arterial venous fistula created remotely not only increases graft blood flow but also augments native arterial blood flow between the distal anastomosis and fistula and thus may improve limb perfusion. A comparative study was carried out to assess the role of intraoperative angioscopy compared with completion arteriography after femoral distal bypass, and, although it lacks sensitivity and specificity, angioscopy can provide valuable information about the distal anatomy. Actual arterial graft patency, limb salvage, and patient survival of 82%, 87%, and 80%, respectively, at 18 months was reported for diabetic patients undergoing dorsal-pedal bypass for limb salvage. Revascularization procedures have been applied with success to treat chronic, nonhealing fractures in ischemic limbs.

Cardiopulmonary bypass, pulmonary bypass, and deep hypothermic circulatory arrest have aided significantly in the management of large retroperitoneal tumors and associated large vena caval thrombi. Reconstruction of the vena cava and its primary tributaries can be achieved preferentially using the spiral saphenous vein graft of the superior vena cava and the expanded polytetrafluoroethylene grafts in the abdomen. Although statistically significant data are not available, the impression is presented that venous thrombectomy plus temporary arteriovenous fistula seems to improve the long-term outcome after acute iliofemoral thrombosis. Anticoagulation treatment remains an acceptable alternative.

Esophagus

A case is made for esophagectomy performed either transhiatally or transthoracically for esophageal disruption occurring in the presence of preexisting disease. Conservative procedures such as direct repair, diversion, or drainage for perforation with preexisting disease often inflict more morbidity than esophageal resection. In patients with reflux-induced esophageal stricture, preoperative dilatation and total fundoplication gastroplasty provide significant improvement and esophageal resection is rarely required. The controversial question regarding the indications for esophagectomy in nonmalignant Barrett's esophagus has once again been addressed. Most patients can be managed with antireflux procedures, and esophageal resection should be applied to a select group of patients, including those with deep penetrating ulcers, high-grade dysplasia, strong suspicion of cancer, and multiple previous operations. Free jejunal interposition grafts have been applied successfully in reconstruction of the esophagus. This popular method is associated with a decreased incidence of reflux when compared with gastric pull-up procedures.

Although there is no prospective randomized trial comparing radiation therapy vs. surgery in management of squamous carcinoma of the esophagus, one report indicates that the results of radical radiotherapy for operable squamous cell carcinoma of the esophagus are similar to the best results achieved by surgical resection. The study of 2-year survivals indicates that intensive chemotherapy and radiation therapy, combined with transhiatal esophagectomy, produce significant improvement in the survival rate (60% compared to 32%). A prospective randomized trial is required to confirm these figures.

Stomach and Duodenum

Changes in the incidence of causes of major upper gastrointestinal bleeding are emphasized, and the importance of early endoscopy is demonstrated. The long-term clinical results after proximal gastric vagotomy have been assessed; the conclusion is that when the procedure is used to treat duodenal and midgastric ulcers, there is an acceptably low long-term recurrence rate. In contrast, the high incidence of recurrent ulcers after proximal gastric vagotomy for pyloric, prepyloric, or combined ulcers suggsts that alternative operations should be performed for ulcers in these locations.

It has long been appreciated that the incidence of duodenal ulcer increases with age, but acid secretion does not. A recent study shows that the progressive breakdown in mucosal defense mechanisms with increasing age makes plain the age-related increase in incidence of duodenal ulcer disease.

A Swedish study reports a dramatic decline in elective peptic ulcer surgery in that country that began long before the advent of fiberoptic endoscopy, highly selective vagotomy, or H_2-receptor antagonists. A comparable decline in emergency procedures suggests that true changes in the incidence of severity of the disease have occurred. The field of laparoscopic management of surgical patients has been extended to the treatment of perforated peptic ulcers in a small series, but its role in the management of this circumstances has not been defined.

The complication of gastrocolic fistula occurring as a consequence of benign gastric ulcer has been reviewed, and it is emphasized that the fistulas often arise in close association with the intake of steroidal and nonsteroidal anti-inflammatory agents. The relationship between peptic ulcer and gastric cancer was investigated in a large series, and the results suggest that gastric ulcers rarely become malignant. A retrospective assessment of a large series of cases with early gastric cancer reveals that the incidence of recurrence resulted in a mortality rate of approximately 2% for mucosal cancer and 8% for submucosal cancer. Studies of the pattern of lymph node metastases from gastric cancer indicated that deposits were most common in perigastric nodes, related to the location of the tumor. More extensive resections for cancer invading beyond the submucosal was advocated.

The cause of malnutrition recurring as a consequence of total gastrectomy despite appropriate caloric and protein intake was investigated. The preoperative deficiencies of body weight, protein, and fats were not corrected, but further deterioration was prevented. It appears that preserving duodenal transit should be the main consideration in gastric replacement after total gastrectomy. Patients undergoing jejunal interposition lose significantly less weight and regain a higher percentage of preoperative body mass index than do those having Roux-en-Y esophagojejunostomy. Although there is a lack of significant difference in the 5-year survival rates between total and subtotal gastrectomy, it appears that total gastrectomy remains a safe and accepted procedure. The number and frequency of lymph node metastases were both parameters of prognostic significance for gastric carcinoma.

Small Bowel

Duodenojejunostomy is proposed as a method of managing constriction of the upper part of the alimentary tract and is considered preferable to gastric jejunostomy or end-to-end duodenojejunostomy. The long-term outcome of reversal of small intestinal bypass operations was studied. Gastroplasty performed simultaneously produced no benefit in alleviation of metabolic complications but decreased body weight when compared with results in patients who had reconstruction without gastroplasty. Prophylactic reversal of the small intestine bypass is not indicated in symptomatic patients with jejunoileal bypass. It is concluded that hydrostatic barium reduction remains the treatment of choice for intussusception during childhood, and abdominal exploration should be reserved for those patients in whom the barium enema is unsuccessful.

The course of approximately 200 patients with Crohn's disease was evaluated. A clinical relapse rate of 27% after 2 years and 38% after 4 years was noted. The patients operated on had a lower relapse rate than the patients treated conservatively (20% vs. 51%). In non-Hodgkin's lymphomas of the gastrointestinal tract, paraffin-reactive antibodies can reliably identify most B cell lymphomas but may be unreliable in detection of lymphomas of T cell origin. Short-bowel syndrome in infants remains a difficult problem. It is believed that until bowel transplant becomes a viable alternative, operative intervention and nutritional support may prolong survival but will not change the outcome of these infants. In pigs it has been shown that short-segment jejunal allografts significantly improve mortality and morbidity rates from surgically created short-bowel syndrome.

Colon—Rectum

The Centers for Disease Control reported that the risk of appendicitis is 8.6% for males and 6.7% for females. The life-time risk of appendectomy is 12% for males and 23.1% for females. Review of 13 cases of primary appendicular carcinoma indicated that the procedure of right hemicolectomy did not confer any clear-cut survival advantage. A series of patients has been reported in whom acute appendicitis was diagnosed, leading to operation. A cecal mass attributable to cecal diverticulitis was found. In most of the patients the cecal mass could be separated from the cecum in a conservative operation; either diverticulectomy or wedge resection was performed.

An analysis of the morbidity and mortality associated with closure of loop end colostomy demonstrated that the mortality rates were not significantly different and complication rates were identical. Endometriosis of the colon remains a rare lesion and almost always involves the sigmoid or rectosigmoid colon. Endoscopic evaluation does not provide a diagnosis. Surgical resection offers the best chance for relief of symptoms. The National Polyp Study includes a database of more than 3,000 adenomas. Adenoma size and the extent of villus, a component, were the major independent polyp risk factors associated with high-grade dysplasia.

A surveillance program, carried out on patients with ulcerative colitis to assess the risk factors for cancer, indicated that all patients with mucosal dysplasia had pancolitis for at least 8 years. Older age at symptom onset was predictive of dysplasia in cancer. It has been suggested that close surveillance and even prophylactic proctocolectomy should be recommended for patients given a diagnosis of pancolitis, especially those who are younger than 15 years at diagnosis. Carcinoma of the colon and rectum has been reported in patients younger than 20 years. In this age group, most patients present with rectal bleeding, and most have advanced disease at the time of diagnosis.

It has been demonstrated that there is no difference in the local recurrence of cancer in patients subjected to low anterior vs. abdominoperineal resection as a method of managing midrectal tumors. In what may represent an exciting breakthrough, it has been shown that in patients with stage C colon carcinoma, therapy with levamisole plus fluorouracil reduces the risk of recurrence by 41% and of mortality by 33%. The median follow-up time at publication was 3 years. Prognosis for anorectal melanoma remains grave, with 83% of the patients dying of the disease and none surviving for more than 6 years. Perineal wounds developing after abdominoperineal resection are generally unresponsive to conservative medical and surgical therapy, and a single-stage muscle flap procedure has provided effective closure.

Liver and Spleen

A series of patients with focal nodular hyperplasia of the liver underwent resection. It has been our contention that this does not represent a surgical lesion, with very rare exceptions. The question has been raised whether transformation to fibrolamellar carcinoma occurs. There is an excellent review of mesenchymal hematoma. Excision of the tumor is advised in all patients, and a complete recovery is to be expected. Although curative surgery cannot be carried out, there is a subset of patients with systematic polycystic disease who benefit from selective resection or fenestration. Repeat hepatectomy is applicable to some patients who have recurrent malignant tumors; morbidity is acceptable, and long-term survivals have been achieved.

In a review of literature, it is stressed that recurrent liver mestastases from colorectal carcinoma can be removed safely; the operation is associated with a long-term disease-free survival in up to 38% of highly selected patients. An aggressive approach is proposed for patients in whom sclerotherapy fails; this includes either portosystemic shunt or a devascu-

larization procedure. A report from China emphasizes that a distal splenorenal shunt is a safe and effective method of treating esophagogastric
varices and is proposed as a prophylactic shunt in Child's A and Child's
B patients. Another article suggests that peritoneovenous shunts provide
a cost-effective method of managing patients with truly intractable ascites.

Clinical experience with 11 patients undergoing ex situ operation on
the liver, or surgery on an in situ hypothermic profused liver after vascular isolation, was reported. This provides a method of removing tumors
that otherwise would not be resectable. A large series of patients with
Budd-Chiari syndrome, treated surgically, demonstrates that the majority
do well after decompressive shunting procedures. Another report concluded that orthotopic liver transplantation is a most effective method of
treating patients with Budd-Chiari syndrome and end-stage liver disease.

A multicenter experience with classes I, II, or III splenic injuries after
blunt trauma indicates that if certain criteria are met, a significant number of adults and children can be managed nonoperatively. Application
of standard splenic salvage techniques resulted in splenic preservation in
100% of children and 93% of adults. The criteria for splenectomy applied to patients with idiopathic thrombocytopenic purpura with HIV
positivity should be essentially the same as those applied to patients without evidence of HIV, AIDS, or AIDS-related complex. Splenectomy represents appropriate treatment for hypersplenism and chronic lymphocytic
leukemia or malignant Hodgkin's lymphoma. Elective subtotal splenectomy is particularly applicable in patients with Gaucher's disease in an
attempt to prevent the postsplenectomy sepsis.

Biliary Tract

A series of 200 consecutive outpatient cholecystectomies done over a
4-year period were analyzed. All patients were discharged within 10
hours after the procedure. No wound infections or serious complications
occurred, and the rate of morbidity seemed similar to that of laparoscopic cholecystectomy. Choledochoscopy is a clinically efficacious
method of obtaining a stone-free duct, but the cost effectiveness has not
been defined. Extracorporeal shock wave lithotripsy with ursodiol is
more effective than lithotripsy alone for the treatment of symptomatic
gallstones. Even in the most favorable series, only 35% of patients receiving ursodiol and lithotripsy remained stone free for 6 months.

A case has been made for biliary drainage as an initial approach to the
management of patients with severe acute cholangitis. Classification of
the Mirizzi syndrome is proposed. During cholecystectomy, partial resection of the gallbladder is recommended to extract stones and to define the
location of the fistula. Endoscopic sphincterotomy and stone extraction
are valuable tools in the management of patients with common duct
stones who have previously undergone cholecystectomy. The spectrum of
surgical procedures applicable to patients with sclerosing cholangitis have
been assessed and a case has been made for orthotopic liver transplanta-

tion as the procedure of choice for patients with refractory cholangitis, portal hypertension, and/or progressive liver failure.

A detailed review of the reported 50 cases of cystic hepatobiliary neoplasm is presented. The lesion known as Edmonson's tumor occurs uniquely in young females and develops from nests of primitive embryonal cells. It has the potential for malignant transformation and therefore should always be removed. Data from one series support the view that a one-stage procedure is, when feasible, a valid option for the management of patients with gallstone ileus when local and surgical conditions argue against common cholecystectomy. In answer to the question, does radical resection improve the outcome of patients with carcinoma of the gallbladder, one must respond with no. Results remain poor for patients with carcinoma of the main hepatic duct junction, with a 5-year actuarial survival rate of about 19%. Adenocarcinoma of the ampulla of Vater represents a unique biologic lesion in which, unlike carcinoma of the pancreas, the 5-year survival rate is independent of the presence or absence of lymph node metastases.

Pancreas

Nineteen percent of patients in whom acute pancreatitis was diagnosed by CT scan had a normal serum amylase level on admission. This occurred more commonly in patients with alcoholic pancreatitis than in patients with a longer duration of symptoms before admission. In the normal amylasemic cases the lipase content was elevated in 68%. There was little gain in diagnostic sensitivity when the peritoneal values were added to the serum determinations. Pancreatic fistula formation associated with acute pancreatitis occurred most frequently in patients after necrosectomy or drainage of the pancreatic abscess or pseudocyst. Spontaneous closure generally occurred with a low-output fistula; operative intervention was needed only for high-output fistulas.

Anterior pancreatography has been extremely helpful in planning the operative strategy for patients with pancreatic disease. In assessing the natural history of pancreatic pseudocysts it was demonstrated that size of the pseudocyst is a significant predictor of the need for operative drainage. Cysts larger than 6 cm required surgical treatment in about two thirds of the cases; cysts less than 6 cm required operative treatment in about 40% of the cases. It is concluded that a large proportion of patients with pancreatic pseudocysts without specific indications can be safely managed nonoperatively.

Selective pancreatic pseudocyst drainage percutaneously or transgastroduodenally can avoid exploration. Endoscopic retrograde cholangiopancreatography is a useful tool in the preoperative diagnosis of pancreatic neoplasms associated with cysts. Controversies about the optimal method of palliating patients with pancreatic carcinoma persists. A review of the records of 142 patients indicates that direct choledochal enteric anastomosis is superior to cholecystojejunostomy, and gastrojejunostomy was considered advantageous in view of a 10% incidence of subsequent gastric obstruction in those without gastric bypass.

Endocrine

Follow-up was made of 117 patients with papillary-follicular thyroid carcinoma, 26% of whom had clinically negative findings but pathologically positive lymph nodes. Recurrence developed more frequently in the regional lymph nodes. No deaths were caused by thyroid carcinoma. In the same institution, the mean length of survival of patients with anaplastic carcinoma of the thyroid was 7 months. Radical surgery did not significantly increase the survival duration over that after less radical surgery. An evaluation of more than 500 patients with sporadic primary hyperparathyroidism indicated that renal stone formation is especially prevalent in younger patients with slight hypercalcemia and parathyroid chief cell hyperplasia, whereas neuromuscular and psychiatric disturbances occur more commonly in older women with higher serum calcium levels. In patients with hyperplasia and more markedly enlarged glands it appeared sufficient to remove only the enlarged gland, whereas the findings suggested improved results using subtotal 3- to 3.5-gland resection in patients with more symmetric or less enlarged hyperplastic glands.

Angiographic ablation of cervical parathyroid adenomas can be considered for selected cases of primary hyperparathyroidism in whom operation has failed or is contraindicated. Adrenocortical carcinoma continues to carry a very poor prognosis. Mitotane therapy offers only transient benefit. The concurrent prospective cure rate for gastrinoma is higher than previously appreciated, and tumors within lymph nodes do not preclude curative resection. Accurate preoperative assessment for insulinomas can be accomplished with CT and angiography. In healthy donors, hemipancreatectomy resulted in deterioration of insulin secretion and glucose tolerance for at least 1 year; studies should be carried out to determine whether development of clinical diabetes mellitus represents a risk.

1 General Considerations

Elective Surgery Without Transfusion: Influence of Preoperative Hemoglobin Level and Blood Loss on Mortality
Spence RK, Carson JA, Poses R, McCoy S, Pello M, Alexander J, Popovich J, Norcross E, Camishion RC (Univ of Medicine and Dentistry of New Jersey, Camden; East Tennessee State Univ, Johnson City)
Am J Surg 159:320–324, 1990   1–1

In the past, preoperative blood transfusion was routine. However, concerns about scarce supplies, rising costs, and the possibility of transmitting fatal diseases have made it desirable to reevaluate this practice. The influence of preoperative hemoglobin levels and operative blood loss on survival after elective surgery was studied prospectively in patients who were Jehovah's Witnesses who refused blood transfusions.

In all, 113 elective surgeries were performed on 107 consecutive Jehovah's Witness patients. The age range was 8–88 (mean, 47 years). Preoperative hemoglobin levels ranged from 6 to 16.7 g/dL (mean, 11.4 g/dL). All patients had blood loss and/or anemia for at least 2 weeks. Surgery was performed on the basis of need, regardless of the hemoglobin level.

Ninety-three patients had preoperative hemoglobin levels of more than 10 g/dL, and 20 had levels between 6 g/dL and 10 g/dL. Estimated blood loss ranged from 0 to 5,600 mL, with a median loss of 500 mL and a mean loss of 750 mL. Fifty-two percent of patients had blood losses of less than 500 mL, and 78% had blood losses of less than 1,000 mL. Volume resuscitation during surgery was principally crystalloid.

Four of the 113 patients died, for a mortality rate of 3.5%. Mortality was unaffected by preoperative hemoglobin levels but was significantly increased by a blood loss of more than 500 mL. Regardless of preoperative hemoglobin levels, there was no mortality among patients whose estimated blood loss was less than 500 mL. The 4 who died had preoperative hemoglobin levels ranging from 6.1 g/dL to 15.2 g/dL, and levels in 3 were above 10 g/dL. However, all 4 had operative blood losses ranging from 800 mL to 5,600 mL.

Mortality in elective surgery seems to be dependent more on estimated blood loss than on preoperative hemoglobin levels. Elective surgery can be performed safely in patients with preoperative hemoglobin levels as low as 6 g/dL if the estimated blood loss does not exceed 500 mL.

▶ In an era of increasing concern about the transmission of viral diseases by blood and blood products, this article has particular meaning. As the authors point out, the chronically anemic patient is already compensated by increasing the stroke volume, and when significant blood loss is not anticipated, it is probably safer to withhold transfusion. The major role for blood replacement relates to acute blood loss before compensation can occur.— S.I. Schwartz, M.D.

Postoperative Myocardial Infarction and Cardiac Death: Predictive Value of Dipyridamole-Thallium Imaging and Five Clinical Scoring Systems Based on Multifactorial Analysis

Lette J, Waters D, Lassonde J, Dubé S, Heyen F, Picard M, Morin M (Maisonneuve-Rosemont Hosp; Montreal Heart Inst; Saint Luc Hosp; Univ of Montreal)
Ann Surg 211:84–90, 1990
1–2

Cardiac complications are important causes of postoperative morbidity and mortality after vascular and major general surgery in patients with coexisting coronary artery disease. It is generally agreed that a patient can safely undergo surgery if the exercise stress test is clinically and electrically negative at 85% of the maximal predicted heart rate. However, many patients cannot achieve an adequate exercise level because of peripheral vascular disease, old age, neurologic or locomotor problems, or β blocker use.

The predictive value of individual clinical parameters, 5 clinical scoring systems, and dipyridamole-thallium imaging for postoperative cardiac events was assessed in 66 patients with suspected or known coronary artery disease who could not attain an adequate exercise level on the treadmill. End points were limited to postoperative myocardial infarction or cardiac death before hospital discharge.

Nine postoperative cardiac events occurred, resulting in 7 deaths. No correlation was found between cardiac events and preoperative clinical descriptors, including individual clinical parameters, the Dripps-American Surgical Association score, the Goldman Cardiac Risk Index score, the Detsky Modified Cardiac Risk Index score, Eagle's clinical markers of low surgical risk, and the probability of postoperative events determined by Cooperman's equation. No cardiac events occurred in 30 patients with normal dipyridamole-thallium scans or in 9 with fixed myocardial perfusion defects. In 9 of 21 patients with reversible perfusion defects undergoing surgery a postoperative cardiac event occurred. In another 6 patients with reversible defects, a preoperative angiography revealed severe coronary disease or cardiomyopathy.

Postoperative outcome cannot be predicted clinically before major general and vascular surgery in patients who are unable to complete a standard exercise stress test. However, dipyridamole-thallium imaging identified all patients who had a postoperative cardiac event in this series.

▶ The predictive value of indices and tests assumes increasing importance as the population ages. Cardiac complications occur in a large number of patients undergoing vascular surgery. Lane et al. (1) reported that a statistically significant prediction of risk is not achieved with simple assessment of thallium results. Quantification of the total number of reversible defects, as well as assessment of ischemia and the distribution of the left anterior descending coronary artery, were required for optimum predictive accuracy. The present paper substantiates the findings of Leppo et al. (2), who showed that dipyridamole-thallium imaging is superior to exercise testing and clinical variables for predicting cardiac events in patients undergoing peripheral vascular surgery.—S.I. Schwartz, M.D.

References

1. Lane SV, et al: *Am J Cardiol* 64:1275, 1989.
2. Leppo J, et al: *J Am Coll Cardiol* 9:269, 1987.

Partial Ileal Bypass for Hypercholesterolemia: 20- to 26-Year Follow-Up of the First 57 Consecutive Cases
Buchwald H, Stoller DK, Campos CT, Matts JP, Varco RL (Univ of Minnesota)
Ann Surg 212:318–331, 1990   1–3

In 57 patients who underwent partial ileal bypass from 1963 to 1968 because of primary hypercholesterolemia, the mean preoperative total plasma cholesterol level was 363 mg/dL. The small bowel was transected

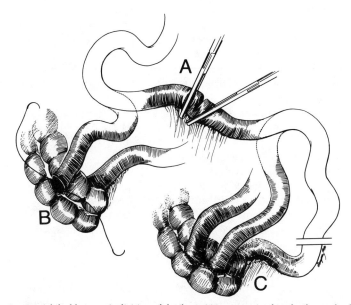

Fig 1–1.—Partial ileal bypass. **A,** division of the ileum 200 cm proximal to the ileocecal valve or one third of the total small bowel length proximal to the ileocecal valve if the total small intestinal length is greater than 600 cm; **B,** end-to-side anastomosis of the proximal segment into the anterior taenia of the cecum, 6 cm distal to the appendiceal stump; **C,** tacking of the closed distal segment to the anterior taenia of the cecum midway between the anastomosis and the appendiceal stump. (Courtesy of Buchwald H, Stoller DK, Campos CT, et al: *Ann Surg* 212:318–331, 1990.)

200 cm proximal to the ileocecal valve, or at a point one third of the small bowel length proximal to the valve if total length exceeded 600 cm (Fig 1–1). Clamps and hand-sewn 2-layer anastomoses were preferred to stapling instruments. The proximal segment was joined end-to-side with the cecum about 6 cm distal to the inverted appendiceal stump.

The total cholesterol level fell significantly to 231 mg/dL within a year of surgery. The 49 patients followed for 2–5 years postoperatively had a mean total cholesterol level of 258 mg/dL, and in 26 patients reexamined at 6–10 years the mean value was 209 mg/dL. Cholesterol levels remained significantly reduced 20 years after partial ileal bypass. Triglyceride levels were lowered but less impressively than the total plasma cholesterol. Many surviving patients had clinical atherosclerotic disease. Eighty percent of deaths were caused by coronary heart disease. The overall actuarial survival was 88% at 5 years and 41% at 25 years from the time of bypass.

Partial ileal bypass leads to a highly significant reduction in the total plasma cholesterol level that persists for at least 2 decades. Prospective randomized trials are needed to confirm a beneficial effect of such a reduction on the course of coronary heart disease.

▶ The results of this unique study are most meaningful. Whether cholesterol lowering has a significant effect on survival or atherosclerosis has not been determined. The rise in high-density lipoprotein cholesterol is relatively low. It is somewhat disturbing that the cholesterol level seems to be significantly correlated with myocardial infarction. A randomized comparison of the effects of drug therapy (such as lovastatin) and bypass is needed.— S.I. Schwartz, M.D.

Perioperative Antibiotic Prophylaxis for Herniorrhaphy and Breast Surgery

Platt R, Zaleznik DF, Hopkins CC, Dellinger EP, Karchmer AW, Bryan CS, Burke JF, Wikler MA, Marino SK, Holbrook KF, Tosteson TD, Segal MR (Harvard Med School; Brigham and Women's Hosp; Beth Israel Hosp; New England Deaconess Hosp; Massachusetts Gen Hosp, Boston; et al)
N Engl J Med 322:153–160, 1990   1–4

Although perioperative antibiotic prophylaxis can reduce the risk of postoperative infection in many clinical settings, its value in relatively simple, clean procedures has not been thoroughly investigated. The efficacy of perioperative antibiotic prophylaxis was assessed in a randomized, double-blind trial of 1,218 patients undergoing herniorrhaphy or breast surgery.

The prophylactic regimen involved a single dose of the long-acting antibiotic cefonicid, 1 g, administered intravenously 30 minutes before surgery. Patients were followed for 4–6 weeks after surgery. Those patients who received antibiotic prophylaxis had 48% fewer infections than controls. Among the breast surgery patients, infection occurred in 6.6% of antibiotic recipients and 12.2% of placebo recipients. Among the herniorrhaphy patients, infection occurred in 2.4% of those receiving antibiotics and 4.2% of those receiving placebo. There were reductions in wound infection, pus drainage, urinary tract infections, postoperative antibiotic therapy, nonroutine physician visits, and readmissions because of problems with wound healing among patients receiving antibiotic prophylaxis.

Perioperative antibiotic prophylaxis with cefonicid is useful for herniorrhaphy and breast surgery. Other clean surgical procedures may also benefit from perioperative antibiotic therapy.

▶ This article was selected because it sets a standard for the practice of surgery related to these 2 frequently performed operations. Recognizing that this article is available to provide support in a litigious society, it is hard to argue against providing perioperative antibiotic coverage for all patients undergoing these procedures. I have changed my practice in accordance with the data provided and now treat my patients with antibiotics if they are undergoing breast or hernia procedures.—S.I. Schwartz, M.D.

2 Fluid, Electrolytes, and Nutrition

Protein Malnutrition Predisposes to Inflammatory-Induced Gut-Origin Septic States

Deitch EA, Ma W-J, Ma L, Berg RD, Specian RD (Louisiana State Univ, Shreveport)

Ann Surg 211:560–568, 1990   2–1

Studies showing impairment or loss of intestinal barrier function under certain circumstances have led to an increased interest in the etiologic role of such impairment in the development of adult respiratory distress syndrome and multiple organ failure. The role of zymosan-induced systemic inflammation on intestinal barrier function was investigated in normally nourished (NN) and protein malnourished (PM) mice. Animals from both groups were challenged intraperitoneally with zymosan (.1 mg/g); controls received saline. The animals were killed 24 hours after zymosan challenge and their organs cultured for translocating bacteria.

Within 16–24 hours, zymosan caused systemic signs of stress in the challenged mice. Unlike the saline-injected controls whose organs were sterile, bacterial translocation to the mesenteric lymph node complex was observed in the zymosan-treated mice. Because cecal bacterial populations did not differ significantly in the 2 groups, zymosan appears to induce bacterial translocation by injuring the intestinal mucosa rather than by disrupting the ecology of the normal intestinal microflora. Although bacterial spread was limited to the mesenteric lymph node in NN mice, the liver, spleen, and bloodstream were involved in PM animals.

Thus PM mice were more susceptible to zymosan-induced bacterial translocation than NN mice. The longer the animals were on the protein-free diet, the more weight they lost and the higher their mortality rate. Patients who are at increased risk of becoming bacteremic from clinically occult foci tend to be malnourished and immunocompromised, and to have received therapeutic agents that alter the normal ecology of the gut flora. Therapeutic strategies that maintain intestinal barrier function may help to prevent the development of potentially fatal gut-origin septic states during a period of systemic inflammation.

▶ This article is from the group that reintroduced the idea of the importance of bacterial translocation as a cause of morbidity and mortality after trauma and sepsis. This study indicates that the increased risk from bacterial translocation may be attributable to the patient's malnourished and immunocompromised condition, or to their treatment with agents that alter bowel flora. Increasingly, therapeutic strategies are being developed that will maintain intestinal barrier function and may help to prevent the development of potentially fatal gut-origin septic states.—G.T. Shires, M.D.

Use of Selected Visceral Protein Measurements in the Comparison of Branched-Chain Amino Acids With Standard Amino Acids in Parenteral Nutrition Support of Injured Patients

Kuhl DA, Brown RO, Vehe KL, Boucher BA, Luther RW, Kudsk KA (Univ of Tennessee, Memphis)

Surgery 107:503–510, 1990   2–2

Modified amino acid formulas enriched with branched-chain amino acids are thought to help restore the nitrogen balance faster than standard amino acid formulas (STD) when used as parenteral nutritional support (PNS) in critically ill and injured patients. However, recent studies have been inconclusive. In a prospective, randomized clinical trial the effects of PNS using either STD or branched-chain amino acid, and 10 (mean age, 40.4 years) were given the STD formula containing 21% of the branched-chain amino acid formula. All 20 patients successfully completed at least 7 days of PNS. Both regimens were designed to be isocaloric, isovolemic, and isonitrogenous. Laboratory studies, including determination of serum levels of somatomedin-C/insulin-like growth factor I, circulating fibronectin, and prealbumin, were done before PNS was initiated and on days 4, 7, 14, and 21 of PNS.

Both groups had significantly improved nitrogen balance after 1 day of PNS, but there was no difference between the 2 groups. Somatomedin-C/insulin-like growth factor I increased significantly from baseline on day 4 in the STD group, day 7 in the branched-chain amino acid formula group, and days 14 and 21 in both groups. There was no significant difference in the level of somatomedin-C/insulin-like growth factor I between groups on any study day. Prealbumin levels increased significantly from baseline in both groups on days 7, 14, and 21, but there were no significant differences between the groups. Circulating fibronectin increased significantly from baseline on day 7 in the STD group, day 14 in both groups, and day 21 in the STD group. Branched chain amino acid formula-treated patients had significantly higher circulating fibronectin levels on day 14 compared with STD-treated patients on day 14. Nitrogen balance increased significantly from baseline in both groups on all days. There appears to be no significant difference in the effects on nitrogen balance in trauma patients whether STD or branched chain amino acid formulations are used as part of PNS.

▶ Several studies during the past 2 years have critically examined the possible benefit of adding branched-chain amino acid formulas for PNS in injured patients. Like the previous studies, no definitive benefit could be found from the addition of branched-chain amino acids to the standard amino acid formulas used. This is particularly critical in view of the cost of branched-chain amino acid formulas.— G.T. Shires, M.D.

Glutamine or Fiber Supplementation of a Defined Formula Diet: Impact on Bacterial Translocation, Tissue Composition, and Response to Endotoxin

Barber AE, Jones WG II, Minei JP, Fahey TJ III, Moldawer LL, Rayburn JL, Fischer E, Keogh CV, Shires GT, Lowry SF (Cornell Univ, New York)
J Parenter Enteral Nutr 14:335–343, 1990   2–3

Enteral feeding with a defined formula diet (DFD) provides sufficient calories for growth but also leads to bacterial translocation, fatty infiltration of the liver, and increased susceptibility to endotoxin in rats. These deleterious effects may be caused by the loss of intestinal barrier integrity resulting from bowel atrophy. The addition of substances to a DFD, which may help to maintain intestinal mass and thus prevent bowel atrophy, remains controversial.

The impact of glutamine or fiber supplementation of a DFD on bowel structure and bowel function was assessed in male Wistar rats. The animals were randomized to DFD containing neither glutamine nor fiber, DFD plus 2% glutamine, or DFD plus 2% psyllium hydrophilic mucilloid. Control rats were given standard rat chow isocalorically pair-fed to DFD. All animals were killed after 2 weeks of the dietary regimen and were analyzed for nutritional status. Additional animals fed the same experimental diets were subsequently challenged with endotoxin and observed for mortality.

All diets resulted in equivalent weight gain and other nutritional parameters. The addition of glutamine or fiber to DFD maintained bowel mass, but only glutamine-enriched DFD preserved normal jejunal mucosal architecture. Neither fiber nor glutamine supplementation prevented cecal bacterial overgrowth or translocation that resulted from feeding with a DFD. In the endotoxin challenge study, mortality was similar in all 3 groups that received DFD, although glutamine enrichment was associated with a significantly lower incidence of bacteremia. Both glutamine and fiber supplementation of DFD prevent the loss of bowel mass, but neither substance protects against spontaneous or endotoxin-induced bacterial translocation, or mortality.

▶ This study examined the hypothesis that glutamine and fiber supplementation of DFDs would protect against bacterial translocation. Although both glutamine and fiber supplementation prevented loss of bowel mass in the experimental animal, neither substance protected against spontaneous bacterial translocation, endotoxin-induced bacterial translocation, or mortality. It would appear that influences on bacterial translocation are not specifically the result of lack of glutamine or fiber in DFDs.— G.T. Shires, M.D.

Total Parenteral Nutrition and Energy Expenditure in General Surgery, Trauma, and Sepsis

Nespoli A, Padalino P, Marradi C, Chiara O, Bosari S, Pallavicini J, Bisiani G (Instituto de Chirurgia d'Urgenza; Univ of Milan; Ospedale Maggiore, Milan)
Surg Res Comm 5:83–91, 1989   2–4

The belief that sepsis and trauma increase energy expenditure has led to the suggestion that energy intake via total parenteral nutrition must be markedly increased. A large caloric intake, however, may produce such complications as hepatic dysfunction, relative respiratory insufficiency, and hyperglycemia with osmotic diuresis.

Resting energy expenditure (REE) was measured by indirect calorimetry in 9 patients who were injured or were scheduled for major surgery and in 11 septic patients. Resting energy expenditure was compared with basal energy expenditure (BEE), as defined using the Harris-Benedict formula. A hypermetabolic state existed when REE exceeded 125% of predicted and a hypometabolic state when it was less than 75% of predicted.

About half of the septic patients had normal metabolism and approximately one third, hypermetabolism. Hypometabolic patients had lower cardiac outputs and impaired cardiac contractility compared with the other groups. Correlations between caloric intake and oxygen consumption, CO_2 production, and REE were weaker in septic patients than in those who had surgery.

The Harris-Benedict formula does not accurately predict energy expenditure in many septic patients. Direct estimates of REE will help to plan energy intake while preventing complications in these patients.

▶ This study reexamines the premise that energy expenditure is markedly increased in sepsis and trauma. Apparently, there is a variety of responses to sepsis and trauma, and defined formulas and multiplication factors for formulas to correct or to supply an increased REE are probably inadequate. It would appear that direct estimates of REE are needed to rationally plan energy intake while minimizing complications from supplying what could well be excessive caloric therapy.—G.T. Shires, M.D.

A Physiologic Basis for the Provision of Fuel Mixtures in Normal and Stressed Patients

Long CL, Nelson KM, Akin JM Jr, Geiger JW, Merrick HW, Blakemore WS (Baptist Med Ctrs, Birmingham, Ala; Med College of Ohio, Toledo)
J Trauma 30:1077–1086, 1990   2–5

Lipid reportedly is a preferred fuel in stressed patients. Glucose oxidation was assessed in 19 patients with sepsis who were given total parenteral nutrition at a rate of 5.65 mg of glucose per kg per minute. Eighteen control patients who were not hypermetabolic or hypercatabolic also were studied. The respiratory quotient (RQ) was measured by indirect calorimetry. The percent VCO_2 arising from glucose oxidation was estimated using $[U-^{14}C]$ glucose.

All patients had an RQ of 1 or higher, indicating that nonprotein energy was derived wholly from glucose. Kinetic data, however, showed that glucose contributed only 55% to 60% of the VCO_2. Protein oxidation contributed less than 20%, as calculated from the urinary nitrogen content. The difference presumably was derived from fatty acid oxidation. Glucose turnover that was not oxidized was presumably converted to lipid at an RQ of 8.6.

Stressed patients do not favor lipid or glucose. The RQ is limited in defining rates of oxidation. The energy needs of hospitalized patients can be defined on the basis of a normal physiologic response rather than by the type of disease that is present.

► This study challenges the concept that lipids reportedly are the preferred fuel in severely stressed patients. In this study, assessment of glucose oxidation, along with the RQ and other variables, in patients given total parenteral nutrition indicates that the energy needs of hospitalized patients can be defined on the basis of a rather normal physiologic response as opposed to the type of disease present. This is an interesting conclusion insofar as the mechanism of energy requirements in the injured patient is concerned.—G.T. Shires, M.D.

Metabolic Effects of Recombinant Human Growth Hormone: Isotopic Studies in the Postabsorptive State and During Total Parenteral Nutrition
Douglas RG, Humberstone DA, Haystead A, Shaw JHF (Auckland Hosp; Ruakura Agricultural Research Ctr, Hamilton, New Zealand)
Br J Surg 77:785–790, 1990   2–6

Accelerated protein breakdown impairs cardiopulmonary performance, immune function, and wound healing in critically ill surgical patients. To determine the metabolic effects of administering recombinant human growth hormone (rHGH) a series of isotopic studies was conducted in 25 critically ill patients; 12 were receiving total parenteral nutrition and 13 were eating a normal hospital diet. All were studied post absorption. Baseline measurements were made before and after a 3-day course of rHGH, 20 units daily subcutaneously.

In the group receiving total parenteral nutrition the net rate of protein loss was decreased by almost half after administration of rHGH. The rate of appearance of leucine was unchanged, which implied that the improved nitrogen balance resulted from enhanced protein synthesis rather than reduced catabolism. In the postabsorptive group, net protein loss and appearance of leucine decreased significantly. No significant changes in glucose concentration, rate of clearance, or rate of oxidation were seen. The amount of free fatty acids and oxidation increased significantly.

Administration of a short-term course of rHGH to critically ill surgical patients appears to be valuable in reducing the net rate of protein loss. This study may not reflect a consistent response to rHGH infusion, given the short period during which isotopic measurements were made. It is also of note that no patient achieved a mean positive nitrogen balance. The protein-sparing effect in postabsorptive patients appears to result from oxidation of fat in preference to protein.

▶ This is one of a host of papers examining the possible utility of rHGH in patients who are receiving total parenteral nutrition. The short-term course of rHGH that was given may not truly reflect a consistent response. However, it does appear that there is a protein-sparing effect in patients that may well result from oxidation of fat in preference to protein. Studies such as this with longer term follow-up are needed.— G.T. Shires, M.D.

3 Shock

Evaluation of an Intraosseous Infusion Device for the Resuscitation of Hypovolemic Shock
Halvorsen L, Bay BK, Perron PR, Gunther RA, Holcroft JW, Blaisdell FW, Kramer GC (Univ of California, Davis)
J Trauma 30:652–658, 1990

3–1

Inadequate delivery of fluid volume and failure to establish vascular access are problems in prehospital fluid resuscitation. Hypertonic saline dextran (HSD) and intraosseous infusion into red bone marrow are thought to be possible solutions to these problems. A new sternal intraosseous infusion device designed for prehospital administration of HSD was evaluated in a study of all 15 sheep subjected to hemorrhagic shock.

Resuscitation was attempted with the intraosseous infusion device in 8 animals and with a central venous catheter in 7. Hemodynamic variables were measured every half hour before and during hemorrhage and more often during resuscitation. Monitoring included vascular pressures, cardiac output, hematocrit value, plasma level of sodium, and blood gases. After being observed for a few days or weeks after intraosseous infusion

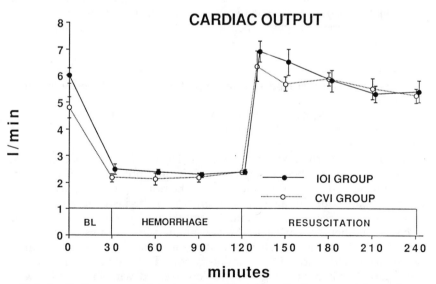

Fig 3–1.—Cardiac output rapidly returned to baseline or better after intraosseous infusion of 7.5% sodium chloride-6% dextran-70 solution. This response was no different from that of control animals resuscitated through a central venous line (means ± standard error of mean). (Courtesy of Halvorsen L, Bay BK, Perron PR, et al: *J Trauma* 30:652–658, 1990.)

13

animals were killed and histologic analysis of their sternums was performed to confirm sternal puncture.

Cardiac output fell by 40% to 50% during hemorrhagic shock. Hemodynamic measurements quickly returned to normal in both groups. There was no significant difference in cardiac output or blood pressure (Fig 3–1). Pulmonary vascular resistance and total peripheral resistance did not return fully to baseline with either method. The hematocrit decreased and the plasma concentration of sodium rose after infusion in both groups. There were no significant pulmonary emboli in the intraosseous infusion group, and histologic study showed no violations of the inner cortical bone table. There was some difficulty in placing the interosseous infusion device.

Intraosseous infusion was used successfully to resuscitate sheep from hemorrhagic shock. Placement of the intraosseous infusion device may be easier and safer than venous catheterization in prehospital resuscitation. The device could allow incorporation of early fluid replacement therapy into the "scoop and run" philosophy.

▶ This article reports on the use of an intraosseous infusion device for resuscitation of hemorrhagic shock. This self-tapping unit is placed in the marrow space of the sternum, where it is held in place by a spring.

This study in sheep shows that fluids can be administered rapidly via intraosseous infusion with recovery of mean arterial blood pressure and cardiac output similar to that after the intravenous administration of the same amount of fluid. A similar device has been advocated for intraosseous infusion in children, particularly when venous access is limited or difficult. Although this device might be useful in delivering small volumes of fluid, it has not yet been adequately investigated either in humans or with larger volumes of fluid.—G.T. Shires, M.D.

Treatment of Uncontrolled Hemorrhagic Shock With Hypertonic Saline Solution

Gross D, Landau EH, Klin B, Krausz MM (Hadassah Univ Hosp, Jerusalem)
Surg Gynecol Obstet 170:106–112, 1990   3–2

Although hypertonic saline solution (HTS) has been recommended as initial treatment for hemorrhagic shock, it may not be safe for patients with "uncontrolled" shock. Uncontrolled hemorrhagic shock, as induced in an animal model by incision of branches of the ileocolic artery, leads to continuous free intra-abdominal hemorrhage. The effect of HTS on uncontrolled hemorrhagic shock was evaluated in 2 groups of rats.

In group 1, the abdomen was closed immediately after induction of hemorrhage and before HTS administration. The animals were then divided into 6 subgroups; 1 group was not treated with HTS and 5 were treated at times ranging from 5 minutes to 120 minutes after closure of the abdomen. In group 2, divided into identical subgroups, the abdomen was kept open to observe the bleeding response after HST therapy.

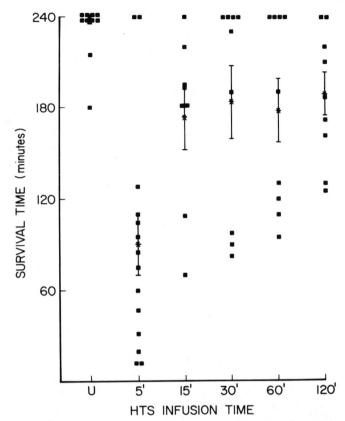

Fig 3–2.—Survival time of rats in uncontrolled hemorrhagic shock after abdominal closure, treated by hypertonic saline solution, *HTS*, at different time periods after injury. (Courtesy of Gross D, Landau EH, Klin B, et al: *Surg Gynecol Obstet* 170:106–112, 1990.)

In group 1, uncontrolled hemorrhagic shock was followed by a fall in mean arterial pressure from 99 mm Hg to 46 mm Hg in 5 minutes, with a gradual rise to 63 mm Hg after 30 minutes. The survival rate was 80% (Fig 3–2). Treatment with HTS led to further falls in mean arterial pressure and increased mortality. In group 2 the response of mean arterial pressure was similar to that of group 1, which received HTS infusion after 5, 60, and 120 minutes. The amount of shed blood was greater at those periods than after 15 minutes and 30 minutes.

The increase in arterial blood pressure and peripheral vasodilation brought about by HTS treatment may increase blood loss. Although HTS restores arterial blood pressure and prevents mortality in controlled hemorrhagic shock, its use in treating victims in hemorrhagic shock after abdominal trauma should be reconsidered. The adverse response to HTS occurs as late as 2 hours after the hemorrhagic insult.

▶ This is another article from a group that continues to study the treatment of uncontrolled hemorrhagic shock with HTS. In the present work, the studies were extended to include uncontrolled bleeding from the ileocolic artery with and without an open abdomen to observe the free and continuing intra-abdominal hemorrhage. Several subgroups of rats were studied to vary the time of administration of HTS after onset of bleeding.

The increase in arterial blood pressure accompanied by peripheral vasodilation brought about by HTS did in fact increase blood loss. This subsequently resulted in a fall in mean arterial blood pressure and early mortality when HTS was given within 2 hours of the hemorrhagic insult. This study of uncontrolled hemorrhagic shock continues to shed doubt on the efficacy of hypertonic fluids, even when used in the early prehospital setting.— G.T. Shires, M.D.

Effect of Different Degrees of Hypothermia on Myocardium in Treatment of Hemorrhagic Shock

Meyer DM, Horton JW, With the technical assistance of Walker P (Univ of Texas, Dallas)
J Surg Res 48:61–67, 1990
3–3

The use of hypothermia in treating hemorrhagic shock is controversial. Previous studies have suggested that moderate hypothermia of 33° C has a protective effect on cardiovascular function and myocardial metabolism. The effects of using hypothermia in treating hemorrhagic shock were examined in 25 dogs.

Hypothermia was established by instillation of chilled saline solution in the peritoneal cavity (group I, 33° C, 7 dogs; group 2, 28° C, 12 dogs). The third group of 6 dogs was maintained at normal body temperature in hemorrhagic shock. The hypothermic dogs were rewarmed after 2 hours. Hemodynamic measurements were made during and after the period of hypothermia.

Four dogs in group 2 died before rewarming. In all of the other dogs blood pressure returned to baseline. During shock, significantly lower heart rates were seen in groups 1 and 2. After hemorrhage, decreases in cardiac output were similar in all groups and returned to baseline with volume replacement. During shock, the stroke volume fell in all, but it remained significantly higher in groups 1 and 2. Total body oxygen consumption was significantly lower in groups 1 and 2, compared to group 3, during hemorrhagic shock and after fluid resuscitation, but this difference was ablated by rewarming. Arterial pH and respiratory rate were significantly lower in hypothermic dogs. Dogs with the lowest body temperature had the lowest arterial pH.

Moderate hypothermia decreases myocardial metabolism at the same time that it maintains hemodynamic status and myocardial perfusion. Severe hypothermia often leads to fatal arrhythmias. The benefits of reduced body temperature in trauma victims therefore appears to depend on the level of hypothermia. Maintenance of acid-base status, ventilatory support, and temperature monitoring seem to be important in maximizing the clinical benefits of hypothermia.

▶ The authors examined the controversial question of the value of hypothermia as therapy for hemorrhagic shock. This article was interesting in that it compared 2 different levels of hypothermia after a standard hemorrhagic shock model was developed. The data show that moderate hypothermia (body temperature no less than 33° C) during hemorrhagic shock increased coronary perfusion, enhanced cardiac contractile performance, and reduced myocardial oxygen requirements. However, severe hypothermia (body temperature of 28° C) in the canine preparation was associated with increased ventricular irritability and fatal arrhythmia.

This study confirms data from other investigators indicating that significant hypothermia is of no value in the treatment of hypovolemic shock. However, the modest hypothermia that generally occurs during hemorrhagic shock may, in fact, be a protective mechanism.—G.T. Shires, M.D.

Organ Distribution of Radiolabeled Enteric *Escherichia Coli* During and After Hemorrhagic Shock
Redan JA, Rush BF, McCullough JN, Machiedo GW, Murphy TF, Dikdan GS, Smith S (UMDNJ–New Jersey Med School, Newark)
Ann Surg 211:663–668, 1990   3–4

Intestinal bacteria may translocate to the blood during hemorrhagic shock. The path of translocated intestinal organisms was followed in a murine model of hemorrhagic shock. The animals were gavaged with viable ^{14}C-oleic acid-labeled *Escherichia coli* and 48 hours later were bled to a mean arterial pressure of 30 mm Hg for 5 hours or until 80% of maximum shed blood was returned. Resuscitation was with Ringer's lactate.

Most translocated bacteria were present in the kidneys and liver 24 hours after resuscitation from shock. In contrast, immediately after shock most of the bacteria were in the lungs. Animals surviving to 48 hours were able to eliminate a majority or organisms from their major organ systems. Positive cultures for *E. coli* were obtained in the blood as well as in the lungs, liver, and kidneys.

The gut flora are translocated during hemorrhagic shock and are present in the lungs and kidneys. The process appears not to continue long after resuscitation from shock, and surviving animals are able to eliminate translocated bacteria from their organs.

▶ There is a whole host of articles appearing in relation to bacterial translocation. This study traced the path of translocated intestinal bacteria in a murine hemorrhagic shock model. Carbon-14-labeled *E. coli* were instilled into the intestine and 48 hours later the animals were bled into shock. Abdominal and thoracic organs were harvested and cultured, and the radioactive content measured a variable period of hours after the shock preparation. Interestingly, translocated enteric bacteria were found primarily in the lung immediately after shock, with redistribution to the liver and kidney 24 hours later. Animals surviving to 48 hours were capable of eliminating most of these bacteria from their major organ systems. This study adds to the increasing body of evidence that sepsis and multiple organ failure after shock and trauma may well be the result of endogenous translocated intestinal bacteria.—G.T. Shires, M.D.

The Role of Intestinal Barrier Failure and Bacterial Translocation in the Development of Systemic Infection and Multiple Organ Failure

Deitch EA (Louisiana State Univ, Shreveport)
Arch Surg 125:403–404, 1990   3–5

Intestinal bacteria can, under some circumstances, escape from the gut and produce systemic infection. Factors promoting such bacterial translocation include disruption of the normal microflora leading to overgrowth, impaired host immunity, and physical disruption of the gut mucosal barrier. Patients with bacteremia of this type tend to have altered intestinal function, to have had major blood loss or hypotension, and to be immunocompromised and/or malnourished. In addition, they often have received drugs that alter the gut flora such as broad-spectrum antibiotics or histamine 2-blockers.

Selective gut decontamination attempts to lower the risk of systemic infection in high-risk patients by the oral administration of nonabsorbable antibiotics active against gram-negative enteric bacilli. Clinical studies to date have given encouraging results, although patient survival has not generally improved. Additional means of boosting local and systemic antibacterial defenses are needed.

Many patients dying of sepsis and multiple organ failure have enteric bacteremia unrelated to a septic focus. Gut barrier failure may be a factor in these deaths. Clinical studies are needed to determine whether preventing gut barrier failure will avoid multiple organ failure.

▶ This is a general statement of the current emphasis on the role of intestinal barrier failure and bacterial translocation, particularly relative to the development of systemic infection and multiple organ failure. This summary nicely points out some of the various circumstances that influence translocation in patients. This includes such things as patients being immunocompromised, having had blood loss or hypotension, and, in addition, possibly being malnourished. Further, drug therapy, which may have altered the flora of the intestine, may have been ongoing at the time of the insult. Studies on selective decontamination of the gut have not been carried out with control of enough variables to truly define the indications or value of reduction of gram-negative enteric bacilli.—G.T. Shires, M.D.

Are the Catabolic Effects of Tumor Necrosis Factor Mediated by Glucocorticoids?

Mealy K, van Lanschot JJB, Robinson BG, Rounds J, Wilmore DW (Brigham and Women's Hosp, Boston)
Arch Surg 125:42–48, 1990   3–6

There is evidence that tumor necrosis factor (TNF) is a major mediator of gram-negative endotoxic shock. In vitro data, however, suggest that the cytokine has little effect in initiating skeletal muscle proteolysis, and its role in regulating in vivo protein metabolism is not clear.

Three series of experiments were undertaken in rats to determine whether the catabolic effects of TNF are mediated by glucocorticoids. The first part of the study examined the effect of TNF on the hypothalamic-adrenal stress response. In a further series of experiments the metabolic effects of TNF were compared with those of corticosterone, the predominant glucocorticoid in the rat. Nitrogen loss was then compared in adrenalectomized animals receiving basal corticosterone infused with TNF and sham adrenalectomized controls.

In the first experiments, parenterally fed male Wistar rats received infusions of TNF at 0, 2×10^5, and 4×10^5 units per kg per 24 hours during a 1- to 6- day period. Adrenal weight was increased with increasing dosage of TNF. The higher dosage of TNF significantly increased the plasma corticotropin level for 24 hours. In the next experiments, rats given corticosterone (75 mg subcutaneously) or TNF (2×10^5 units per kg per 24 hours) showed decreased nitrogen balance and carcass nitrogen content for a 6-day period. In comparison with control and corticosterone groups, however, TNF alone brought about a significant increase in liver nitrogen content and diminished jejunal mucosa DNA and protein levels. In the final experiments, urinary nitrogen loss was significantly diminished in the adrenalectomized animals, indicating that an intact adrenal stress response is necessary for the increased nitrogen loss after TNF infusion.

Administration of TNF results in skeletal muscle proteolysis and diminished nitrogen balance resembling that after severe injury or infection. A similar alteration occurs after the administration of corticosterone alone. Tumor necrosis factor also exerts visceral alterations not reproduced by glucocorticoid administration.

▶ This is one of many, many articles investigating the exact role of TNF as a major mediator of gram-negative endotoxic shock. This study was undertaken to determine whether the catabolic effects of TNF are mediated by glucocorticoids.

In this rat model, corticosterone brought about decreased nitrogen balance and carcass nitrogen content during a 6-day period. In a comparison of control and corticosterone groups, TNF alone significantly increased the liver nitrogen content and diminished jejunal mucosa DNA and protein levels. Thus the administration of TNF resulted in skeletal muscle proteolysis and diminished nitrogen balance resembling that after severe infection or injury. The visceral alterations, however, were not reproduced by glucocorticoid administration and were therefore unique to TNF.

The findings tend to confirm the postulation that the efflux of amino acids from the periphery to the liver, and the subsequent synthesis of acute-phase proteins, are required to support the metabolic demands of immune proliferation and the healing wound. Certainly, TNF elaboration is one of a number of stress hormone response to shock and trauma, but TNF seems to be a major mediator of gram-negative endotoxic shock.— G.T. Shires, M.D.

Tumor Necrosis Factor Induces Adult Respiratory Distress Syndrome in Rats

Ferrari-Baliviera E, Mealy K, Smith RJ, Wilmore DW (Brigham and Women's Hosp, Boston)
Arch Surg 124:1400–1405, 1989   3–7

Sepsis is often associated with deterioration in pulmonary function that may lead to adult respiratory distress syndrome (ARDS). Although a number of circulating factors have been implicated in the etiology of ARDS, the specific cause of the syndrome in sepsis remains unclear. Tumor necrosis factor (TNF) has been identified as one of the mediators of sepsis. Furthermore, in animals given lethal doses of TNF, pulmonary alterations are seen that resemble those present in the lungs of patients with ARDS. The effect of TNF on lung structure and pulmonary function was examined in experimental animals.

After venous catheter placement for administration of TPN, 69 adult rats were divided into 3 groups. Twenty-three rats were given TPN infusion only, another group received TPN and low-dose TNF infusion, and the third group was given TPN and hig-dose TNF infusion. After 24 hours of TNF infusion, all animals were killed. Volume-pressure measurements were determined in excised lungs, using both air and saline to eliminate surface tension forces. Total lung wet and dry weight, nitrogen level, and DNA and protein content also were evaluated.

The lungs of TNF-treated rats accepted significantly smaller volumes of air and saline at all pressures than did the lungs of untreated controls. Both total wet and dry lung weights were significantly increased with TNF infusion, suggesting that the increased weight could not be accounted for by an increase in fluid retention alone. Protein content and DNA values also were increased with TNF infusion which, suggested an increased cellularity in the TNF-infused lungs. Lungs of TNF-treated rats were stiffer and had reduced compliance compared with lungs of untreated control animals. Thus TNF infusion clearly affects pulmonary mechanics in experimental animals.

Tumor necrosis factor may be involved in the activation of a cascade of events leading to functional and structural alterations in the lungs of experimental animals. These events appear to be similar to those observed in human ARDS.

▶ This look at TNF was directed specifically at the pulmonary response, particularly TNF-induced ARDS, in rats. This study shows clearly that the lungs of TNF-treated rats accepted smaller volumes of air and saline at all pressures than did the lungs of untreated controls. Wet and dry lung weights were significantly increased with TNF infusion, suggesting that the increased lung weight could not be accounted for by an increase in fluid retention alone. Lungs of TNF-treated rats were stiffer and had reduced compliances compared with lungs of untreated controls. This is one more article indicating that the ARDS seen in patients after trauma is related to the mediator TNF in association with sepsis.—G.T. Shires, M.D.

Tumor Necrosis Factor-α Mediates Acid Aspiration-Induced Systemic Organ Injury
Goldman G, Welbourn R, Kobzik L, Valeri CR, Shepro D, Hechtman HB (Brigham and Women's Hosp, Boston; Harvard Med School; Boston Univ)
Ann Surg 212:513–520, 1990   3–8

Acid aspiration-induced injury to systemic organs involves the sequestration of activated neutrophils. Because cytokines increase neutrophil-endothelial adhesion in other settings, an attempt was made to determine whether tumor necrosis factor (TNF)-induced synthesis of an adhesion protein mediates systemic leukosequestration and increased permeability after aspiration.

A cannula was placed in the anterior segment of the left lung in anesthetized rats, and either .1 N HCl or saline was instilled in a volume of .1 mL. Pulmonary leukosequestration ensued and permeability edema developed, as evidenced by an increased protein concentration in bronchoalveolar lavage fluid on the aspirated side. Generalized pulmonary edema also was noted. Myeloperoxidase activity increased in both heart and kidney in association with edema of these organs. Administration of anti-TNF-α antiserum 20 minutes after aspiration effectively countered the effects of acid aspiration. Treatment with cycloheximide, which inhibits protein synthesis, also was effective.

Tumor necrosis factor has a role in mediating local and systemic injury secondary to acid aspiration. A mechanism involving the expression of endothelial adhesion protein probably is involved.

▶ This study looked at TNF in relation to systemic organ injury after acid aspiration. Specifically, this study examined whether TNF induced synthesis of an adhesion protein mediating systemic leukosequestration and increased permeability after aspiration. Certainly, the most convincing proof of this study was that administration of anti-TNF antiserum 20 minutes after aspiration was able to counter the effects of acid aspiration. It is interesting that treatment with cycloheximide, which inhibits protein synthesis, also was effective.

The studies indicate quite clearly that TNF has a role in mediating local and systemic injury secondary to acid aspiration. A mechanism involving expression of endothelial adhesion protein is probably the primary mechanism involved. This is just another way of showing the dramatic effects of TNF in relation to a different kind of injury.—G.T. Shires, M.D.

Endotoxin-Induced Procoagulant Activity, Eicosanoid Synthesis, and Tumor Necrosis Factor Production by Rat Peritoneal Macrophages: Effect of Endotoxin Tolerance and Glucan

Moore JN, Cook JA, Morris DD, Halushka PV, Wise WC (Medical Univ of South Carolina, Charleston; Univ of Georgia, Athens)
Circ Shock 31:281–295, 1990
3–9

Macrophages appear to release pro-inflammatory substances that can enhance the intravascular coagulopathy associated with endotoxemia. The effects of *Salmonella enteritidis* endotoxin on procoagulant activity, eicosanoid metabolism, and production of tumor necrosis factor (TNF) by rat peritoneal macrophages were examined. Tumor necrosis factor was assayed using a murine fibrosarcoma cell line.

Endotoxin produced dose-dependent increases in immunoreactive thromboxane B_2, 6-ketoprostaglandin $E_{1\alpha}$, and TNF. More marked increases in thromboxane B_2 and prostaglandin were produced by calcium ionophore. Endotoxin also increased procoagulant activity in macrophage lysates, but the calcium ionophore had little effect on it. Tolerance to endotoxin, produced by repeated sublethal doses, rendered the macrophages resistant to endotoxin-induced production of prostaglandin, TNF activity, and procoagulant activity. Opposite effects were achieved by pretreating rats with glucan, a macrophage stimulant that enhances the lethality of endotoxin. Endotoxin leads to the in vitro production of eicosanoids and TNF by rat peritoneal macrophages, as well as the expression of procoagulant activity by these cells.

▶ This nicely done study studied the effects of *Salmonella* endotoxin on procoagulant activity and the production of TNF by rat peritoneal macrophages. The authors show that some tolerance to endotoxin produced by repeated sublethal doses rendered the macrophages resistant to production of TNF. However, this is a good model for in vitro production of TNF by rat peritoneal macrophages in response to endotoxin.—G.T. Shires, M.D.

Elevated Tumor Necrosis Factor$_\alpha$ Production Concomitant to Elevated Prostaglandin E_2 Production by Trauma Patients' Monocytes

Takayama TK, Miller C, Szabo G (Univ of Massachusetts, Worcester)
Arch Surg 125:29–35, 1990
3–10

Patients with severe traumatic or thermal injuries have elevated serum levels of tumor necrosis factor$_\alpha$ (TNF$_\alpha$) that correlate with injury severity. Posttrauma monocytes are the primary source of TNF$_\alpha$. Prostaglandin E_2 (PGE$_2$) production is also increased in posttrauma monocytes. However, previous studies have found that high levels of PGE$_2$ downregulate monocyte TNF$_\alpha$. Thus the increase in monocyte TNF$_\alpha$ levels after trauma seems to be an anomaly. The relationship between PGE$_2$ production and TNF$_\alpha$ production was assessed in posttrauma monocytes.

Blood samples were obtained from 11 patients with burns of more than 20% total body surface area, 11 patients with major trauma, and 26 normal controls. Monocytes were isolated from the blood samples, cultured for 24 hours, and suboptimally stimulated to increase TNF_α production. Tumor necrosis factor-α levels and PGE_2 levels in the supernates of the monocyte cultures were measured by enzyme-linked immunosorbent assay.

Patients with sepsis had significantly greater total TNF_α levels 3 days before septic episodes developed, compared with normal controls. Further increases in patients' total monocyte TNF_α levels to more than 30 $ng/10^6$ monocytes per mL correlated with septic episodes. Total monocyte TNF_α levels increased during septic episodes despite a concomitant increase in PGE_2 levels. Patients with sepsis had simultaneous massively elevated monocyte TNF_α levels and massively elevated monocyte PGE_2 levels.

Monocyte TNF_α production may be resistant to PGE_2 downregulation. Further, TNF_α apparently can be induced concomitantly with the induction of PGE_2.

▶ This study examined the monocyte as a source for the increased production of TNF in severe injury. The authors concluded that posttrauma monocytes are a primary source of TNF-α. They further examined the relationship between prostaglandin production and TNF-α production in posttrauma monocytes and found them to be essentially independent variables, although both levels were massively elevated in monocytes with onset of sepsis.

This is another of the continuing investigations into the details of the activity of the cascades that are turned on by the presence of sepsis.—G.T. Shires, M.D.

Serum Tumor Necrosis Factor Levels in Patients With Infectious Disease and Septic Shock
Offner F, Philippé J, Vogelaers D, Colardyn F, Baele G, Baudrihaye M, Vermeulen A, Leroux-Roels G (State Univ, Ghent, Belgium; IRE-Medgenix, Fleurus, Belgium)
J Lab Clin Med 116:100–105, 1990   3–11

Much evidence suggests that tumor necrosis factor (TNF-α) is a mediator in the pathogenesis of septic shock in animal models. To examine the role of TNF-α in the pathophysiology of septic shock in human beings, 60 patients admitted to the medical intensive care unit with severe infection were studied. All were at risk for sepsis and septic shock. Each patient was assessed daily for clinical condition using APACHE II scoring and for serum levels of TNF-α by a commercial immunoradiometric assay.

Sepsis was diagnosed in 34 of the 60 patients, and 24 of the 34 died (6 within the first 24 hours). At the time of admission the serum level of TNF-α in patients who did not later have sepsis was significantly lower than that in those who did later have septic shock (median, .5 vs. 79 pg/

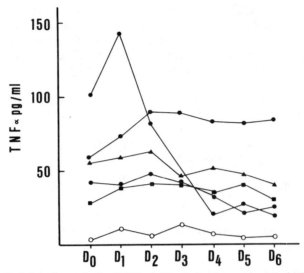

Fig 3–3.—Evolution of serum levels of TNF-α in 5 typical patients with septic shock on 7 consecutive days from day of admission. Evolution of single typical nonsepsis patient is added for comparison *(open circles)*. (Courtesy of Offner F, Philippé J, Vogelaers D, et al: *J Lab Clin Med* 116:100–105, 1990.)

mL). The patients who died within the first 25 hours had significant higher levels of TNF-α than patients who later had sepsis (median, 917 vs. 58 pg/mL). In most patients who survived for more than 24 hours the levels of TNF-α tended to remain rather constant over a period of several days (Fig 3–3); the onset of septic shock was neither accompanied nor followed by sudden changes in levels of TNF-α. The APACHE II scores of patients in whom sepsis occurred were significantly correlated with levels of TNF-α.

Serum levels of TNF-α were not useful predictors of the survival of individual patients because there were large overlaps between TNF-α values of patient groups that did and did not have septic shock. It is likely that other cytokines in addition to TNF-α are involved in the occurrence of septic shock.

► This article only confirms what has previously been shown in relation to the serum levels of TNF after injury. It is increasingly clear that TNF, although generated from monocytes systemically, probably has its major effect as a paracrine or autocrine substance, i.e., at the site of local production, rather than being correlated as a serum level.—G.T. Shires, M.D.

Beneficial Effect of Enhanced Macrophage Function in the Trauma Patient
Browder W, Williams D, Pretus H, Olivero G, Enrichens F, Mao P, Franchello A
(Tulane Univ; Univ of Torino, Italy)
Ann Surg 211:605–613, 1990   3–12

Sepsis remains a major problem during recovery in trauma patients. Host immunosuppression after trauma has a major role in the development of sepsis. Altered macrophage function is a key factor in the increased susceptibility to sepsis after trauma. Because glucan is a potent macrophage stimulant in animal models, a prospective, randomized, double-blind study was done to determine whether glucan administration during the early post trauma period could prevent the subsequent development of sepsis.

During a 2-year period, 38 patients were entered into the trial, 21 of whom were randomly allocated to receive intravenous glucan for 7 days; 17 were given placebo. Delayed hypersensitivity skin testing was performed on days 1 and 7 after trauma. Serum interleukin-1 (IL-1) and tumor necrosis factor levels also were measured. Blunt trauma from automobile accidents was the most common mechanism of injury, accounting for 12 of the 21 injuries in the glucan-treated group and 15 of the 17 injuries in the placebo-treated group. Most of the other patients had sustained penetrating injuries caused by gunshots or stabs.

The total mortality rate was 0% among glucan-treated patients and 29% in the placebo-treated group. There were 3 deaths caused by sepsis in the placebo-treated group, but the difference in mortality from sepsis did not reach statistical significance. However, the morbidity from sepsis was 49% in the placebo-treated group and 9.5% in the glucan-treated group, a statistically significant difference. Glucan-treated patients had a greater increase in serum IL-1 levels than placebo-treated patients had on day 3 after trauma, but there was no difference between the groups thereafter. Tumor necrosis factor levels did not differ between groups. Furthermore, neither IL-1 nor TNF levels were reliable indicators of future sepsis. Although the increase in IL-1 production after glucan therapy in the early posttrauma period is an encouraging finding, why glucan therapy did not enhance IL-1 levels beyond day 3 remains to be investigated.

▶ This article discusses an attempt to modify the response to trauma insofar as immunosuppression is concerned. In this study, a macrophage enhancer was given in the form of glucan. Although glucan is a potent macrophage stimulant, the downstream cascade of production of interleukins was quite variable when the macrophages were stimulated in such a nonspecific way.—G.T. Shires, M.D.

Endotoxin (LPS) Increases Mesenteric Vascular Resistance (MVR) and Bacterial Translocation (BT)
Navaratnam RLN, Morris SE, Traber DL, Flynn J, Woodson L, Linares H, Herndon DN (Univ of Texas, Galveston; Thomas Jefferson College of Medicine, Philadelphia)
J Trauma 30:1104–1115, 1990   3–13

Endotoxin produces many of the cardiovascular changes seen in septic patients. Reduced intestinal blood flow could promote the release of toxic products of ischemia and also lead to breakdown of its immune barrier, allowing the entrance of enteric organisms and their toxins into the circulation.

Hemodynamic function in the gastrointestinal tract was assessed in sheep given either *Escherichia coli* endotoxin or Ringer's lactate by infusion. Mesenteric blood flow declined by more than half in endotoxin-treated sheep, and mesenteric vascular resistance increased. Nonmesenteric vascular resistance declined at the same time. Positive bacterial cultures were obtained consistently from the mesenteric lymph nodes of endotoxemic sheep.

Endotoxin promotes mesenteric vasoconstriction, thereby diverting intestinal blood to the nonintestinal systemic circulation. If, as a result, bacterial translocation is increased, sequential organ failure could ensue. There seems to be a level of mesenteric arterial perfusion at which the gut mucosal barrier is no longer maintained.

▶ This article looks at another factor reducing the gut barrier to bacterial translocation. In this instance, the measured reduction of intestinal blood flow did seem to result in greater bacterial translocation, which would then, of course, help to explain subsequent multiple organ failure. The authors suggest that there seems to be a level of mesenteric arterial perfusion at which the gut mucosal barrier is no longer maintained. Although other studies have shown that this is clearly not the only factor in bacterial translocation, in early response to injury it may be one of the many factors involved.—G.T. Shires, M.D.

4 Trauma

Critical Care Air Transportation of the Severely Injured: Does Long Distance Transport Adversely Affect Survival?
Valenzuela TD, Criss EA, Copass MK, Luna GK, Rice CL (Arizona Health Sciences Ctr, Tucson; Harborview Med Ctr, Seattle)
Ann Emerg Med 19:169–172, 1990   4–1

The success of air evacuation of wounded soldiers led to a proliferation of civilian air transport services for trauma victims. Few studies, however, have examined the risks and benefits of such services. Data from the first 2 years of operation of Airlift Northwest, a critical care air transportation system serving the Pacific Northwest and southeast Alaska, were collected and analyzed.

During the study period, 118 of 620 transported patients met the entry criteria, including age (15 years or older), and time of trauma (24 or fewer hours before flight). A fixed wing aircraft staffed by a physician and an intensive care unit registered nurse was used for the flights. The mean 1-way flight distance was 340 miles. A control population of 50 patients was transported to the same trauma center by a ground paramedic unit. The 2 groups did not differ significantly in age, Glasgow Coma Score, or Injury Severity Score.

In-hospital mortality was 18% for ground-transported patients and 19% for the air-lifted population. Age, Injury Severity Score, and type of trauma were the most powerful predictors of mortality. Among the air-transported patients, these same 3 variables were the best predictors of mortality. Subsequent death or survival was not significantly affected by the magnitude of the distance flown.

Injured patients were not adversely affected by long-distance air transport designed to deliver an "intensive care unit" level of care. Trauma patients are known to have better outcomes when treated in a trauma center, and Airlift Northwest extends the benefits of a regional trauma center up to 800 miles.

▶ This is one of the few of badly needed studies revealing outcome data substantiating the benefit of air medical transportation system. This particular study used comparisons with rapid ground transport as opposed to fixed wing aircraft transport for an average distance of 340 miles, the range being from 100 to 800 miles. The 2 groups of patients transported were comparable in that they did not differ significantly in age, Injury Severity Score, or Glasgow Coma Score.

The results clearly indicate that death or survival was not significantly affected by the magnitude of the distance flown when the fixed wing aircraft transport was designed to deliver an intensive care unit level of treatment.

When one combines this study with previously documented data showing that patients have a better outcome when treated in a trauma center, the benefits of this form of transport become quite impressive.—G.T. Shires, M.D.

APACHE II Score Does Not Predict Multiple Organ Failure or Mortality in Postoperative Surgical Patients

Cerra FB, Negro F, Abrams J (Univ of Minnesota)
Arch Surg 125:519–522, 1990   4–2

Use of the acute physiology and chronic health evaluation (APACHE) II system in the surgical intensive care unit (ICU) has been proposed on the assumption that physiologic abnormalities present within 24 hours of surgical ICU admission accurately reflect the later course and outcome. The ability of this system to predict the development of multiple organ failure syndrome was studied in 92 patients seen in 1 year.

Sixty-nine patients had multiple organ failure syndrome and 68 of these died. The APACHE II scores failed to a clinically useful extent to predict either multiple organ failure or death (Fig 4–1). Scores signifi-

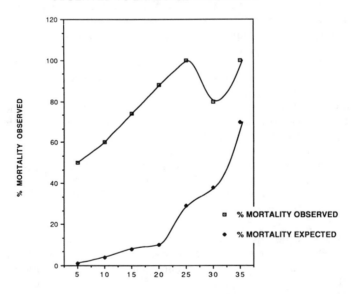

ADMISSION APACHE II SCORE:
OBSERVED VS EXPECTED MORTALITY

Fig 4–1.—The observed *(squares)* and expected *(diamonds)* mortality in each score range. The admission APACHE I score consistently under-estimated the subsequent development of multiple organ failure syndrome and mortality. (Courtesy of Cerra FB, Negro F, Abrams J: *Arch Surg* 125:519–522, 1990.)

cantly underestimated the potential for organ failure syndrome to develop. Factors that did help to predict multiple organ failure syndrome and mortality included the ratio of PaO_2 to inspired oxygen fraction, the serum lactate level, and the creatinine and bilirubin levels.

In multiple organ failure syndrome, the extent of organ injury is manifest several days after ICU admission. A useful predictive severity index would have to take into account the particular disease process, previous treatment used to stabilize the patient, and the time required for injury to become physiologically apparent.

▶ This is another approach to evaluating a system of patient scoring (APACHE II) in predicting the outcome of severely ill patients treated in an ICU. Once again, the APACHE II score failed to predict either multiple organ failure or death to a clinically useful extent. The authors point out that a useful predictive severity index would have to take into account the particular disease process, the previous treatment used to stabilize the patient, and the time required for the injury to become apparent physiologically.—G.T. Shires, M.D.

Evaluation of APACHE II for Cost Containment and Quality Assurance
Civetta JM, Hudson-Civetta JA, Nelson LD (Univ of Miami)
Ann Surg 212:266–276, 1990   4–3

The acute physiology score and chronic health evaluation (APACHE II) system has been proposed for use in limiting admissions to the intensive care unit (ICU) and in judging surgical outcomes. The performance of APACHE II was assessed in a 6-month study of 372 surgical ICU patients. The total score consists of age, chronic health evaluation, and the acute physiology score, the latter comprising 11 variables.

For patients with APACHE II scores below 10, mortality increased from 1% for short-stay cases to 19% for long-stay cases. Among those with scores exceeding 24, mortality declined from 94% (short stay) to 60% (long stay). Grouped APACHE II scores failed to correlate with either total hospital charges or number of days in the ICU. These findings call into question the use of APACHE II, either for cost containment or for quality assurance.

▶ This credible study evaluated the use of the APACHE II system in limiting admission to ICUs and in judging surgical outcome. This study of a significant number of surgical ICU patients examined all of the related variables and concluded that the APACHE II score was not useful either for cost containment, quality assurance, or uniformity of prediction of mortality rates. Furthermore, the duration of ICU stay had no relation to the APACHE II score.

This is one of the very few definitive studies looking at a variety of scoring system that have been proposed for use in relation to the level of care to be afforded severely ill patients.—G.T. Shires, M.D.

Evaluation of the Pediatric Trauma Score

Kaufmann CR, Maier RV, Rivara FP, Carrico CJ (Univ of Washington; Harborview Injury Prevention and Research Ctr, Seattle)
JAMA 263:69–72, 1990   4–4

The Revised Trauma Score (RTS) is an accepted triage score that is applicable to all ages. A recently developed triage tool, the Pediatric Trauma Score (PTS), is rapidly gaining acceptance for use in prehospital triage of the injured child. The 2 scoring systems were compared to determine the value of the PTS.

The study group included 376 patients younger than 15 years who were admitted consecutively to a level 1 trauma center in a 30-month period. Motor vehicle collisions accounted for 50% of the injuries and falls for 24%. Charts were reviewed for a number of variables, including the Glasgow Coma Scale. An APACHE II score was calculated for each patient using initial vital signs and laboratory data. The Injury Severity Score was calculated at discharge.

The PTS is a combination anatomical and physiologic scoring system. Resulting scores can range from −6 to +12, with the most severe injuries assigned the lowest scores. In the RTS, a physiologic score, results can range from 0 to 12, and like the PTS, the lowest scores represent the most serious injuries. Using scene data, rates of overtriage, undertriage, and triage accuracy were calculated.

Overtriage was significantly greater using the PTS, whereas undertriage was greater with the RTS. Overall accuracy was significantly greater for the RTS (78.8%) compared with the PTS (68.3%). The PTS had no statistical advantage over the RTS, even in the youngest children.

Both systems were significantly correlated with survival, the Injury Severity Score, APACHE II score, Glasgow Coma Scale, hematocrit, need for an operation, and number of days in an intensive care unit. But the PTS has no advantage over the RTS and is more complicated to use. Miscalculation of 1 of the 6 variables in the PTS can result in significant undertriage or overtriage.

▶ This is another sophisticated study comparing various means of injury scoring. This particular study compared the RTS and the PTS, along with APACHE II scoring. As with most scoring systems, there is correlation with survival, but the value of these injury severity scores in predicting specific therapeutic needs, including the need for operation or the need for the number of days to be in intensive care, simply could not be demonstrated. This is appearing in more and more evaluations of injury severity scoring scales.— G.T. Shires, M.D.

Emergency Department Deaths

Webb GL, McSwain NE Jr, Webb WR, Rodriguez C (Louisiana State Univ, Shreveport; Tulane Univ; New Orleans Police Dept)
Am J Surg 159:377–379, 1990   4–5

An efficient ambulance system with well-trained attendants that delivers patients to a regional trauma center can dramatically lower morbidity and mortality among trauma patients. The incidence of prehospital or hospital emergency department (ED) problems and preventable deaths was determined.

During a 2-year period, 186 trauma deaths occurred in the ED of Charity Hospital of Louisiana at New Orleans, a level I trauma center that serves a large inner-city population. All patients who died were autopsied. Patients ranged in age from 1 month to 81 years. Sixty-five patients were aged 20–29 years, and 73% were younger than 40 years. Black men accounted for 51% of the deaths. Gunshot wounds comprised 59% of the injuries; motor vehicle accidents, 11%; stab wounds, 7%; pedestrian injuries, 7%; falls, 5%; motorcycle accidents, 2%; and other injuries, 7%.

No deaths were attributable to inappropriate prehospital care of patients transported by the New Orelans police ambulance services. The average response time was 5.8 minutes and ranged from less than 1 to 16 minutes. Time at the accident scene averaged 16.2 minutes. The total interval between the time the call was received and arrival at the ED averaged 27.4 minutes. In contrast, patients brought in by private vehicles or transferred from other hospitals arrived after longer periods. Death was attributable to head injury in 44% of the cases, cardiac injury in 16%, multiple trauma in 13%, aortic injury in 8%, hemorrhage in 8%, and other causes in 11%.

Autopsy results revealed that the injuries in 180 of the 186 patients were unsurvivable. Of the 6 patients who had injuries compatible with survival, 3 were late arrivals by transfer or self-imposed delay, and these patients died of protracted hemorrhage. Only 3 ED deaths were potentially preventable.

Very few deaths in this well-established trauma center were preventable. The favorable outcome is attributable to proper supervision and monitoring of care. Maximizing survival of trauma patients requires rapid transport by an experienced emergency medical ambulance service to a well-staffed trauma center where immediate, appropriate, and rapid evaluation, quick diagnosis, resuscitation, and definitive therapy are always available.

▶ This study of ED deaths is one of the few outcome data studies in relation to initial care and is the first to appear since the articles from Southern California approximately 10 years ago. This study showed quite clearly that if survival from trauma is to be maximized, rapid transport by an experienced medical ambulance service to a well-staffed trauma center, where immediate, appropriate, and rapid evaluation, quick diagnosis, resuscitation, and definitive therapy are available, will certainly minimize preventable deaths. In this series there were 6 potentially preventable deaths among a total of 186. Three deaths were related to delay in transport; the other 3 were potentially preventable in the ED.—G.T. Shires, M.D.

Prophylactic Antibiotics in Trauma: The Hazards of Underdosing

Ericsson CD, Fischer RP, Rowlands BJ, Hunt C, Miller-Crotchett P, Reed L II
(Univ of Texas, Houston; Queen's Univ of Belfast, Northern Ireland)
J Trauma 29:1356–1361, 1989   4–6

The optimal regimen of antibiotics in trauma patients who require laparotomy remains controversial. Because prophylactic antibiotic regimens in trauma patients may be significantly altered by large fluid shifts and hyperdynamic physiologic responses, the effects of duration of coverage, dosing interval, and dose of prophylactic amikacin and clindamycin in abdominal trauma patients who require laparotomy were assessed. After receiving intravenous doses of clindamycin (1,200 mg) and amikacin (7.5 mg/kg) in the emergency room, 150 patients received at random additional doses of clindamycin and amikacin 12 hours later (24-hour therapy), clindamycin and amikacin every 12 hours for 5 doses (72-hour therapy), or clindamycin (600 mg) every 6 hours for 11 doses and amikacin (7.5 mg/kg) for 5 doses (72-hour therapy) (table). The patients were followed for 30 postoperative days to detect development of wound or intra-abdominal infection.

The rates of infection did not differ significantly between the 24-hour and 72-hour antibiotic coverage (21% vs. 19%). Acceptable serum concentrations were achieved with clindamycin, 1,200 mg every 12 hours, and infection rates with this regimen were not significantly higher than those achieved with 600 mg every 6 hours (21% vs. 12%). In some patients who received amikacin, 6.7–7.5 mg/kg, the observed peak concentrations of the drug were lower than generally accepted peak values, which correlated with higher volumes of distribution; also, the half-life of amikacin was shorter than expected. Raising the amikacin dose to 11

Comparison of Infection Rates in Three Antibiotic Regimens

Subject Characteristics	Antibiotic Regimen †		
	I	II	III
All subjects	9/47 (19)	11/52 (21)	6/51 (12)
Gunshot wounds	7/26 (27)	9/33 (27)	4/27 (15)
Knife wounds	1/9 (11)	1/6 (17)	1/9 (11)
Blunt trauma	1/12 (8)	1/13 (8)	1/15 (7)
Colon penetrated	4/13 (31)	6/14 (43)	3/18 (17)
High blood loss *	7/20 (35)	9/23 (39)	4/27 (15)
Injury Severity Score ≥20	4/15 (27)	4/13 (31)	4/22 (18)

*Defined as ≥ median (6 units) blood loss.
†Numbers in parenthesis are percentages. Regimens I–III are defined as 1,200 mg of clindamycin plus 7.5 mg/kg or 11 mg/kg of amikacin followed by: I—additional doses of clindamycin (1,200 mg) and amikacin 12 hours later (i.e., 24-hour therapy); II—clindamycin (1,200 mg) and amikacin repeated every 12 hours for 5 additional doses each (i.e., 72-hour therapy); and III—clindamycin (600 mg) every 6 hours for 11 additional doses, and amikacin every 12 hours for 5 additional doses (i.e., 72-hour therapy.)

(Courtesy of Ericsson CD, Fischer RP, Rowlands BJ, et al: *J Trauma* 29:1356–1361, 1989.)

mg/kg significantly lowered the infection rate in patients with high blood loss and high Injury Severity Scores, and in patients without colon penetration. In trauma patients who require laparotomy, high doses of antibiotics are more effective than long courses of antibiotics in reducing the incidence of infection.

▶ This is another article in the continuing studies of the value of antibiotics in trauma patients. The authors use the word *prophylactic,* but in a technical sense, because antibiotics were not present at the time of injury, the description should be *presumptive,* i.e., antibiotics given as soon as possible after the injury.

These studies indicate that in specific cases, e.g., patients with severe loss of blood or high injury severity scores, or patients without colon preparation, the use of high-dose antibiotics may be far more effective. Longer courses of the same antibiotics were not nearly as effective in reducing the incidence of infection as was the short-term use of high-dose antibiotics.—G.T. Shires, M.D.

Trauma in the Elderly: Determinants of Outcome
Smith DP, Enderson BL, Maull KI (Univ of Tennessee, Knoxville)
South Med J 83:171–176, 1990   4–7

Patients older than 65 years have a lower incidence of injury than other age groups but are more likely to die of their injuries. As the elderly population grows in the United States, trauma in this age group will become an increasingly important health care issue. Data on trauma in the elderly were examined and an attempt was made to outline those factors that influence outcome.

The study group included 456 patients aged 65 or older who were treated at a level I trauma center in a 3-year period. Factors considered were cause of injury, injury severity score, preexisting disease, complications, hospital and intensive care unit (ICU) length of stay, and mortality. Death rates were compared with those of 985 patients younger than 65 years who were admitted to the trauma center during the last year of the study.

The patients had a mean age of 76.1 years; there were 268 women and 188 men. Most of the injuries resulted from falls (61.8%) or accidents involving motor vehicles (25.4%). Thermal injuries accounted for only 2.2% of the cases but had the highest mortality rate (50%). Overall mortality was 8.6% for older patients and 6% for those younger than 65. Except for the severely injured who died, the ICU and hospital length of stay increased with severity of injury. Patients with more than 1 complication had a higher mortality rate (30%) than those with no complications (5.4%). Preexisting risk factors were not significantly associated with outcome.

Elderly trauma patients, even those with moderate injuries, should be cared for aggressively to prevent complications. A lower threshold should be used for admission of these patients to an ICU. The injury severity score at which the probability of death was 10% was 17.3 in the elderly group and 24.9% in the younger patients.

▶ The data generated by this study confirm the impression that many have had concerning determinants of outcome after treatment of trauma in the elderly. As the authors point out, the incidence of trauma in patients older than 65 years of age is decreased, but the morbidity and mortality rates are increased. There were several interesting things about this study, particularly the observation that preexisting risk factors were not significantly associated with outcome, contrary to what is generally thought concerning the elderly patient. Nevertheless, in the severely injured patients, the ICU and hospital length of stay increased with the severity of injury, and patients with more than one complication had a much higher mortality rate than those with no complications. The injury severity score at which the probability of death was 10% was 17% in the elderly group and 25% in the younger patients, indicating a higher mortality per severity of injury in the older group. Because these patients were treated in the same trauma center during the same period of time, it is likely that this is a valid comparative study.— G.T. Shires, M.D.

Bayesian Analysis of the Reliability of Peritoneal Lavage
Velanovich V (Letterman Army Med Ctr, Presidio of San Francisco)
Surg Gynecol Obstet 170:7–11, 1990   4–8

Peritoneal lavage is widely used as a diagnostic test in assessment of abdominal trauma. However, there is some disagreement over the "accuracy" of the test. The confusion stems from the fact that accuracy in this context means that the test can produce positive results when a given disease is present and negative results when that disease is absent. However, the accuracy of a test does not indicate what the chance is that a patient has the disease if the results from a particular test are positive or negative for that disease. Bayesian analysis does answer this question.

Data from 29 studies of peritoneal lavage, published in 1965–1986, were analyzed using the bayesian method. The information recorded from each study included the number of patients tested, whether the trauma was blunt or penetrating, whether an open or closed technique of peritoneal lavage was used, whether standard or other criteria were used to determine a positive test result, the frequencies of disease and nondisease, and the frequencies of true positive, false positive, true negative, and false negative test results.

The probability of an intra-abdominal injury being present if findings from peritoneal lavage are positive ranged from .448 to 1. The probability of an intra-abdominal injury being present if findings from lavage are negative ranged from 0 to .286. The reliability of peritoneal lavage, as determined by bayesian analysis, varied with type of trauma, technique of lavage used, and the criteria used to define positivity. In general, the findings from peritoneal lavage were most reliable when the procedure was used to diagnose blunt trauma, with the use of standard criteria to define positivity, and when open peritoneal lavage was used.

▶ This interesting mathematical analysis of the validity of peritoneal lavage tends to confirm the previous impressions of many trauma surgeons. This comparative analysis showed that the open technique of peritoneal lavage was the most reliable, and that the procedure was far more accurate when used to diagnose blunt abdominal trauma. The reliability of a strongly positive and completely negative peritoneal lavage was also reaffirmed.— G.T. Shires, M.D.

Is Diagnostic Peritoneal Lavage for Blunt Trauma Obsolete?
Hawkins ML, Bailey RL Jr, Carraway RP (Med College of Georgia, Augusta; Carraway Methodist Med Ctr, Birmingham, Ala)
Am Surg 56:96–99, 1990   4–9

Since it was first introduced in 1965, diagnostic peritoneal lavage (DPL) has been a mainstay in evaluation of severely injured patients. Computed tomography is highly accurate in detecting intra-abdominal injuries after blunt trauma. Whether the continued use of DPL is justified was examined in a 5-year study during which 414 trauma patients underwent 415 DPLs. (One patient had a repeat study several hours after admission.) Diagnostic peritoneal lavage was considered grossly positive if 10 mL of blood was aspirated and microscopically positive if more than 100,000 red blood cells per mm^3, more than 500 white blood cells per mm^3, elevated amylase or bilirubin levels, or bacteria or vegetable fibers were found in the effluent.

None of the patients had elevated levels of bilirubin, amylase, or bacteria in the effluent. Of the 415 DPLs, 117 (28%) were true positive, 286 (69%) were true negative, 7 (2%) were false positive, and 5 (1%) were false negative, for a 97% accuracy rate. Rare vegetable fibers, found in 4 cases, were falsely positive. Three of the 5 patients with false negative lavages had a ruptured diaphragm as the only intra-abdominal injury. The only complication in this study population was an inadvertently penetrated urinary bladder that was treated successfully with Foley catheter drainage.

The hospital charge for peritoneal lavage was $94.50, compared to $350 for abdominal CT scanning exclusive of the radiologist's fees. Because DPL is accurate, rapid, safe, avoids the disruption of patient care that results in the radiology suite, and is much less expensive than CT, it remains the procedure of choice for evaluating blunt abdominal trauma in adults at the authors' institution.

▶ This was another of many attempts in the past severel years to assess the diagnostic accuracy, sensitivity, and specificity of DPL. This study showed once again that DPL is a very highly sensitive diagnostic test that is low in cost, rapid, accurate, safe, and avoids disruption in patient care; it remains the procedure of choice for evaluating blunt abdominal trauma in the adult population.—G.T. Shires, M.D.

Diagnostic Peritoneal Lavage: Is an Isolated WBC Count ≥500/mm³ Predictive of Intra-Abdominal Injury Requiring Celiotomy in Blunt Trauma Patients?
Soyka JM, Martin M, Sloan EP, Himmelman RG, Batesky D, Barrett JA (Univ of Illinois College of Medicine, Chicago; Cook County Hosp, Chicago)
J Trauma 30:874–879, 1990   4–10

The predictive value of an isolated lavage white blood cell (WBC) count of 500/mm³ or higher was assessed in a series of 3,503 patients, 13% of whom had counts on this order. The mean lavage WBC count in this group was 1,646. Twenty patients were observed and discharged without morbidity and 28 were operated on.

Eleven of the patients operated on had an intra-abdominal injury requiring drainage or repair, for a true positive rate of 39%. None of these patients had more than 1 intra-abdominal injury. The rate of false positive lavage was 35%. The mean lavage WBC count was 1,677/mm³, compared with 2,020/mm³ in the true positive group. The positive predictive value of an isolated high WBC count for injury requiring drainage or repair was only 23%.

Many patients will undergo laparotomy unnecessarily if an isolated lavage WBC count of 500/mm³ or more is used as a criterion of exploration in patients who sustain blunt abdominal trauma. Raising the criterion WBC count will not significantly improve its predictive ability. Blunt injuries of solid or hollow viscus organs and gynecologic processes also can produce an elevated lavage WBC count.

▶ This paper evaluated the isolated, elevated WBC count in diagnostic peritoneal lavage as to its predictive value in detecting significant intra-abdominal injury in patients with blunt trauma. The positive predictive value of an isolated high WBC count for injury requiring drainage or repair was only 23%.

I believe that this is another study confirming what most have concluded, i.e., the only true indicator of a positive diagnostic peritoneal lavage is the presence of 100,000 red blood cells per mm³.—G.T. Shires, M.D.

Emergency Endotracheal Intubation in Pediatric Trauma
Nakayama DK, Gardner MJ, Rowe MI (Children's Hosp of Pittsburgh; Univ of Pittsburgh)
Ann Surg 211:218–223, 1990   4–11

Timely endotracheal intubation in trauma care provides a therapeutic margin that may ensure survival under critical circumstances. It is often recommended that patients with severe head injuries undergo early endotracheal intubation because it assures optimal gas exchange and allows controlled hyperventilation to decrease intracranial pressure through cerebral vasoconstriction.

To determine the effectiveness and examine the associated problems of emergency intubation in head-injured children, data were reviewed on 63 infants and children who underwent endotracheal intubation at the scene of injury, at a referring hospital, or in the emergency department during 1987. Fifty-seven of the 63 children (90.4%) had head injuries and 39.7% had multiple injuries. Indications for intubation included coma (74.6%), shock (28.6%), apnea (22.2%), and airway obstruction (3.2%).

When intubations at the scene of injury were successful, more often more than 1 attempt was required, compared to when intubations were done at the referring hospital or at the emergency department. Six of 14 intubations attempted at the scene (42.8%) were unsuccessful; 4 of the 6 were subsequently successful at the referring hospital or at the emergency department. Two other children underwent unsuccessful needle cricothyroidotomy and both died of their injuries, 1 before ventilation was established.

Sixteen patients had airway-related complications and 13 were immediately life threatening, including 5 main-stem intubations, 2 massive barotraumas, 2 failures of adequate preoxygenation, 1 massive aspiration, 1 esophageal intubation, 1 attempt at nasotracheal intubation in an open facial fracture, and 1 extubation during transport. There were 3 late complications, including 2 cases of vocal cord paresis and 1 of subglottic stenosis. There were 4 complication-associated fatalities, all at the scene of injury.

Twenty-eight of the 63 children (44.4%) had problems in respiratory management after arrival at the emergency department, including major airway complications, hypoxemia, or hypercarbia. These factors were significantly more common with scene intubations. Despite endotracheal intubation, head-injured children remain at considerable risk for secondary brain injury from hypoxia and intracranial hypertension.

▶ This interesting article shows the necessity for early airway control in pediatric trauma. This study was particularly slanted toward head trauma, because 90% of the patients had significant head injury. What is apparent from the details of the study, however, are that the major complications of endotracheal intubation occur at the scene of the injury, where many attempts were unsuccessful and led to immediate or subsequent problems. This article should serve to alert everyone caring for the trauma patient about the vital necessity of airway and breathing control in patients with head injury, particularly children.— G.T. Shires, M.D.

Comparison of Conventional Mechanical Ventilation and High-Frequency Ventilations: A Prospective, Randomized Trial in Patients With Respiratory Failure

Hurst JM, Branson RD, Davis K Jr, Barrette RR, Adams KS (Univ of Cincinnati; Children's Hosp Med Ctr, Cincinnati)
Ann Surg 211:486–491, 1990   4–12

There have been many reports attesting to the advantage of high-frequency ventilation (HFV) in treating acute respiratory failure. Conventional mechanical ventilation was compared with percussive HFV in a prospective series of 100 patients admitted to surgical intensive care who were at risk of acute respiratory failure. The therapeutic end point consisted of a pH above 7.35, an arterial carbon dioxide pressure of 35–45 torr, and an arterial oxygen pressure–forced inspiratory oxygen ratio exceeding 225.

Acute respiratory failure occurred in 60 of the 100 patients, including 32 on HFV and 28 who were conventionally ventilated. Patients on HFV reached the therapeutic end point at lower levels of continuous positive airway pressure and mean airway pressure, but there were no differences between the 2 management groups in mortality, time in the surgical intensive care unit, cardiovascular interventions, or incidence of barotrauma. Four patients failed to reach the therapeutic end point, and 3 died despite transfer to the alternate mode of ventilatory support.

High-frequency ventilation offers no clear advantage over conventional mechanical ventilation in patients with adult respiratory distress syndrome. Its use should be limited to patients who are resistant to conventional ventilatory measures.

▶ This is one of several articles appearing in the past 3 years comparing conventional mechanical ventilation with HFV. In this study, HFV was compared with conventional therapy in a randomized trial in patients with established respiratory failure.

As in most of the other series reported, there was in fact no clear advantage for HFV over conventional mechanical ventilation in patients with adult respiratory distress syndrome. It is believed, therefore, that HFV should probably be limited to patients who have been resistant to conventional mechanical ventilatory support.—G.T. Shires, M.D.

Principles of Management of Shotgun Wounds

Walker ML, Poindexter JM Jr, Stovall I (Morehouse School of Medicine, Atlanta)
Obstet Gynecol 170:97–105, 1990   4–13

Patients with shotgun wounds are frequently seen in urban trauma centers. At short distances the destructive capacity of the shotgun can equal that of a high-velocity missile injury. No radical changes in the design of the weapon have occurred since Browning patented a semiautomatic shotgun in 1905. The 12-gauge shotgun is most commonly used in the United States today. The 3 main types of ammunition are birdshot, buckshot, and slugs.

Type I shotgun wounds result when the target distance is more than 7 yd and the subcutaneous tissue and deep fascia are penetrated. In type II wounds, from a target distance of 3–7 yd, there is penetration of structures deep to the deep fascia. Type 3 wounds, from target distance of 2–3 yd, cause massive local destruction. Blast-injury wounds from less than 3 yd are equivalent to high velocity wounds. Because pellets rarely exit the body, all the kinetic energy of the blast is transferred to the victim.

Initial treatment for a shotgun injury should be that given any victim of penetrating trauma, with attention to an adequate airway, breathing, and circulation. Cefoxitin is a good choice of antibiotic therapy. Direct pressure can best control obvious bleeding. Further treatment is then determined by the site of the wound: the head and neck, chest, abdomen, or extremities. The basics of ballistics, ammunition, and clinical presentation provide the information needed to manage these complex wounds. Careful application of these data, together with the fundamental principles of trauma therapy, should improve morbidity and mortality in victims of shotgun wounds.

▶ This is a valiant effort at developing algorithms for the treatment of shotgun wounds. The authors correctly point out the extreme variability of the resultant injury, depending on the distance of the patient from the shotgun at the time of discharge. Specifically, low-velocity distant injuries in selected instances can obviously be managed safely without operative intervention. On the contrary, the algorithms for close-range shotgut injuries would therefore approximate high-velocity missiles and demand operative intervention.— G.T. Shires, M.D.

Diagnosis and Management of Penetrating Neck Trauma
Garramone RR Jr, Jacobs LM, Sahdev P (Hartford Hosp, Hartford, Conn)
Contemp Orthop 21:153–162, 1990   4–14

Penetrating neck injuries are a significant source of morbidity and mortality. However, their significance may be obscured by the benign appearance of the neck wound.

Man, 24, was transported by air ambulance to a level I trauma center after sustaining 2 gunshot wounds to the left neck. On arrival he was unresponsive and had a Glasgow Coma Scale of 3. Radiographs of the cervical spine revealed a bullet posterior to the third cervical vertebra with a fracture of the vertebral body. Computed tomography of the cervical spine confirmed that the bullet had traversed the spinal canal. Four-vessel angiography demonstrated an isolated irregularity in the lumen of the left internal carotid artery. Immediate surgical exploration of the neck revealed a contusion of the left internal carotid artery. After ar-

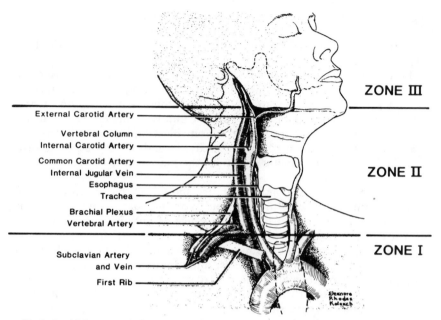

Fig 4–2.—Major anatomical structures and zones of the neck. (Courtesy of Garramone RR Jr, Jacobs LM, Sahdev P: *Contemp Orthop* 21:153–162, 1990.)

teriotomy the injured segment was excised, and vascular continuity was reestablished with an interposition saphenous vein graft using an intraluminal shunt. However, the patient remained quadriplegic and was discharged to a rehabilitative facility.

Classification of the neck wound based on its depth and zone of penetration is of primary importance in anticipating organ injury. Based on bony and superficial landmarks, the neck can be divided into 3 zones that are important in defining the management and likely clinical course of penetrating neck injuries (Fig 4–2). Injuries in zone I are associated with the highest mortality. Nonsurgical diagnostic investigations are more helpful in zone I and zone III injuries because they may indicate the need for an alternate surgical approach to gain access to the injury. Indications for preoperative investigation in zone II injuries are less well established because surgical exploration can usually be accomplished through a neck incision alone. However, preoperative angiography is still recommended by many physicians even in zone II injuries. Hemodynamic stability will determine the need for immediate surgical intervention vs. preliminary diagnostic investigation.

▶ This article illustrates the still unresolved issue of intelligent management of penetrating neck injuries. The well-described zones of injury in the neck are evaluated in terms of structures. However, the decision to operate beyond immediate bleeding is still obscured in this discussion. However, it does appear more and more that the safest, shortest course of action that causes the least morbidity is mandtory exploration of the neck, particularly in zone II if the platysma muscle has been penetrated.— G.T. Shires, M.D.

Periportal Tracking in Hepatic Trauma: CT Features
Macrander SJ, Lawson TL, Foley WD, Dodds WJ, Erickson SJ, Quiroz FA (Med College of Wisconsin, Milawukee)
J Comput Assist Tomogr 13:952–957, 1989   4–15

Dynamic contrast-enhanced CT of the abdomen in 51 patients with hepatic trauma was analyzed for types and distributions of hepatic injuries and presence of periportal tracking and its rate of resolution. Periportal tracking was considered present when low attenuation was identified circumferentially about peripheral subsegmental portal venous branches.

Periportal tracking was evident in 7 of 8 (87%) hepatic fractures, 6 of 10 (60%) hematomas, 8 of 19 lacerations, and 2 of 5 contusions; it was the only abnormality in about 18%. Overall, periportal tracking was evident in 62% of the cases. It usually occurred in the right lobe (63%), only rarely in the left lobe (3%). Both lobes were commonly affected in pediatric patients. Follow-up CT in 16 cases of hepatic trauma showed resolution of the periportal tracking within the first week in 8 patients.

In hepatic trauma, disruption of small trigonal vessels and adjoining hepatic parenchyma is common and results in bleeding. Blood tracks along the sheath of connective tissue surround the portal triads, mainly because it is a low-resistance tissue plane. Periportal tracking occurs secondary to the tracking of blood and not to the development of periportal lymph edema. The presence of periportal tracking may be an important sign of subtle liver injury.

▶ This article illustrates some of the subtle ways of tracking hepatic trauma. It has been established by these and other authors that the finding of periportal zones of decreased attenuation, presumably representing blood, will be seen in a large number of patients following injury. Although this is a useful sign, it is still difficult to differentiate which patients may need operative intervention from those who can by managed safely by careful observation. The most difficult patients are those with intrahepatic injury with confined hematoma. It would appear that many of these patients can be managed even more safely by repeated scanning with magnetic resonance imaging.— G.T. Shires, M.D.

The Use of Segmental Anatomy for an Operative Classification of Liver Injuries
Buechter KJ, Zeppa R, Gomez G (Univ of Miami)
Ann Surg 211:669–675, 1990   4–16

The lack of a standard classification for liver injuries makes an accurate comparison of reports on the subject somewhat difficult. A 3-grade classification of injuries based on the segmental anatomy of the liver as described by Couinaud was applied in evaluating a group of 95 patients. Grade I included injuries that required no operative intervention or operative intervention limited to a segment or less. Grade II injuries required operative intervention that involved 2 or more segments. Grade III injuries involved associated juxtahepatic or retrohepatic vein injury.

Fifty-six patients had penetrating trauma and 39 had blunt trauma. Grade I injuries were observed in 69 patients. Many of these patients were treated by suture and drainage (20) or drainage only (23). The mortality rate associated with grade I injuries was 1% and the morbidity rate, 9%. Six of 13 patients (46%) with grade II injuries died. The morbidity rate in this group was 57%. Nine of 13 patients (69%) with grade III injuries died and 50% had complications.

The scheme introduced by Couinaud in 1954 divides the liver into 8 segments based on the end distribution of the portal vein. By using this scheme the amount of liver parenchyma involved, either through injury or surgery, is related to subsequent mortality. Liver injuries that involve the retrohepatic veins cause significant mortality regardless of associated parenchymal injury. A classification based on these 3 grades of injuries will provide a simple and reliable means of reporting and comparing liver injuries.

▶ This is an interesting proposal of a classification for recording the management of significant hepatic injuries. Based on anatomical segments of the liver, 3 grades of injuries are described: those requiring repair of less than 2 or more than 2 segments of the liver, as opposed to those in which there is an associated juxtahepatic or retrohepatic vein injury.

This proposal will be useful if trauma surgeons in future reporting would use a classification such as this, which seems to be a good predictor of results in hepatic injury surgery.— G.T. Shires, M.D.

Evaluation of Splenic Injury by Computed Tomography and Its Impact on Treatment

Malangoni MA, Cué JI, Fallat ME, Willing SJ, Richardson JD (Univ of Louisville; Humana Hosp Univ, Louisville)
Ann Surg 211:592–599, 1990   4–17

An increased understanding of the role of the spleen in the immunologic defense against infection has led to the development of surgical techniques to salvage the injured organ. Also, the availability of noninvasive imaging procedures now allows splenic injuries to be graded so that surgery is often avoided. The accuracy of the CT scan in classifying splenic injuries was assessed in 37 cases of blunt trauma to the spleen.

The study group included 16 adults (18 years of age or older) and 21 children. All were hemodynamically stable and had undergone CT scanning. The average Splenic Injury Score (with 1 the least serious and 5 the most severe injury) assessed by CT scan was 2.5 for adults and 2.8 for children.

Twenty-five patients (19 children and 6 adult) were treated initially by observation; their mean Splenic Injury Score was 2.3. The mean score for those operated on initially was 2.6. Observation alone was successful in 80% of all patients—84% of children and 67% of adults. Four of the 5 patients who subsequently required surgery underwent splenectomy and 1 had successful splenic repair. Overall, 13 patients had splenectomy and 4 had splenic repair.

The value of CT in splenic injury lies in its ability to identify patients whose injuries are likely to stop bleeding spontaneously. Computed tomography accurately determines the presence of splenic injury but often underestimates its severity: CT underestimated the degree of injury in 9 of 17 (53%) patients who underwent operation. Observation is most successful in children with grades 1 through 3 injuries. Adults with more minor injuries may require surgery. Computed tomography may fail to detect coexisting abdominal injuries.

▶ This article follows on the heels of a similar one in 1989 showing the inability of CT scanning to predict the severity of splenic injury after trauma. In many patients in this series and in the previous one, relatively small injuries to the spleen subsequently bled profusely. Conversely, rather large injuries to the spleen were self-contained and could either be observed or undergo splenorrhaphy. Consequently, it is becoming more and more clear that CT scanning is an unreliable predictor and should not be used to estimate the need for operation in splenic injury.—G.T. Shires, M.D.

Benefits of Intra-Abdominal Pack Placement for the Management of Non-mechanical Hemorrhage
Saifi J, Fortune JB, Graca L, Shah DM (Albany Med College; Albany VA Med Ctr)
Arch Surg 125:119–122, 1990   4–18

Patients who continue to bleed from injuries to the liver despite treatment with standard techniques for securing hemostasis have a poor prognosis. The use of intra-abdominal packs to control bleeding fell out of favor because of the high risk of infection with packs. Recent studies have shown, however, that intra-abdominal packs can effectively control hemorrhage and allow time for correction of metabolic disturbances.

The benefits of intra-abdominal pack placement were assessed in 7 men and 2 women (mean age, 25 years). Two liver injuries were classified as grade IV and 5 as grade V. When other treatment methods failed and the onset of coagulopathy was confirmed, a decision was made to pack the liver. Patients were then taken to the intensive care unit for aggressive resuscitation with crystalloids and blood products. Once their hemodynamic values, coagulopathy, acidosis, and hypothermia were corrected, patients were returned to the operating room for pack removal. The mean interval between the procedures was 46 hours.

No patient rebled after the packs were removed and no patient died of hemorrhage. Two patients died of a combination of sepsis, intra-abdominal abscess, and multiple-organ failure. Although the study group was small, the data suggest that hypothermia and a low intraoperative hematocrit value may indicate a poor outcome.

In patients with massive nonmechanical bleeding after severe liver injury, intra-abdominal pack placement may be an effective means of controlling hemorrhage and preventing the continuation of severe metabolic disturbances. The packs should be removed soon after these disturbances are corrected.

▶ This article confirms the conclusions reached in an article reviewed in the 1990 YEAR BOOK. Both agree that there are probably 2 times when intra-abdominal packing is useful for several days after liver injury: (1) when transporting patients with exsanguinating liver injury from one hospital to another if inadequate facilities are available at the primary hospital, and (2) when coagulopathies develop in a patient with severe bleeding from liver injury who requires great replacement of blood and other fluids. In the latter case, packing may well be the only way to control the nonmechanical bleeding resulting from such coagulopathy.

In either instance, these packs are temporary and should be removed as soon as possible (within 2–3 days usually) to avoid the very high mortality that will ensue from subsequent sepsis.—G.T. Shires, M.D.

Intestinal Injuries Missed by Computed Tomography
Sherck JP, Oakes DD (Stanford Univ; Santa Clara Valley Med Ctr, San Jose, Calif)
J Trauma 30:1–6, 1990   4–19

Isolated intestinal injuries from blunt trauma often are difficult to diagnose using physical examination and routine laboratory studies only, but delayed diagnosis may increase morbidity and the risk of death. A total of 36 patients with small bowel injury were seen in an 8-year review period. Data on 10 of these patients whose small bowel injuries were missed by CT examination were reviewed.

The patients had an average age of 31 years, and all were injured in motor vehicle accidents, 4 while wearing a seat belt. All 10 patients had physical findings suggestive of possible abdominal trauma, but in no case was the plain abdominal radiograph abnormal. The patients were observed initially but eventually underwent laparotomy, 7 within 24 hours of admission. All had intestinal injuries that required surgical treatment; 9 patients had free perforation. One patient died.

The results of 3 CT studies were suboptimal. Two scans were diagnostic of perforation on review and careful review of the remaining scans demonstrated other abnormalities. Five patients had free intraperitoneal fluid not explained by a liver or spleen abnormality.

Patients having abdominal CT should be stable enough to receive sedation, if required, to limit motion. Gastric contrast should always be used but in dilute solution. The proper diagnosis and management of bowel injuries still rely on serial evaluation by an experienced surgeon.

▶ It is now well established that the failure of CT scanning to detect abdominal injuries is extremely high when intestinal injuries are present. Another group of patients are reported here in whom the intestinal injuries were missed, and all had free perforation requiring surgical treatment. The conclusion of these studies was that proper diagnosis and management of bowel injuries still depend on serial evaluations by an experienced surgeon.—G.T. Shires, M.D.

Venous Thromboembolism in Patients With Major Trauma
Shackford SR, Davis JW, Hollingsworth-Fridlund P, Brewer NS, Hoyt DB, Mackersie RC (Univ of California, San Diego)
Am J Surg 159:365–369, 1990   4–20

Patients with major trauma are believed to be at high risk of venous thromboembolism (VTE); the reported incidence has varied between 20% and 90%. To determine which patients were at risk for VTE, the need for prophylactic measures, and the frequency of complications associated with prophylaxis in patients with major trauma, all 719 patients admitted to a regional trauma center in a 5-month period were evaluated for 9 risk factors of VTE. One hundred seventy-seven patients had at least 1 risk factor and were placed in the high-risk group. This group received prophylaxis with heparin or pneumatic compression hose (PCH). The PCH alone was used in 46% of patients, 30% received PCH and heparin, 10% received heparin only, and 14% received no prophylaxis because of contraindications to both PCH and heparin.

Efficacy and Complications of Prophylaxis in 177
High-Risk Patients

Type of Prophylaxis	n	VTE (%)	Complications
None	25	1 (4)	1 Hct drop
Heparin only	18	1 (6)	1 Hct drop
Heparin + PCH	53	5 (9)	1 GI bleed
			2 wound hematomas
			2 Hct drop
PCH	81	5 (6)	1 Hct drop
			1 GI bleed

Abbreviations: GI, gastrointestinal; *Hct drop,* hematocrit decrease of 75%.
(Courtesy of Shackford SR, Davis JW, Hollingsworth-Fridlund P, et al: *Am J Surg* 159:365–369, 1990.)

Twelve patients had VTE, including 1 who had no prophylaxis. When the frequency of VTE for each risk factor alone and in combination with the others was analyzed, age older than 45 years was the only factor that increased risk predictably. Patients who had more than 1 risk factor were also at higher risk. Patients who received prophylaxis showed no significant reduction in the incidence of VTE, compared to those who did not receive prophylaxis (table). Bleeding complications were more common in patients who received heparin, but the difference was not significant.

Patients older than age 45 years who have more than 3 days of enforced bed rest and those with more than 1 risk factor are at higher risk of VTE than other trauma patients. These patients should receive prophylaxis if possible. Current prophylactic measures are contraindicated for some patients.

▶ This interesting study indicated that in the traumatized patient the only significant across-the-board factor increasing the risk for VTE was age alone, and the cutoff age was at 45 years. Other factors were identified, the presence of any one of which increased the risk. This included such things as venous repair, long bone fractures of the lower extremity, pelvic fractures, and spine fractures. A rational program of prophylaxis in patients with one risk factor was evolved that was not accompanied by a significant bleeding complication.— G.T. Shires, M.D.

Nonoperative Management of Adult Blunt Splenic Trauma: Criteria for Successful Outcome

Longo WE, Baker CC, McMillen MA, Modlin IM, Degutis LC, Zucker KA (Yale Univ)
Ann Surg 210:626–629, 1989   4–21

Nonoperative treatment of blunt splenic trauma in adults is controversial, although many physicians have advocated such management. A retrospective review of adult splenic injuries was done to better define criteria that may predict a successful outcome. Data were examined on all cases of splenic injury seen at 1 center from 1980 to 1988. The injuries were documented by scintillation studies or CT scanning, or at laparotomy.

Sixty of 252 patients with splenic injuries (24%) were treated initially without surgery. Management included bed rest, intensive care unit monitoring, frequent physical examinations, nasogastric tubes, serial hematocrits, and follow-up splenic imaging. Five of these 60 patients subsequently required interval laparotomy. Treatment failure was attributed to blood loss of more than 4 units, enlarging splenic defects, or increasing peritoneal signs. Predictors of successful outcomes were localized trauma to the left flank or abdomen, hemodynamic stability, transfusion requirements of less than 4 units, rapid return of gastrointestinal function, patient age younger than 60 years, and early resolution of splenic defects on imaging studies. None of the patients died or had complications as a result of delayed surgery. Blunt splenic trauma can be managed successfully without surgery in carefully selected adults.

▶ This thoughtful study attempted to identify those adult patients with splenic injury who could possibly be treated successfully without surgery. The criterion was applied initially to less than 25% of the patients. In addition, it is clear that a significant portion of these subsequently did require surgery.

One of the more compelling recent arguments in favor of a decision to do splenorrhaphy or splenectomy is the unwillingness of many to accept the risk blood loss, the replacement of which is associated with a significant risk for blood-transmitted diseases. As a consequence, insofar as managing splenic injuries is concerned, it is becoming very clear that, for the overwhelming majority of adults, the decision should be made in the operating room.— G.T. Shires, M.D.

Silent Deep Vein Thrombosis in Immobilized Multiple Trauma Patients
Kudsk KA, Fabian TC, Baum S, Gold RE, Mangiante E, Voeller G (Univ of Tennessee, Memphis)
Am J Surg 158:515–519, 1989   4–22

Severely injured patients who are immobilized by multiple fractures, spinal cord or head injuries, or life support systems are at risk for unrecognized deep vein thrombosis (DVT) and potentially fatal pulmonary embolism. An autopsy study assessing the incidence of unrecognized DVT in immobilized multiple trauma patients reported an increased incidence of DVT without PE, but the study population consisted mostly of elderly patients and DVT was only indirectly related to the type of injury.

The incidence of silent DVT in immobilized multiple trauma patients was evaluated in 39 patients aged 19–78 years (average age, 37 years). All had been immobilized for at least 10 days. Contrast venograms of the lower extremities were obtained successfully in 38 patients; satisfactory cannulation of veins was not possible in 1. The injured extremity was studied first. A venogram of the contralateral lower extremity was obtained only if the injured extremity showed no DVT. Twenty-four of the 38 patients had no DVT in the injured leg and thus underwent bilateral studies.

Eighteen men (69%) and 6 women (50%) immobilized for 10 days or longer after multiple trauma had silent DVT, 12 with thrombi extending above the knee. Only 1 patient had clinical evidence of DVT. Thrombi were isolated to the calf veins only in 12 patients, the thigh veins only in 5, and both the calf and thigh veins in 7. Increasing age correlated with the incidence of DVT. All 5 patients older than age 60 years had positive venograms. However, the frequency of DVT correlated poorly with injury severity. None of the patients had clinical evidence of pulmonary embolism. The 60% incidence of silent DVT in patients immobilized for at least 10 days with multiple trauma is in line with that reported in earlier studies.

▶ This study confirms a significant and high instance of DVT, but without pulmonary embolism, in patients sustaining prolonged immobilization after trauma. The interesting part of the correlation was the lack of influence of multiple injuries or severity of injury on the incidence of DVT. The only positive correlation was with increasing age.

The question is still not answered as to how many injured patients should receive prophylactic anticoagulation. This study, as have several others previously, showed a significant incidence of thrombosis when venograms were obtained, as well as the significant absence of pulmonary embolism. The complications occurring from anticoagulation remain significant. Consequently, a routine recommendation concerning anticoagulation after trauma is still not possible.—G.T. Shires, M.D.

Traumatic Hemipelvectomy: A Catastrophic Injury
Beal SL, Blaisdell FW (Univ of California, Davis)
J Trauma 29:1346–1351, 1989   4–23

Traumatic hemipelvectomy is a catastrophic injury resulting from extremely violent blunt forces. During a 3-year period, 8 patients were brought to the University of California at Davis General Surgery Trauma Service after sustaining traumatic hemipelvectomy; only 3 survived. Since 1915 only 39 patients have survived traumatic hemipelvectomy, including the latter 3.

The 39 survivors of hemipelvectomy ranged in age from 7 to 34 years. Thirty-one patients were involved in motor vehicle accidents and 8 were injured in industrial accidents. In 17 patients the hindquarter was completely avulsed and brought in as a separate specimen. The limb was still attached in 21 patients. Hemipelvectomy wounds consistently included degloved abdominal and flank skin with contusions and lacerations. The peritoneum was exposed, often with lacerations and bowel evisceration.

Treatment involved control of the massive hemorrhage and completion of the hemipelvectomy. All patients required multiple operations for débridement that ranged from 3 to 17 acute surgical procedures. Thirty-two patients required colostomies, and 8 underwent reanastomoses of urethral transections. The most commonly reported complications were intractable pain, skin flap necrosis, systemic sepsis, and vesico- or urethrocutaneous fistula.

At follow-up, 34 patients were able to walk, 18 with a modified Canadian hip disarticulation prosthesis and 16 with crutches. Two patients remained bedridden. The outcome of the remaining 3 patients was not known. Twelve patients were able to return to work. One patient had married since the accident and given birth to 3 children. Another patient was sexually active at follow-up.

Traumatic hemipelvectomy is a near-lethal injury because of massive hemorrhage and subsequent sepsis. Although hemipelvectomy is a devastating injury, patients not only survive, but survivors can be successfully rehabilitated to an active, productive, and independent life.

▶ This is an excellent review of an extensive experience with traumatic hemipelvectomy. This study indicates once again that traumatic hemipelvectomy is a near-lethal injury most of the time. However, this study also reveals that, while this is a devastating injury, some patients do survive and can be successfully rehabilitated to an active, productive, and independent life. This should go a long way to settle the issue of whether or not posttraumatic hemipelvectomy should be performed.— G.T. Shires, M.D.

Penetrating Injuries of the Abdominal Aorta
Frame SB, Timberlake GA, Rush DS, McSwain NE Jr, Kerstein MD (Naval Hosp, San Diego; Univ of South Carolina, Columbia; Tulane Univ)
Am Surg 56:651–654, 1990   4–24

Although trauma care may have improved over all, no benefit is apparent for patients with penetrating abdominal aortic injuries. Data were reviewed on 56 such cases seen between 1973 and 1985. More than 90% of the patients were men, and the average age was 28 years. Gunshot wounds caused 82% of injuries; usually, a weapon of .38 caliber or larger was responsible.

Initial systolic blood pressure averaged 87 mm Hg in surviving patients and 40 mm Hg in nonsurvivors, not a significant difference. The overall mortality rate was 73%. Nearly two thirds of the deaths were attributed to exsanguination. Six deaths each were caused by coagulopathy and sepsis, and 4 by multiple organ system failure. Two of 6 patients having thoracotomy before celiotomy to gain proximal vascular control survived. Survival did not correlate significantly with the number of associated injuries.

Exsanguination was the chief cause of death in this series of penetrating abdominal aortic injuries. Associated injuries were not a significant prognostic factor. It may be that the use of higher-energy firearms is neutralizing attempts to improve trauma care for these patients.

▶ This article indicates the continuing concern for the extremely high mortality rate associated with abdominal aorta injuries. As documented again here, exsanguination is the chief cause of death in most such injuries rather than the associated injuries. This article simply emphasizes the need for extremely rapid transportation, diagnosis, and intervention if this high mortality rate, approaching 75% of all such patients, is to be lowered at all.— G.T. Shires, M.D.

Successful Atrial Caval Shunting in the Management of Retrohepatic Venous Injuries

Beal SL, Ward RE (Univ of California, Sacramento)
Am J Surg 158:409–413, 1989   4–25

Traumatic retrograde bleeding from a hepatic vein or a retrohepatic vena caval laceration is almost impossible to treat surgically because these veins are the most inaccessible of the vascular system. The atrial caval shunt (ACS) was first described in 1967, but its use was not successful until 1976. However, the mortality associated with the ACS remains prohibitively high, and some surgeons will not attempt this procedure. Experience with the ACS at a level I trauma center was evaluated.

During a 3-year period, 519 patients underwent laparotomy for liver injuries, of whom 7 men and 2 women aged 18–42 years had an ACS inserted for hemostasis. All 9 patients arrived at the emergency department in shock with a blood pressure of 80 mm Hg or less. Six patients had sustained blunt trauma and 3 had penetrating trauma. When hemorrhage could not be controlled with conventional surgical techniques, midline laparotomy incisions were extended into a median sternotomy for shunt placement. Shunts were passed through a right atriotomy after placement of a pursestring suture.

In 3 patients the shunt arrested the hemorrhage. Injured veins were exposed by hepatotomy, using the finger fracture technique. The exposed hepatic vein or vena caval injuries were repaired or ligated under direct visualization. A patients who survived initially later died of necrotizing fasciitis.

From this experience and that in other reported series, it is clear that, for a successful outcome, the nature of the liver injury should be determined quickly. Because it is time-consuming to assemble the proper shunt tubing and vascular instruments, a prepackaged, sterilized atrial caval shunt tray that contains all of the required equipment has now been assembled to be on hand when the need arises.

▶ This is the third year in a row in which an article has appeared reporting increased survival with some sort of vena cava shunting in management of retrohepatic venous injuries. Some authors have reported dismal results from such a technique, but the details of the technique, including the immediate availability of a bypass catheter and necessary instrumentation, is well pointed out in this article. My own experience suggests that, when this particular injury is encountered, this may be the only way to improve survival.—G.T. Shires, M.D.

Pediatric Chance Fractures: Association With Intra-Abdominal Injuries and Seatbelt Use

Reid AB, Letts RM, Black GB (Univ of Manitoba, Winnipeg)
J Trauma 30:384–391, 1990   4–26

Since mandatory seat belt legislation was enacted, numerous trauma centers have reported an increased frequency of seat-belt-related injuries, particularly in the number of flexion-distraction, or Chance fractures, of the spine. The association of the "seat belt sign" with intra-abdominal injuries is also seen more often, especially in the pediatric population. A previous study reported that 21% of the patients who had evidence of the seat belt sign also had flexion-distraction fractures of the spine. The association of these 2 injuries is now recognized as the seat belt syndrome.

A 10-year review of the medical records of children who were injured in motor vehicle accidents yielded 7 patients (5 boys and 2 girls aged 7–17 years) with the flexion-distraction spinal injury of Chance fracture. Six children were wearing seat belts, 4 of the lap variety and 2 of the shoulder harness variety. Six children sustained injuries of the lumbar spine. The seat belt sign was seen in 5 of the 6 children who wore a seat-belt restraint. Three children had concomitant abdominal injuries, including jejunal transection or perforation and late small bowel stenosis secondary to infarction.

Only 1 patient underwent operative stabilization of the spine because of progressive refractory kyphosis. The other 6 patients were treated with bedrest and a total body cast, and all had satisfactory healing of the fractures. At follow-up, kyphosis progression averaged 3 degrees. The incorrect positioning of lap and shoulder restraints, and the not-universal availability of shoulder restraints in the rear passenger seats of North American automobiles, puts patients, especially children, at increased risk of sustaining Chance fractures, intra-abdominal injury, or both.

▶ This is another in a series of articles in the past few years highlighting the seat belt syndrome. Since mandatory seat belt legislation has been enacted, it is clear that the mortality rate from frontal crashes has been lowered. However, one of the prices paid for increased use of the seat belt has been the development of the "seat belt sign," which is a broad ecchymotic band across the lower abdomen; now the "seat belt syndrome" has been identified, which includes a Chance fracture of the spine. This entity is becoming more commonly recognized and therefore better handled.— G.T. Shires, M.D.

Superiority of Closed Suction Drainage for Pancreatic Trauma: A Randomized, Prospective Study
Fabian TC, Kudsk KA, Croce MA, Payne LW, Mangiante EC, Voeller GR, Britt LG (Univ of Tennessee, Memphis)
Ann Surg 211:724–730, 1990   4–27

Pancreatic injuries cause significant illness and death. Although sump drainage is generally recommended after pancreatic trauma, closed-suction drainage minimizes the risk of colonization. To evaluate the effects of the 2 types of drainage on the postoperative course in patients who had sustained pancreatic injury, all 65 patients with pancreatic trauma who were admitted to a regional trauma center in a 42-month period were randomly assigned to sump or closed-suction drainage.

Patients with grade I or II injuries had drainage alone; most of those with grade III or IV injuries had distal pancreatectomy. Appropriate injury scores were calculated for both groups. Drainage and complications were evaluated on an ongoing basis. Twenty-four patients with sump drainage and 35 with closed-suction drainage survived and had evaluable drainage.

Patient profiles were not significantly different between the 2 groups, including injury scores. There were more grade II injuries in the closed-suction group. Twelve patients in each group had pancreatic resections. Five patients in the sump drainage group had abscesses, compared to 1 patient in the closed-suction group. The volume of drainage was similar in the 2 groups.

The occurrence of an abscess in 21% of patients in the sump group, compared to 3% in the closed-suction group, appears to favor closed suction. Sump drainage catheters seem to be a major source of bacterial contamination after pancreatic trauma, even though patients with grade I or II injuries are at lower risk of sepsis.

▶ This is the second year in which a comparison has been made of the closed-suction drainage (Jackson-Pratt) as opposed to a sump type drain. It was fairly clear that closed-suction drainage was superior to Jackson-Pratt drainage, at least in this series of patients. As the authors point out, the difference may well be the easier access of bacteria in the presence of an open sump type drainage.—G.T. Shires, M.D.

Management of Traumatic Retroperitoneal Hematoma
Feliciano DV (Univ of Rochester)
Ann Surg 211:109–123, 1990   4–28

The management of retroperitoneal hematoma is complex and continues to evolve. From 20% to 33% of these injuries result from penetrating trauma and are secondary to contact with a knife, a missile or its fragments, or cavitation from a high-velocity missile. In blunt trauma a moving or stationary victim strikes or is struck by a moving or stationary object.

Victims of blunt abdominal trauma who may have retroperitoneal hematoma often undergo peritoneal lavage as an adjunct to CT evaluation. Laparotomy is indicated if there are signs of significant intra-abdominal blood loss, or overt peritonitis. Stable patients with mild symptoms or without symptoms may be managed without operation. When surgery is necessary, the presence of a rupture or pulsatile hematoma calls for proximal control of the infrarenal abdominal aorta and inferior vena cava. A retrohepatic hematoma should be left alone if active bleeding is not present, once an overlying liver injury is treated.

A stable patient with hematuria after penetrating injury near the kidney should undergo pyelography followed by CT if the findings at pyelography are abnormal. Laparotomy is recommended for signs of significant intra-abdominal blood loss, overt peritonitis, significant evisceration, hematemesis, or proctorrhagia. Laparotomy often can be avoided in stable patients with no more than mild symptoms, even if a gunshot wound has produced peritoneal penetration. Certain retroperitoneal hematomas found at laparotomy after penetrating trauma should be opened, but this is not always necessary. The treatment for patients with traumatic retroperitoneal hematomas is based on the mechanism of injury, location of the hematoma, hemodynamic status of the patient, and the presence of associated injuries.

▶ This is a review article of the management of a major problem in surgery following trauma, i.e., retroperitoneal hematomas. The main message of the majority of such studies is that most retroperitoneal hematomas should be explored, for those arising at or below the brim of the pelvis. Experienced trauma surgeons believe that, although many hematomas will be opened to no avail, potentially lethal injuries can be left if such hematomas are not explored.—G.T. Shires, M.D.

The Role of Pancreaticoduodenectomy in the Management of Traumatic Injuries to the Pancreas and Duodenum
Heimansohn DA, Canal DF, McCarthy MC, Yaw PB, Madura JA, Broadie TA (Indiana Univ, Indianapolis)
Am Surg 56:511–514, 1990   4–29

The value of pancreaticoduodenectomy as a treatment for combined pancreatic and duodenal trauma was assessed in 6 young males whose mean injury severity score was 15.4. Four patients had penetrating and 2 had blunt injuries causing pancreatic duct disruption and significant duodenal damage. Four patients underwent primary pancreaticoduodenectomy and 2 initially had drainage and diverticulization.

The mean hospital stay after primary pancreaticoduodenectomy was 28 days. The patients required no further surgery, and all were well within 6 months to 9 years afterward. There were no problems with biliary sepsis or stricture of the biliary-enteric anastomosis. One patient has occasional abdominal bloating, which resolves spontaneously. Two other patients required further surgery for pancreatic leakage, enterocutaneous fistula, or drainage of abscesses. They ultimately required pancreaticoduodenectomy and survived. No patient has yet had evidence of diabetes or exocrine pancreatic insufficiency. Pancreaticoduodenectomy remains an option in some cases of combined pancreatic and duodenal injury.

▶ This is one more article attesting to the benefit of pancreaticoduodenectomy in the management of certain severe combined injuries of the pancreas and duodenum. In most series the limiting factor is the ability to control blood loss from retroperitoneal and major vascular structures. If blood loss can be controlled, the rapid performance of pancreatic and duodenal resection is a safe and satisfactory way to handle such a devastating injury.— G.T. Shires, M.D.

Elevated Production of Neutrophil Leukotriene B$_4$ Precedes Pulmonary Failure in Critically Ill Surgical Patients
Davis JM, Meyer JD, Barie PS, Yurt RW, Duhaney R, Dineen P, Shires GT (Cornell Univ; Beth Israel Hosp, Boston)
Surg Gynecol Obstet 170:495–500, 1990   4–30

Leukotriene B$_4$ (LTB$_4$) is a potent neutrophil chemotactic factor that is also produced by neutrophils. The relationship between LTB$_4$ production and adult respiratory distress syndrome (ARDS) has not been defined. Neutrophil function was examined in 12 patients at risk for development of ARDS. Peripheral blood neutrophils were tested for chemotaxis to f-met-leu-phe (fMLP) and leukotriene B$_4$ and for production of LTB$_4$, Plasma was assessed for C3a desArg levels.

In 5 of the 12 patients ARDS developed within 3 days of hospital admission. Neutrophil production of LTB$_4$ was significantly enhanced on day 1 in these patients as compared with those who did not have ARDS. Chemotaxis to fMLP and LTB$_4$ was significantly reduced in all 12 patients. Neutrophil chemotaxis improved in patients who did not have ARDS and worsened in those who did. Plasma C3a desArg levels were significantly elevated on day 1 in those patients who subsequently had ARDS.

The production of LTB$_4$ by neutrophils increases simultaneously with complement activation in patients in whom ARDS develops subsequently. Leukotriene B$_4$ may play a role in the development of pulmonary failure in patients with ARDS.

▶ This article, along with many others, indicates that the leukotrienes from neutrophils may well be one of the several pathways, including cytokines, that are responsible for ARDS in severely ill surgical patients.— G.T. Shires, M.D.

Monocyte HLA-DR Antigen Expression Characterizes Clinical Outcome in the Trauma Patient
Hershman MJ, Cheadle WG, Wellhausen SR, Davidson PF, Polk HC Jr (Univ of Louisville)
Br J Surg 77:204–207, 1990   4–31

Whether or not a surgical patient has infection seems to be determined by his or her immunologic response. Histocompatibility leukocyte antigen (HLA)-DR-bearing monocytes play a central role in the generation of the immune cascade. Whether the behavior of these monocytes is related to the clinical outcome of severely injured patients was studied. Sixty consecutive patients admitted to a trauma service were monitored daily

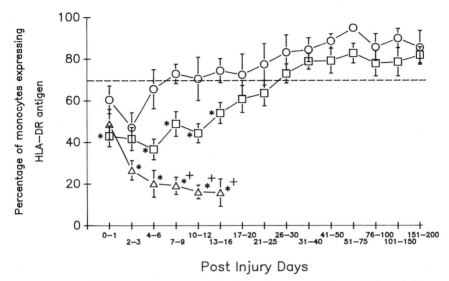

Post Injury Days

Fig 4–3.—Percentages of monocytes that expressed HLA-DR antigen after severe injury: *circle*, uneventful recovery group; *square*, major sepsis group; *triangle*, group of patients who died. Error bars refer to the standard error of the mean. *Statistically significant difference from uneventful recovery group;–statistically significant difference from major sepsis group. (Courtesy of Hershman MJ, Cheadle WG, Wellhausen SR, et al: *Br J Surg* 77:204–207, 1990.)

for clinical parameters and expression of HLA-DR antigen on peripheral blood monocytes. Overall, 17 had an uneventful recovery, 27 recovered after major sepsis, and 16 died. For comparison, 77 asymptomatic volunteers were also studied.

Among patients, relative monocytosis developed, but this was accompanied by an overall reduction in monocytes expressing surface HLA-DR. All 3 patient groups had reduced percentages of monocytes that expressed HLA-DR (Fig 4–3). Patients who had an uneventful recovery took only 1 week for a return to normal HLA-DR antigen expression, whereas those who recovered after major sepsis took 3 weeks. No normalization occurred in those patients who died. No significant difference in HLA-DR antigen expression was seen between patients who received 10 or more units of blood and those who received less than 10 units. Patients who subsequently died had significantly lower levels of HLA-DR expression in response to incubation with lipopolysaccharide stimulation than those who survived.

Upward trends in HLA-DR expression on the surface of monocytes was highly predictive of recovery in these patients; conversely, downward trends were seen in patients who died. Measurement of monocyte HLA-DR antigen expression may be useful to identify patients at high risk of infection and death who should receive early therapeutic intervention.

▶ This is a new approach to early immunologic assessment to characterize host defense response in the traumatized patient. Such assessment may also predict the development of significant infection earlier than any other known means. Expression of HLA-DR antigen may well be one of the ways in which an early severity assessment score could be improved in terms of prediction of outcome.

This type exploration may also pave the way for some sort of immunologic manipulation in the traumatized patient.—G.T. Shires, M.D.

5 Wound Healing

A Multivariate Analysis of Determinants of Wound Healing in Patients After Amputation for Peripheral Vascular Disease

van den Broek TAA, Dwars BJ, Rauwerda JA, Bakker FC (Free Univ Hosp, Amsterdam)

Eur J Vasc Surg 4:291–295, 1990   5–1

Primary healing does not occur in up to 20% of patients who have amputations for peripheral vascular disease. More than 8% of patients require reamputation, and the mortality rate is between 7% and 15%. Because better preoperative methods of assessment might improve outcome, a comparison was made of clinical criteria, pulse volume recording (PVR), Doppler pressure, and a new noninvasive technique—photoplethysmographic assessment of skin-perfusion pressure (PPG/SPP)—for their effectiveness in predicting amputation wound healing.

Investigators studied 45 amputations in 42 patients. Nine amputations were above the knee, 22 were below the knee, 5 were knee disarticulations, and 9 were foot amputations. Sixty-nine percent of patients were men, and 44% were diabetic.

The only technique that was able to predict skin healing was PPG/SPP. When measured anteriorly, PPG/SPP was very reliable in helping to select the level of amputation. Angiography also correlated significantly with successful results.

The findings suggest that surgeons should not rely on clinical evidence to select the amputation level. If a reliable noninvasive test is not available, angiography may be useful. However, PPG/SPP is a noninvasive procedure that will enable the surgeon to choose an optimal level for amputation that will reduce complications and improve rehabilitative outcome. A combination of angiography and PPG/SPP can be used to assess blood flow both at the level of large arteries and at the skin level.

▶ This prospective series demonstrates the usefulness of PPG/SPP as a noninvasive predictor of healing ability of amputation stumps (1). The technique may also be a good predictor of chronic vascular ulcers such as the venous stasis ulcer and diabetic ulcer. The study demonstrates that if the methodology is unavailable, the best predictor is angiography.—M.C. Robson, M.D.

Reference

1. Brock TAA, et al: *J Vasc Surg* 8:10, 1988.

Stimulation of Repair in Chronic, Nonhealing, Cutaneous Ulcers Using Platelet-Derived Wound Healing Formula

Knighton DR, Ciresi K, Fiegel VD, Schumerth S, Butler E, Cerra F (Univ of Minnesota; Minneapolis VA Hosp)
Surg Gynecol Obstet 170:56–60, 1990   5–2

Current treatments for chronic, nonhealing, cutaneous ulcers are not designed to stimulate active wound repair. However, a recently developed autologously prepared platelet-derived wound healing formula (PDWHF) offers a method of actively stimulating the formation of granulation tissue and epithelialization. A prospectively randomized, blinded trial was undertaken to evaluate PDWHF in 32 patients.

All had chronically nonhealing ulcers in a lower extremity and a normal peripheral blood platelet count. Half were treated with PDWHF and half received placebo. Patients applied the wound dressings twice a day and returned to the clinic for evaluation every 2 or 3 weeks during the 8-week study period.

Thirteen patients in the treatment group and 11 in the control group completed the trial. After 8 weeks 17 of the 21 wounds in the treatment group achieved 100% epithelialization. The remaining 4 wounds decreased in size, although they did not heal fully. In contrast, in the control group only 2 of 13 wounds achieved 100% epithelialization and 7 increased in size. When the control patients were treated subsequently with PDWHF, all achieved 100% epithelialization in an average of 7.1 weeks.

Topical administration of PDWHF in microcrystalline collagen significantly accelerated the healing of chronic cutaneous ulcers in these patients. The formula contains at least 5 locally active growth factors, each with a different cellular function: platelet-derived growth factor, platelet-derived angiogenesis factor, platelet-derived epidermal growth factor, transforming growth factor-beta, and platelet factor 4.

▶ Much publicity has surrounded the use of this autologous platelet-derived formula. Early studies were neither randomized nor blinded. This trial is randomized and blinded but suffers other errors in design. The ulcers were not divided into homogeneous subgroups, so that a greater number of arterial ischemic ulcers were treated by placebo. This would bias the results toward the agent-treated group. Also, bacteriology of tissue biopsy specimens was not performed to be sure that the 2 groups were similar. It is difficult to perform good clinical trials, but it is an absolute necessity when assessing agents claiming to improve wound healing.—M.C. Robson, M.D.

PDGF and FGF Stimulate Wound Healing in the Genetically Diabetic Mouse

Greenhalgh DG, Sprugel KH, Murray MJ, Ross R (Univ of Washington; Zymo-Genetics Inc, Seattle)
Am J Pathol 136:1235–1246, 1990   5–3

Patients with wound complications usually have an underlying condition such as diabetes or malnutrition or have undergone treatment with steroids, chemotherapy, or radiation. Recent research directed at improving wound healing has centered on growth factors. In an experiment using genetically diabetic mice, the effects of recombinant growth factor on wound healing were examined.

The C57BL/KsJ-db/db mice have characteristics similar to those of human-onset diabetes. Compared with their littermates without diabetes, significant delays in the formation of granulation tissue and wound closure occur in these mice. Wounds created in mice with and without diabetes were examined during a 6-week period.

Whereas wounds of the animals without diabetes closed completely within 10–16 days, 4–6 weeks were required for closure in the animals with diabetes. In many cases new epithelium had completely covered the wound in mice without diabetes by 10 days. At this same time, only minimal cellular infiltrates and granulation tissue developed in the animals with diabetes.

When mice with diabetes received recombinant human platelet-derived growth factor (rPDGR-BB, 1 or 10 μg), recombinant human basic fibroblast growth factor (rbFGF, 1 μg), or combinations of both applied topically to the wound for 5 days after surgery, all parameters of healing were improved (table).

At 10 days mice with diabetes treated with either dose of rPDGF-BB or with rbFGF had thicker and more erythematous wounds than vehicle control mice. By 21 days application of either growth factor resulted in an 80% to 90% reduction in open wound area. Controls, in contrast, had only a 50% reduction.

Application of a single growth factor appeared to have the same effect as the 2 applied together, and application of either for 5 days had the

Effects of 5 Days of Treatment With rPDGF-BB and/or
rbFGF on Diabetic Wounds Evaluated at 21 Days

Treatment*	Histologic score†	% Wound closure‡	N
Vehicle	5.1 ± 0.5	48.0 ± 5.1	17
10 μg rPDGF-BB	9.7 ± 0.7§	90.6 ± 5.5‖	9
1 μg rbFGF	8.2 ± 0.4§	79.5 ± 3.7‖	16
rPDGF-BB/rbFGF	8.0 ± 0.7§	78.7 ± 5.7‖	8

*Full-thickness skin wounds on diabetic mice were treated with vehicle, rPDGF-BB (10 μg/day), rbFGF (1 μg/day), or a combination of both for 5 days.

†Histology scores were assigned to each coded specimen by 2 investigators. Values are expressed as mean ± SEM.

‡Values are expressed as mean ± SEM.

§$P < .05$ when compared to vehicle treatment by ranking the histologic specimens and determining statistical significance using the Kruskal-Wallis test with individual comparisons performed using Dunn's procedure.

‖ $P < .05$ when compared to vehicle treatment by analysis of variance (ANOVA) and individual comparisons by Tukey's procedure.

(Courtesy of Greenhalgh DG, Sprugel KH, Murray MJ, et al: *Am J Pathol* 136:1235–1246, 1990.)

same effect as application for 10–14 days. Recombinant growth factors may be of value in treating patients with impaired wound healing.

Recombinant Basic Fibroblast Growth Factor Stimulates Wound Healing in Healing-Impaired db/db Mice
Tsuboi R, Rifkin DB (New York Univ; Beverly Sackler Found Lab, New York)
J Exp Med 172:245–251, 1990   5–4

There is evidence that agents inducing fibroblast or endothelial cell proliferation can promote granulation tissue formation and wound repair when applied to healing-impaired wounds. The effect of recombinant basic fibroblast growth factor (bFGF) on wound healing was studied in healing-impaired *db/db* mice. Full-thickness wounds were made in diabetic *db/db* mice and in their normal littermates by punch biopsy, and recombinant bFGF was applied to the open wound once a day.

Untreated wounds in *db/db* mice exhibited relatively poor reepithelialization and granulation tissue formation. Application of bFGF to the wounds significantly improved these responses, whereas the factor had little effect in normal mice. Heated growth factor and factor pretreated with neutralizing antibody had little stimulatory effect on wound healing. The breaking strength of healed wounds in *db/db* mice was enhanced by bFGF treatment.

Recombinant bFGF can significantly improve dermal healing in healing-impaired mice. It would appear to have potential as a potent, self-limited healing-promoting agent.

Epidermal and Dermal Effects of Epidermal Growth Factor During Wound Repair
Nanney LB (Vanderbilt Univ)
J Invest Dermatol 94:624–629, 1990   5–5

More than 25 years of predominantly in vitro studies have indicated the role of epidermal growth factor (EGF) in wound repair. To evaluate both epidermal and dermal responses to topical application of EGF in a porcine wound repair model, surgical wounds were produced along the dorsal surface of domestic male and female pigs. Topical formulations containing either recombinant EGF or placebo were applied daily to the wounds. After full-thickness removal of the wound, tissues were sectioned and stained for computerized morphometric analysis of histologic sections.

In the EGF-treated wounds epithelialization was complete by day 5. Wounds treated with placebo reached 100% resurfacing by day 6. However, growth-curve patterns in both treatment groups were similar. There was a marked increase in cellularity and thickness in the epidermis when EGF was applied. The degree of keratinocyte differentiation was striking in the EGF-treated wounds. With placebo treatment the epidermis was thin and the cells were pale and poorly differentiated. A dose-responsive increase in the thickness of the granulation tissue was also apparent.

In this porcine model topical application of EGF stimulated epithelialization of partial-thickness wounds and positively affected the underlying dermis during the early phases of wound repair. Treatment with EGF may have clinical application in patients with chronic wounds or burns.

Transforming Growth Factor-β Stimulates Wound Healing and Modulates Extracellular Matrix Gene Expression in Pig Skin: I. Excisional Wound Model
Quaglino D Jr, Nanney LB, Kennedy R, Davidson JM (Vanderbilt Univ; Veterans Affairs Med Ctr, Nashville)
Lab Invest 63:307–319, 1990   5–6

Recombinant transforming growth factor-β1 (TGF-β1) is a multifunctional peptide growth factor that enhances the synthesis of collagen, fibronectin, elastin, and other matrix components in cultured cell populations. The effect of TGF-β1 on matrix gene expression was examined using pigs bearing split-thickness excisional wounds. In situ hybridization studies served to assess the activity and location of cells involved in matrix gene expression after administration of recombinant TGF-β1.

Granulation tissue formation was substantially greater in wounds treated with TGF-β1 than in control wounds, and it was better organized and vascularized. Growth factor treatment increased the expression of

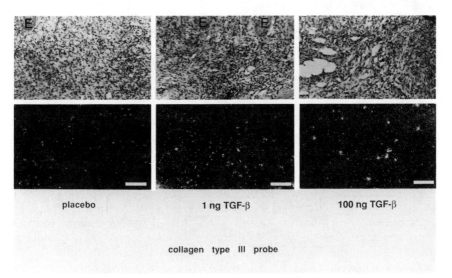

placebo   1 ng TGF-β   100 ng TGF-β

collagen   type   III   probe

Fig 5–1.—In situ hybridization for collagen type III mRNA. Hybridization shows a similar response as described for collagen α(2) I mRNA. Granulation tissue from wounds treated with placebo, 1 ng and 100 ng of transforming growth factor-β (TGF-β1) are shown. Photographs were taken at or near the dermal/epidermal junction. Epidermis *(E)*. Bars, 100 μm. (Courtesy of Quaglino D Jr, Nanney LB, Kennedy R, et al: *Lab Invest* 63:307–319, 1990.)

both collagen type I and collagen type III matrix protein genes (Fig 5–1).There also were increased levels of mRNAs for fibronectin and TGF-β1 itself.

Increased matrix formation after application of TGF-β1 is apparently the result of fibroplasia regulated by mRNAs for several structural matrix proteins. In addition, TGF-β1 is autostimulating in wounds, helping to explain the lasting effects of even single doses of the cytokine.

▶ Recombinant technology has allowed various peptide growth factors to be cloned in large amounts. This had led to their usage both in experimental animals and clinically. To enlarge the window to demonstrate efficacy, impaired wound healing models are often chosen. These include animal models with impairment caused by genetic or chemical diabetes, chemotherapeutic drugs, steroids, radiation, and infection. Some of these models may have little relevance to the clinical situation. In each of the preceding 4 papers (Abstracts 5–3 through 5–6), single combined peptide growth factors were used to affect "wound healing." It is clear from studying these papers that wound healing can no longer be considered a generic form but must be divided into its processes such as angiogenesis, inflammation, fibroplasia, extracellular matrix deposition, contraction, or epithelialization. Each growth factor may affect one or several of these processes. The animals models help to delineate which process or processes a given agent affects. However, it is then necessary to select a human wound that heals predominantly by that given process and test the agent in such a wound. Such trials are just beginning to be done and the papers describing them will be watched for by all surgeons who find these initial animal trials of interest.—M.C. Robson, M.D.

Wound Healing and T-Lymphocytes
Efron JE, Frankel HL, Lazarou SA, Wasserkrug HL, Barbul A (Sinai Hosp of Baltimore; Johns Hopkins Med Insts)
J Surg Res 48:460–463, 1990   5–7

Lymphocytes are involved in the process of wound healing, but their specific role is not fully understood. Although T cell depletion leads to impaired wound healing, depletion of the T suppressor-cytotoxic subset actually enhances it. The effect of simultaneous depletion of T helper-effector and T suppressor-cytotoxic lymphocytes on fibroplasia was examined and compared with the effect of all T lymphocyte depletion.

Young male balb/c mice received a 2.5-cm skin incision followed by subcutaneous implantation of polyvinyl alcohol sponges. One group of mice was treated with 1 mg of 3OH12, a rat anti-mouse monoclonal antibody against the Thy-1.2 antigen present on all T cells. A second group received 1 mg each of GK1.5 (anti-L3T4, CD4; antihelper-effector subset) and 2.43 (anti-Lyt2.1, CD8; antisuppressor-cytotoxic subset). Control animals were given 1 mg of nonspecific rat IgG. All treatments were given the day before wounding and once a week thereafter until death.

The 2 groups had equal depletion of all T- and Th- and Ts- subsets in peripheral blood and spleens. Wound healing was markedly impaired at both 2 weeks and 4 weeks after depletion of T lymphocytes by administration of 3OH12. However, at both 2 weeks and 4 weeks after wounding the combined administration of GK1.5 and 2.43 resulted in statistically significant enhancement of the wound healing parameters. Assessments of healing were based on wound breaking strength and accumulation of hydroxyproline in the implanted sponges.

Wound healing is strongly regulated by immune lymphocytes. Because combined anti-T helper-effector and T suppressor-cytotoxic depletion enhances wound healing, there appears to be a Thy-1.2$^+$, L3T4$^-$, Lyt2$^-$ subpopulation of T lymphocytes that normally stimulates wound healing.

▶ The role of the lymphocyte in wound healing has been debated. Much of the problem has been that the lymphocyte has been considered a single cell. It is now known that there are many subsets of lymphocytes that have significantly different actions. Sophisticated studies such as that reported in this paper will elucidate the role of various subsets of lymphocytes on specific wound healing processes. These experiments will have to be expanded beyond looking at collagen deposition and wound breaking strength before the role of lymphocytes in the summation of processes is understood.—M.C. Robson, M.D.

Tumor Necrosis Factor and Wound Healing
Mooney DP, O'Reilly M, Gamelli RL (Univ of Vermont)
Ann Surg 211:124–129, 1990   5–8

Recent studies have suggested that tumor necrosis factor-α (TNF-α), a product of activated macrophages, may modulate wound healing. The effect on wound disruption strength (WDS) of the topical application of recombinant human TNF-α to both normal and Adriamycin-impaired mice was examined in groups of 12 animals each that were randomized to receive saline (PBS), TNF in PBS, collagen, or TNF in collagen, applied locally. Systemic administration of TNF was used in some of groups of animals. Wound histology was examined 6 months after wounding and local application of TNF.

At 11 days after wounding the effect on WDS produced by local administration of collagen did not differ from that produced by PBS. When compared with animals that received collagen alone, those receiving 10, 50, 100, or 500 ng of TNF in the collagen vehicle had a 14% to 49% increase in WDS 11 days after wounding. The animals that received Adriamycin at the time of wounding and 5, 25, or 50 ng of TNF applied locally to the wound in the collagen vehicle had a 33% to 65% increase in WDS, compared to those receiving collagen alone.

The WDS was not affected significantly when 1, 100, or 250 ng of TNF in collagen was applied to the wound (Fig 5–2). Systemic administration of TNF (25, 50, or 75 μg/kg daily for 11 days) did not significantly increase WDS, even though the white blood cell and monocyte counts were increased and the neutrophil count was decreased. At

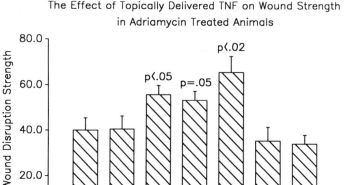

Fig 5–2.—Mean WDS ± standard error of mean for groups of 12 animals each given Adriamycin, 15 mg/kg, intraperitoneally then TNF locally in collagen in doses shown (expressed as percentage of mean WDS of animals given saline intraperitoneally and collagen alone locally). P values are versus animals given Adriamycin intraperitoneally and collagen alone locally. (Courtesy of Mooney DP, O'Reilly M, Gamelli RL: *Ann Surg* 211:124–129, 1990.)

6-month evaluation local TNF in collagen did not induce histologic pathology.

Tumor necrosis factor-α acts on the macrophage and on other cell types present in the wound. In this model dose range and timing were both important in achieving an effect on WDS. Local administration of TNF to the wound resulted in an increase in WDS only when a collagen vehicle was used in the appropriate dose, timing, and vehicle, TNF appears to be present and active in wound-healing processes.

▶ As has been reported elsewhere in this volume, TNF-α appears to have many effects. Some are beneficial and others are detrimental. It may well be a dose-response problem, causing almost a Yin-Yang type activity. If this is true, it will be like many other mediators described. Arachidonic acid metabolites cause almost opposite effects depending on the dose used. The effect shown in this paper of TNF increasing wound disrupting strength when applied topically needs to be further studied in other models because of the potentially dangerous side effects of the agent.—M.C. Robson, M.D.

Studies in Fetal Wound Healing: IV. Hyaluronic Acid-Stimulating Activity Distinguishes Fetal Wound Fluid From Adult Wound Fluid
Longaker MT, Chiu ES, Harrison MR, Crombleholme TM, Langer JC, Duncan BW, Adzick NS, Verrier ED, Stern R (Univ of California, San Francisco)
Ann Surg 210:667–672, 1989   5–9

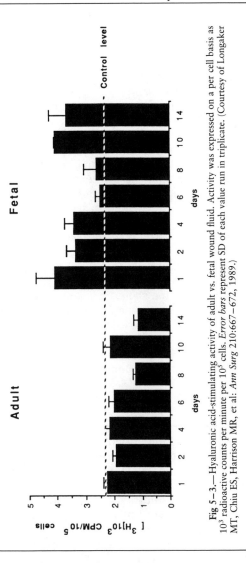

Fig 5–3.—Hyaluronic acid-stimulating activity of adult vs. fetal wound fluid. Activity was expressed on a per cell basis as 10^3 radioactive counts per minute per 10^5 cells. *Error bars* represent SD of each value run in triplicate. (Courtesy of Longaker MT, Chiu ES, Harrison MR, et al: *Ann Surg* 210:667–672, 1989.)

Animal studies and surgery performed on human fetuses have suggested that fetal wounds heal differently from adult wounds. The former heal rapidly and without scarring, inflammation, and contraction, perhaps because of the unique extracellular matrix (ECM) found in the fetus. The fetal ECM has an abundance of glycosaminoglycans, particularly hyaluronic acid (HA).

A study was designed to define the mechanisms by which HA is deposited in the fetal wound and to compare that process with adult wound healing. The wire mesh wound cylinder model, which creates a dead space that fills with wound fluid, was used in the experiment for which the fetal lamb was chosen because of its long gestation period. A wound was also created in 1 nonpregnant adult sheep. Wound fluid was obtained by aspiration at 1, 2, 4, 6, 8, 10, and 14 days after subcutaneous implantation of the wound cylinders.

At each of these time points the adult wound fluid had less HA-stimulating activity than did control samples (Fig 5–3), and levels of HA-stimulating activity in fetal wound fluid were much higher than in adult specimens at each evaluation time. The highest levels of activity were at days 1 and 10.

Fetal and adult wound fluid differed remarkably in their levels of HA-stimulating activity. This difference may underlie the elevated deposition of HA in the fetal wound matrix. The extracellular environment supported by HA fosters cell motility and proliferation that may perhaps account for the unique qualities observed in fetal wound healing.

▶ The study of fetal wound healing may yet give vital information about scar formation in adults. However, if one follows all of the reports, the subject becomes quite murky. It is now obvious that the species studied, the exact period of observation, and the environment affect the conclusions reached. These authors have concentrated on the sheep. It will be useful to see if those who concentrate on the rabbit or on humans can isolate this apparent HA-stimulating substance, and whether it has clinical applicability.—M.C. Robson, M.D.

Keloids and Hypertrophic Scars: A Comprehensive Review
Rockwell WB, Cohen IK, Ehrlich HP (Massachusetts Gen Hosp, Boston; Med College of Virginia, Richmond)
Plast Reconstr Surg 84:827–837, 1989   5–10

Although keloids were first described centuries ago, their exact cause is still not known and a universally effective treatment is not available. Keloid research is hampered by the fact that there is no reliable animal model available, as keloids do not occur in animals. Consequently, most theories are based on in vivo studies that approach the problem indirectly by using wound models. The current knowledge of keloid formation and experience with various treatments were reviewed.

The exact incidence of keloid formation is not known, but individuals of certain races such as blacks and Asians are more susceptible than Caucasians. The observation that keloid formation occurs mainly in parts of the body where melanocytes have the greatest concentration has led to the suggestion that an aberration of metabolism of melanocyte-stimulating hormone may be responsible for keloid formation. Hypoxia may also contribute to the formation of abnormal scars. Increased proline hydroxylase activity has been implicated. Preliminary studies have suggested a role of growth factors in the formation of keloids.

The control of keloid formation remains limited, and no routinely effective method is available. Among the many pharmacologic approaches that have been tried, topically applied herbs and vitamins to soften the lesions have proven ineffective. The use of various enzymes has yielded inconsistent results. Topically applied and intralesionally injected corticosteroids have also proven ineffective. Although preliminary studies suggest that laser surgery may be effective, the results to date have been inconsistent.

▶ Although it is unusual for a review article to be included in the YEAR BOOK, this article is particularly timely and useful. With the explosion of papers suggesting that modulation of wound healing processes may soon be possible, a new look at proliferative scar formation may be possible. Having a good review article of what is presently known about keloids and hypertrophic scars will be helpful to the practicing surgeon.—M.C. Robson, M.D.

Proteoglycan-Lymphocyte Association in the Development of Hypertrophic Scars
Linares HA (Shriners Burns Inst; Univ of Texas, Galveston)
Burns 16:21–24, 1990   5–11

The sulfated forms of the glycosamino occur chiefly as proteoglycans consisting of a central protein core to which many glycan side chains are covalently attached. This component of the extracellular macromolecular matrix reportedly is associated at cell surfaces, as well as intracellularly, with many types of cells, including epithelial and mesenchymal cells, endothelial cells, fibroblasts, mast cells, lymphocytes, and others. In hypertrophic scars there is marked increase in proteoglycans in comparison with that in normal scars and normal skin, and the existence of large amounts of chondroitin 4-sulfate may contribute to the excess of collagen deposition that distinguishes this abnormal healing process.

Surgical specimens of 17 hypertrophic scars and 6 normal scars were taken from patients younger than 16 years who had thermal burns. The age of the hypertrophic scars ranged from 16 months to 23 months post burn, and the age of the normal scars varied from 2 years to 6 years post burn. A few samples of normal skin were studied for comparison. The specimens were fixed in 10% neutral buffered formalin and B-5 fixative, embedded in paraffin at 56° C, and sectioned at 4 μm. Parallel histologic and immunohistologic stains were used in the scar specimens to identify the type of cells and associated proteoglycans present in perivascular cuffs in hypertrophic scars.

Sections from hypertrophic scars had no true epidermal rete ridges. The collagen fibers of the dermis were predominantly in a whorl-like arrangement or in a nodular pattern. In these areas a marked coat of proteoglycans was seen, as well as a network of small vessels with perivascular mononuclear cell infiltration varying from a more dense cuff in younger scars to a much lesser density in older ones. In sections from normal scars the collagen fibers of the dermis had a predominantly parallel orientation with a slight quantity of proteoglycans and no significant perivascular cell infiltration. In normal skin the collagen of the dermis had an orthogonal pattern with a minimal amount of proteoglycans, chiefly in the papillary layer and in the connective tissue surrounding the skin appendages.

Most of the mononuclear cells forming the perivascular cuff in hypertrophic scars are T cells. The role of the T cells in wound healing appears to be regulation of fibroblastic activity at the site of tissue repair. The proteoglycan associated with the perivascular T cell infiltration in hypertrophic scars is mainly chondroitin 4-sulfate. Consequently, it is assumed that the persistence of perivascular lymphoid cells, particularly in the early and active phase of hypertrophic healing, may be an important contributory factor in development of this abnormal scar.

▶ This paper describing perivascular T cells and excess proteoglycans in postburn proliferative scars may well be related to the paper by Efron et al. (Abstracts 5–7) about T lymphocytes and the one by Longaker et al. (Abstract 5–9) about hyaluronic acid reviewed previously. As the knowledge on basic wound healing evolves, understanding the etiology of proliferative scar formation and its eventual control becomes an attainable goal.—M.C. Robson, M.D.

6 Infections

What's in a Name? Is Methicillin-Resistant _Staphylococcus aureus_ Just Another _Staphylococcus aureus_ When Treated With Vancomycin?
McManus AT, Mason AD Jr, McManus WF, Pruitt BA Jr (US Army Inst of Surgical Research, Fort Sam Houston, San Antonio, Tex)
Arch Surg 124:1456–1459, 1989   6–1

Methicillin-resistant _Staphylococcus aureus_ (MRSA) strains, which are resistant to penicillinase-resistant penicillins and aminoglycosides, are common nosocomial pathogens. Their virulence and pathogenicity relative to other _Staphylococcus aureus_ strains causing infections in the same patient population are not clear. The significance of MRSA and methicillin-sensitive _S. aureus_ (MSSA) strains in causing infections was compared in 1,100 consecutively admitted, severely burned patients in whom vancomycin was used to treat staphylococcal infections.

Staphylococcus aureus was isolated in 658 patients, 319 of whom were colonized by MRSA strains. A total of 253 _S. aureus_ infections occurred in 178 patients; MRSA caused 58 infections in 43 patients and MSSA caused 157 infections in 120 patients. The frequencies of bacteremia, pneumonia, and other infections did not differ between these 2 groups. A severity index, based on multiple-regression analysis of mortality adjusted for burn size and age, showed no measurable increase in mortality attributable to MRSA.

There is no significant increase in the risk of death in infections caused by MRSA. These results question the clinical and economic significance of added control practices to control MRSA infections in critical care areas. The universal effectiveness of vancomycin against these organisms strongly favors the concept that MRSA infection is just another staphylococcal infection.

▶ This article is a must on the reading list for all surgeons. Because MRSA has a convenient marker, it has gained a notoriety and pavlovian responses that are not justified. The authors find that it reacts like other staphylococci when treated properly. I have found that it prevents skin graft take or flap closure at the same level (>10^5 organisms per g) as other staphylococci. Methicillin-resistant _S. aureus_ is becoming common in patients even at the time of admission and may not justify the expense presently attributed to it.—M.C. Robson, M.D.

Detection of Surgical Pathogens by in Vitro DNA Amplification: I. Rapid Identification of *Candida albicans* By in Vitro Amplification of a Fungus-Specific Gene

Buchman TG, Rossier M, Merz WG, Charache P (Johns Hopkins Med Insts)
Surgery 108:338–347, 1990   6–2

The increasingly common problems of nosocomial candidemia and disseminated candidiasis must be identified quickly so that therapy can be initiated. Such therapy is often withheld until the diagnosis is certain because of its potential toxicity. To circumvent the need for fungal growth in culture, the polymerase chain reaction (PCR) technique was used to amplify a segment of fungal DNA coding for the cytochrome $P_{450}L_1A_1$ (lanosterol-14-α-demethylase) in vitro.

Clinical specimens of urine, sputum, wound fluid, and blood were collected from patients in whom infections was suspected. Growing *Candida albicans* cultures were diluted serially in blood from healthy volunteers to evaluate the sensitivity of PCR in clinical samples. In this experiment as few as 12 yeasts could be detected in as few as 6 hours. Based on the clinical specimens, 6 patients had correct diagnoses of *C. albicans* infection. Of 17 additional culture-negative specimens, PCR suggested the presence of yeast in 2.

The PCR technique appears to have a role in the early detection and therapy of yeast infection. It may also have a place in evaluation of response to therapy or detection of recurrent disease. The sensitivity of PCR makes it vulnerable to even the slightest contamination. Unexpected amplification patterns are also seen.

▶ The diagnosis of candidemia is difficult but essential. Presumptive diagnosis treated by potentially toxic drugs is less than ideal. These authors suggest that the PCR technique may be more rapid and more accurate than standard fungal cultures. A larger series with reproducibility is needed to demonstrate the usefulness of this test.—M.C. Robson, M.D.

Development of a Bacteria-Independent Model of the Multiple Organ Failure Syndrome

Steinberg S, Flynn W, Kelley K, Bitzer L, Sharma P, Gutierrez C, Baxter J, Lalka D, Sands A, Van Liew J, Hassett J, Price R, Beam T, Flint L (State Univ of New York, Buffalo; Buffalo VA Med Ctr)
Arch Surg 124:1390–1395, 1989   6–3

Multiple organ failure (MOF) is estimated to result in 100,000 deaths each year in the United States. A suitable experimental model has been sought to study the development and progression of this syndrome. Goris and colleagues described a rat model of MOF created by the intraperitoneal injection of zymosan A, an extract of the cell wall of the yeast *Sac-*

charomyces cerevisiae. A set of experiments was designed to assess pathophysiologic and histopathologic alterations in this potential model of MOF.

Wistar rats were randomly assigned to receive no treatment, 4 mL of sterile saline, 4 mL of sterile mineral oil, or 1 mg of zymosan A suspended in 4 mL of mineral oil per gram of body weight. Results were evaluated according to the criteria for a model of MOF: alterations in organ function, changes in hepatocyte metabolism, dysfunction of the gut mucosal barrier to bacteria, and characteristic histopathologic findings.

Bacterial translocation occurred in the animals given zymosan. These animals also had hypoxia, decreased creatinine clearance, and changes in hepatic microsomal cytochrome P450 content and aniline hydroxylase activity. Histopathologic changes were seen in the lungs, liver, and kidneys of the rats ti at received zymosan. Although some effects were seen in the mineral oil g oup, they were not accompanied by any histopathologic findings.

This model fulfills the criteria for a model of MOF and should allow detailed evaluation of potential mechanisms of the syndrome. Although the model had an early mortality rate of 60%, surviving animals were stable and amenable to experimental manipulation.

▶ An experimental model that mimics MOF has been needed. These authors show that such a model is now available to study this syndrome, which is the second leading cause of death in intensive care units. By carefully examining the specific dysfunction of each organ system, they have shown that bacteria are not the primary cause of MOF. This is correlated with clinical series suggesting that inflammatory mediators are the initial cause of dysfunction. Bacterial translocation from the bowel followed other organ dysfunction rather than preceding it.— M.C. Robson, M.D.

Surgical Infection in the Morbidly Obese Patient
Sugerman HJ (Med College of Virginia, Richmond)
Infect Surg 9:18–30, 1990

6–4

Severely obese patients who require abdominal operations are at increased risk for postoperative infections. Consequently, surgeons commonly avoid elective operations on morbidly obese patients. However, it is not appropriate to delay elective procedures because of severe obesity. Cholecystitis is common in obesity. Rather than delay operation, obese patients requiring elective cholecystectomy should be advised of the availability of elective gastric procedures for the reduction of obesity. Both procedures can be performed concomitantly.

Elective gastric operations for morbid obesity were performed on more than 700 patients at one institution. The incidence of wound infection significant enough to delay hospital discharge or require hospital readmission was 4%. The incidence of deep vein thrombophlebitis or pulmo-

---

Signs and Symptoms of Peritonitis in the Morbidly Obese

Symptoms*	Signs†
Abdominal Pain	Fever
Shoulder Pain	Tachycardia
Back Pain	Tachypnea
Shortness of Breath	
Anxiety	

*Guarding, localized, or rebound tenderness, and rigidity are often absent.
†Usually left sided if a gastric reduction procedure has been performed.
(Courtesy of Sugerman HJ: *Infect Surg* 9:18–30, 1990.)

---

nary embolism, or both, was 1%. The early postoperative mortality was .6%

One of the major problems in the postoperative care of morbidly obese patients is the great difficulty in diagnosing complicating peritonitis, as the typical signs and symptoms of peritonitis are usually absent whereas different signs and symptoms are present. In addition to abdominal pain, symptoms of peritonitis may include anxiety, shoulder pain, back pain, shortness of breath, pelvic or testicular pain, urinary frequency, and tenesmus (table). Physical signs of peritonitis may be absent in the early stages, resulting in a delayed diagnosis. However, if intervention is delayed, marked hypotension and tachypnea consistent with septic shock may develop. In addition to an increased risk for peritonitis, morbidly obese patients are also at increased risk for postoperative atelectasis and pneumonia, necrotizing panniculitis, boils, intertriginous infections, and infected venous stasis ulcers.

The weight reduction that follows gastric surgery for obesity will reduce or correct many of the risks for surgical infection in morbidly obese patients. To prevent missing a diagnosis of peritonitis, a high index of suspicion should be maintained throughout the postoperative course.

▶ With an experience of performing elective gastric operations on more than 700 morbidly obese patients, this author has reduced his infection rate significantly. Certainly, every surgeon who operates on the morbidly obese patient can benefit from this article. The author stresses physical examination as the best diagnostic tool to determine peritonitis in these patients and outlines the subtle changes to look for. Interestingly, he does not discuss the pros and cons of various diagnostic techniques such as ultrasound, CT scans, and nuclear magnetic resonance spectroscopy. With the author's experience, this would have been a helpful discussion.—M.C. Robson, M.D.

Single-Stage Management of Sternal Wound Infections
Jeevanandam V, Smith CR, Rose EA, Malm JR, Hugo NE (Columbia Univ; Presbyterian Hosp, New York)
J Thorac Cardiovasc Surg 99:256–263, 1990   6–5

Deep sternal wound infections, which occur in up to 5% of patients undergoing cardiac surgery, have been managed by a number of methods. Several procedures are often required to treat the complication. An approach was developed that combines débridement and bilateral pectoralis major musculocutaneous flap reconstruction in a single operation. The outcome was compared in 31 patients treated with single-stage management (group B) and in 16 treated by previous methods (group A).

Patients in the 2 groups were similar with regard to initial operation, causative organisms, antibiotics used, and interval between surgery and appearance of the sternal wound infection. There were more cardiac transplant patients, however, in group B (5) than in group A (1), and these patients presented a special problem because of immunosuppression.

Group A patients underwent débridement, dressing changes, and closure by secondary intention (3); débridement, sternal reclosure, and antibiotic irrigation (3); or débridement, dressing changes, and delayed muscle flap closure (10). Group B patients underwent débridement and immediate closure with a pectoral musculocutaneous flap. Dissection extended from the clavicle to the inferior ribs and from the medial insertion of the sternum to the anterior axillary line. Flaps were closed over the sternal defect in 2 layers. Although the flaps do not immediately fill the sternal defect, a combination of muscle swelling and suction obliterates the space within several days.

Group B patients had a shorter hospital stay (18 days) after the initial procedure for sternal wound infection than group A patients (42 days). Although 16 patients in group A required reoperation, only 4 patients in group B had additional surgery. Reoperation in group B was for dehiscence or bleeding, not for persistent infection. Infection was eradicated in all group B patients. The success of single-stage management recommends it as the initial treatment of choice for sternal wound infections.

Antibacterial Drug Delivery Into Fibrotic Cavities Using Muscle Flaps
Feller AM, Russell RC, Roth AC, Graham DR (Technical Univ Munich, Germany; Southern Illinois Univ, Springfield)
Eur J Plast Surg 13:105–111, 1990   6–6

Muscle flaps have been used successfully as a cover for infected wounds in a variety of applications. A vascularized muscle can also enhance blood supply and improve antimicrobial delivery. The antibiotic-carrying capacity of a vascularized muscle flap transferred into an artificially produced fibrotic cavity was evaluated in a tissue cage model in rabbits.

Silastic tubes were inserted to create bilateral fibrotic cavities over the animal's dorsal thorax. Three months later a vascularized strip of muscle was placed into the anterior end of the cavity. The animals later received injections of either ceftriaxone (20 mg/kg) or ciprofloxacin (50 mg/kg). Cavity serum samples were withdrawn from experimental and control sites at periods ranging from 2–24 hours after injection.

For several weeks, concentrations of ceftriaxone exceeded 10 μg/mL in both control and muscle chambers. At 1 week the muscle chamber peak concentration exceeded the control chamber by 5 μg/mL. Concentrations in both chambers decreased with time. At 12 weeks, concentrations fell to 8.3 μg/mL in the muscle chamber and 6.4 μg/mL in the control chamber. The peak serum level of ciprofloxacin, 6.91 μg/mL, was less than 10% of the serum peak achieved with a smaller dose of ceftriaxone, indicating very poor absorption of the injection.

Results obtained with ceftriaxone indicate that muscle flaps are able to increase the concentration of antibiotics within a fibrotic cavity. With time, increased scarring around the muscle results in a decreased blood supply to the cavity and decreased delivery of the antibiotic. To achieve highest antibiotic levels, this therapy should be started immediately after the muscle transfer and provided at a higher dose after 6 weeks.

▶ Plastic and reconstructive surgeons have long believed that adequate débridement and primary closure with vascularized tissue is the therapy of choice for infected tissue such as osteomyelitis and sternotomy wounds (1). Others have not been as willing to accept this or to discard their beliefs in serial débridement, continued inflammation, and eventual healing by secondary intention or tertiary closure. The first article (Abstract 6–5) compares single-stage management to serial procedures for infected sternotomy wounds and confirms what others have shown, namely, 1-stage débridement and closure is superior. This is important in these patients, who are often not good risks for multiple procedures. The second article (Abstract 6–6) provides experimental evidence supporting the concept. Vascularized flaps containing muscle increase the ability to deliver antibiotics into an infected cavity. In an infected cavity such as the mediastinum, using flaps to deliver bloodborne antibiotics is rational and effective.—M.C. Robson, M.D.

Reference

1. Mathes SJ, et al: *Plast Reconstr Surg* 69:815, 1982.

Enhanced Effectiveness of Intraperitoneal Antibiotics Administered via Liposomal Carrier
Price CI, Horton JW, Baxter CR (Univ of Texas, Dallas; Univ of Oklahoma)
Arch Surg 124:1411–1415, 1989   6–7

Some surgeons use peritoneal antibiotic instillation or irrigation to treat acute peritoneal contamination or peritonitis. However, the rapid absorption of antibiotics from the large peritoneal surface area can cause unwanted systemic side effects. Moreover, the rapid absorption of antibiotics may decrease their concentration in the peritoneal cavity where therapy is needed. Liposomes are increasingly used as drug delivery systems. They are not rapidly absorbed from the peritoneal cavity as their large size prevents their crossing through capillary membranes. The feasibility of using liposomes for the delivery of antibiotics into the peritoneal cavity was investigated in rats with experimentally induced peritonitis.

Twenty controls were left untreated, 15 rats received intramuscular (IM) cefoxitin injections at the time of peritoneal contamination, 15 were treated with intraperitoneal (IP) cefoxitin at the time of contamination, and 15 were given IP liposome-encapsulated cefoxitin injections at the time of peritoneal contamination. Serum antibiotic levels were studied in an additional 17 rats treated with free or liposome-encapsulated tobramycin given intraperitoneally at the time of peritoneal contamination. Quantitative blood cultures were done on samples drawn at 4 hours and 24 hours after peritoneal contamination. All surviving rats were killed at 7 days.

Blood cultures of samples taken at 4 hours and 24 hours after peritoneal contamination from animals treated with IM or IP free cefoxitin had significantly fewer microorganisms than samples obtained from untreated controls. However, the use of a liposome delivery system significantly enhanced the antibiotic efficacy as compared with that in IM- and IP-treated animals. Survival data paralleled the blood culture results in that survival was only 10% in the control group, 33% in the IM-treated group, 80% in the IP-treated group, and 100% in the liposome-treated group. Liposome delivery of cefoxitin also tended to prevent peritoneal abscess formation compared with routes of administration. Animals treated with free tobramycin had higher serum tobramycin levels at 4 hours than those treated with liposome-encapsulated tobramycin. Liposomal drug delivery into the peritoneal cavity significantly enhances the antibiotic efficacy of cefoxitin in an animal model of fecal peritonitis.

▶ Prolonged sustained release of antimicrobials at the site of infection is the goal of managing chronic infection. The previous article (Abstract 6–6) about muscle flaps into fibrotic cavities describes an approach to reach this goal. Liposomes may well prove to be another approach. Certainly, in sustained active peritonitis, parenteral antibiotics alone have been unsuccessful. Just as the chronic infected burn wound responds to a topical antimicrobial cream, the fibrin-covered infected peritoneal surfaces may best respond to sustained release of antibiotics from a liposomal carrier. Although it would be difficult to accomplish in a rodent model, another arm of the study comparing prolonged intravenous antibiotics to the lysosomal dispersion of antibiotics would be useful.—M.C. Robson, M.D.

Occlusive Dressings: Does Dressing Type Influence the Growth of Common Bacterial Pathogens?

Marshall DA, Mertz PM, Eaglstein WH (Univ of Miami)
Arch Surg 125:1136–1139, 1990
6–8

Occlusive dressings are being used increasingly in the treatment of many types of wounds because they speed healing while reducing pain and scarring. Although an increased incidence of infections has not been observed with the use of these dressings, there is concern about the number and types of bacteria beneath occlusive dressings. That concern arises because occlusive dressings are known to alter a wound's pH, cellular infiltration, moisture content, and oxygen concentration, which may affect the resident flora of intact skin. The effects of 3 occlusive dressings with different permeabilities to oxygen on the proliferation of 4 pathogens with different oxygen requirements, inoculated into superficial skin wounds, were documented.

Twenty-four partial-thickness wounds made in the skin of 8 young Yorkshire pigs were inoculated with *Staphylococcus aureus*, *Clostridium perfringens*, *Bacteroides fragilis*, or *Pseudomonas aeruginosa*. Each animal was inoculated with only 1 pathogen. Six wounds each were covered with either DuoDERM, Opsite, or Vigilon occlusive dressings, and 6 wounds were left exposed to air. At 24, 48, and 72 hours after inoculation, the wounds were cultured by quantitative techniques on selective media.

Staphylococcus aureus was able to survive and proliferate well in air-exposed wounds, as well as under all occlusive dressing-covered wounds. The numbers of the strict anaerobes *C. perfringens* and *B. fragilis* were greatly reduced in air-exposed wounds and slightly reduced in wounds covered with Opsite, an oxygen-permeable dressing. Wounds covered with Opsite or Vigilon had the greatest numbers of *P. aeruginosa*. The permeability to oxygen for Vigilon is uncertain. Although no recommendations for dressing selection can be made on the basis of these limited data, it appears that occlusive dressings should not be used to cover wounds that may contain anaerobic organisms or appear to be grossly contaminated.

▶ The warning suggested by this paper should be carefully heeded. Since the demonstration that clean wounds such as the split-thickness skin graft donor site epithelialize more rapidly in the moist environment beneath an occlusive dressing, surgeons have been using these dressings more widely. Most wounds in need of a dressing are not clean, and this paper demonstrates that covering a contaminated wound can result in bacterial proliferation. I have never understood the rationale for using an occlusive dressing for treatment of a contaminated wound such as a venous stasis ulcer or partial-thickness burn. To me it is like putting an impermeable cover on an abscess.—M.C. Robson, M.D.

The Promotional Effect of Bone Wax on Experimental *Staphylococcus aureus* Osteomyelitis

Nelson DR, Buxton TB, Luu QN, Rissing JP (Med College of Georgia, Augusta)
J Thorac Cardiovasc Surg 99:977–980, 1990   6–9

Bone wax is frequently used for hemostasis, but there have been few reports of its potential role in promoting infection. The role of bone wax in promoting chronic *Staphylococcus aureus* osteomyelitis was examined in rats.

Rats were inoculated with staphylococci in the tibial metaphysis. Sterile bone wax was applied in some of the animals. Inocula of several strengths were used. Animals were killed for evaluation after 21 days. Additional animals were used to evaluate early bone dynamics within 10–30 minutes and 24 hours after inoculation.

Bone wax greatly reduced the amount of bacterial inoculum, as measured in log colony-forming units, required to establish chronic osteomyelitis in 50% and 100% of animals. Without bone wax the 50% infection rate was log 6.9 and the 100% infection rate was log 8.2. With bone wax, the 50% infection rate was significantly reduced to log 2.6 and the 100% infection rate to 4.4. In animals killed within 10–30 minutes after inoculation, tibias that received bone wax yielded more organisms than those without bone wax. In those animals killed 24 hours after inoculation no significant difference was noted.

On the basis of these data and the results of other studies, the routine use of bone wax appears to warrant serious reconsideration. This is especially so in operations such as the sternum-splitting procedure, in which osteomyelitis is an infrequent but serious complication.

▶ For someone who long ago discarded the use of bone wax, this article was refreshing. Surgeons who still use bone wax will benefit from reading this paper and its references, which discuss other complications from bone wax, including pulmonary emboli, inflammatory cysts, fibrosis, inhibition of osteogenesis, and potential nonunion.—M.C. Robson, M.D.

Protective Effects of Recombinant Human Tumor Necrosis Factor α and Interferon γ Against Surgically Simulated Wound Infection in Mice

Hershman MJ, Pietsch JD, Trachtenberg L, Mooney THR, Shields RE, Sonnenfeld G (Univ of Louisville)
Br J Surg 76:1282–1286, 1989   6–10

The most common postoperative surgical complication is wound infection. Because antibiotics, sterile techniques, and mechanical barriers do not completely prevent infection, a biologic response modifier has been sought. Tumor necrosis factor-α (TNF) and interferon γ (IFN-γ), both active in immune response regulation, were assessed for their ability to increase resistance to infection in surgical wound models.

A number of experiments were carried out on adult male mice. The

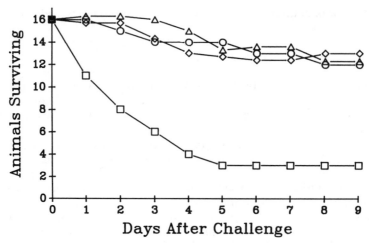

Fig 6–1.—Survival of mice treated with TNF and/or IFN-γ for 5 days before intramuscular *K. pneumoniae* challenge compared with controls: *squares*, controls; *triangles*, TNF; *circles*, IFN-γ; *triangles*, TNF + IFN-γ. TNF, IFN-γ, and TNF + IFN-γ groups had significantly improved survival compared with controls at each day after bacterial challenge. (Courtesy of Hershman MJ, Pietsch JD, Trachtenberg L, et al: *Br J Surg* 76:1282–1286, 1989.)

test bacterium was *Klebsiella pneumoniae*. One model consisted of an intramuscular bacterial challenge and another involved use of a bacterium-laden thigh suture. The experiments were conducted with or without pretreatment with TNF, alone or in combination with IFN-γ therapy.

Mice pretreated with 7,500 units of TNF daily for 5 days survived significantly longer than controls. When TNF and IFN-γ were administered together as a pretreatment, survival was also significantly improved in the treatment group over the control group after bacterial challenge (Fig 6–1). Both methods of treatment also improved survival when initiated 1 hour after infection. Pretreatment with TNF before the suture challenge resulted in the survival of 11 mice; only 3 control animals survived. Quantitative bacterial counts revealed that the TNF-pretreated group consistently had significantly lower systemic blood borne counts than the control group.

Pretreatment with TNF at doses far below those inducing toxic effects afforded protection against bacterial infection in an animal model. A lesser degree of protection resulted when TNF was given after initiation of bacterial infection. Tumor necrosis factor was more potent than IFN-γ, and the latter resulted in no additive or synergistic effect.

▶ Cytokine manipulation of host defense is on the horizon. Several animal reports are suggestive that this approach will be clinically successful. Many reports require pretreatment, a nonfeasible approach clinically. However, this paper suggests that treatment with TNF-α may be successful after the infection-initiating event.—M.C. Robson, M.D.

7 Burns

Hospital and Prehospital Resources for Optimal Care of Patients With Burn Injury: Guidelines for Development and Operation of Burn Centers
American Burn Association
J Burn Rehabil 11:97–104, 1990   7–1

In the United States, burn injuries annually account for more than 500,000 hospital emergency department visits and approximately 70,000 acute inpatient admissions. Whereas most burn injuries are relatively minor with patients being discharged after outpatient treatment at the facility where they are first seen, about 20,000 patients sustain burn injuries requiring their transfer to special burn care centers. The requirements that institutions need to meet to qualify as a burn care center were reviewed. The burn care system is described and the documentation of policies and procedures, staffing needs and staff educational requirements, referral criteria, physical facilities, rehabilitation needs, and quality assurance procedures are listed.

▶ Standards remain something with which many do not wish to deal. However, they are becoming necessary and are best derived by the most knowledgeable professionals. The American Burn Association has provided these guidelines to describe the necessary resources to operate burn centers for optimal patient care. This document should be required reading for all who care for the thermally injured patient.—M.C. Robson, M.D.

Systemic Lipid Peroxidation and Inflammation Induced by Thermal Injury Persists Into the Post-Resuscitation Period
Demling RH, Lalonde C (Brigham and Women's Hosp, Boston; Beth Israel Hosp, Boston)
J Trauma 30:69–74, 1990   7–2

The oxidant-induced systemic lipid peroxidation that occurs in lung and systemic tissues early after burn injury may persist and contribute to hypermetabolism and organ dysfunction. To determine the time course of these initial postburn oxidant changes, lipid peroxidation was measured by circulating, as well as lung and liver tissue, lipid peroxides.

A third-degree burn injury covering 15% of total body surface was produced in 12 anesthetized adult sheep. Circulating lipid peroxides were monitored by malondialdehyde (MDA) and conjugated dienes (CD), verified markers of the peroxidation process, for 3–5 days.

Several hours after the burn there was a significant but transient increase in circulating MDA and CD. There was an increase in venous levels of plasma at 3–5 days post burn with the onset of wound inflammation. At 3 days post burn lung function, blood gases, and lung lymph flow remained at baseline. A 35% increase in oxygen consumption at 3 days was the result of both an increase in cardiac index and an increase in the extraction of oxygen from hemoglobin.

At 5 days lung function and lymph flow were similar to baseline values. Oxygen consumption remained significantly increased, as at 3 days, and venous CD and MDA were further increased. Although lung tissue MDA was not significantly greater than that in control animals, a significant mononuclear cell infiltration was still present in the lungs.

The systemic lipid peroxidation that occurs early after burns is also present at 3 days and 5 days post burn. The mechanism may involve activation of neutrophils via myeloperoxidase activity or from cells, in particular endothelium, with increased xanthine oxidase activity. Thus even a modest burn injury appears to lead to significant systemic oxidant release, which perhaps explains the organ dysfunction observed with an additional septic injury in burned patients.

▶ Lipid peroxidation with generation of oxidants and metabolites is now a well-recognized event following all trauma. Initially, it was believed to be a self-limited event occurring immediately after injury, but it is becoming apparent that the effects of lipid peroxidation may be prolonged. This experimental paper demonstrates that resuscitation alone, with restoration of tissue perfusion, does not abrogate lipid peroxidation and the effects of metabolites.—M.C. Robson, M.D.

Serum Cachectin/Tumor Necrosis Factor in Critically Ill Patients With Burns Correlates With Infection and Mortality

Marano MA, Fong Y, Moldawer LL, Wei H, Calvano SE, Tracey KJ, Barie PS, Manogue K, Cerami A, Shires GT, Lowry SF (New York Hosp-Cornell Med Ctr; Rockefeller Univ)
Surg Gynecol Obstet 170:32–38, 1990   7–3

In burn injuries there are major alterations in physiologic homeostasis during postburn and septic periods. These derangements include cellular dysfunction, cachexia, hypermetabolism, altered immune function, and hypercortisolemia. Cachectin-tumor necrosis factor (TNF) is among the cytokines identified as being produced during sepsis and may be the principal cytokine mediator of both acute and chronic sequelae of infection. Tumor necrosis factor is secreted by macrophages in response to endotoxin-lipopolysaccharide and other invasive stimuli. The frequency of detection of elevated serum levels of TNF during protracted critical burn injury is unknown.

Serial serum samples from 43 critically ill patients with burns were analyzed for TNF by using an enzyme-linked immunosorbent assay. The mean body surface area burned was 33%. Twenty-five patients had concomitant inhalation injury, and 16 patients had sepsis. Blood samples were also obtained from 21 healthy controls.

Serum TNF was present in 20 of 43 injured patients but in only 1 healthy control. At 1 or more time points, TNF was detectable in 69% of patients with sepsis, compared with 33% of injured patients without sepsis and in 71% of patients who died, but in only 31% of survivors.

Serum TNF is detectable with greater frequency and in higher concentrations in patients with sepsis and in those who ultimately die of burn injury. Serum TNF appears transiently and recurrently in the circulation during injury. Higher serum levels of cortisol are correlated with the absence of serum TNF during sepsis and fatal injury.

▶ Cytokines are definitely demonstrable in serum and tissue after trauma and during episodes of sepsis. What these levels mean is difficult to determine. Whether they are responsible for activity or the result of events is like the question of the chicken and the egg. What levels of TNF may be useful in immune defense and what levels are harmful are as yet unknown. Measuring levels in a series of patients as reported in this paper does not answer the questions. Until more specific information is known, these papers can only be read with interest.—M.C. Robson, M.D.

Total Energy Expenditure in Burned Children Using the Doubly Labeled Water Technique

Goran MI, Peters EJ, Herndon DN, Wolfe RR (Shriners Burns Inst, Galveston; Univ of Texas, Galveston)
Am J Physiol 259:E576–E585, 1990   7–4

Patients with burn injury experience elevated rates of resting energy expenditure (EE). Although nutritional therapies have been developed for burn patients, there are no universally accepted guidelines, partly because of limitations in methodologies used to estimate caloric requirements. An attempt was made to define the relationship between total EE and resting EE by using the doubly labeled water technique and indirect calorimetry to assess burned children.

Fifteen burned children were enrolled, but 5 studies were discarded because of potential errors. All patients were given standardized nutritional support. For the doubly labeled water protocol, a nude body weight was recorded and a baseline urine sample collected before isotope administration. Highly enriched $H_2^{18}O$ and ^2H_2O were administered intravenously in saline. For 7 days after isotope administration, daily urine samples were collected for analysis. Resting energy expenditure was measured at least every other day using a Beckman metabolic cart with face mask.

The total EE was 1.33 times the predicted basal EE. When the resting EE was measured simultaneously, the total EE was 1.18 times the resting EE. In turn, the resting was 1.6 times the predicted basal EE. The total EE was significantly correlated with measured resting EE but not with predicted basal EE.

These findings demonstrate that total EE in burned children is much lower than thought previously. Apparently, total EE in these children consists principally of resting EE. It is recommended that optimal predictions of total energy requirements be obtained by adjusting an individually measured rate of resting EE by a suitable activity factor, which in the case of convalescing burned children is 1.2.

▶ Stable isotope technology allows direct measurements of values previously indirectly calculated. The direct measurements reported here are less than previously predicted. This technology will allow surgeons to decrease the amount of nutrition supplied to critically injured patients. It also suggests that maintenance of body composition, and not just body weight, should be the indicator of successful nutritional therapy.— M.C. Robson, M.D.

Hypertonic Saline Dextran Resuscitation of Thermal Injury
Horton JW, White DJ, Baxter CR (Univ of Texas, Dallas)
Ann Surg 211:301–311, 1990   7–5

Thermal injury requires rapid crystalloid volume replacement. To restore cardiocirculatory function after thermal injury, administration of up to 14 L of isotonic crystalloid fluid during the first 48 hours may be required. Several studies have demonstrated impaired myocardial function after burn injury, which may be further exacerbated by the large volumes of crystalloid fluid. Small-volume hypertonic saline dextran (HSD) resuscitation is effective in the treatment of shock. To determine whether an initial bolus of HSD would prevent myocardial dysfunction after a major burn injury and decrease the subsequent volume of isotonic crystalloid resuscitation, 75 guinea pigs received third-degree scald burns comprising 45% of total body surface area using a template device; 25 animals that did not receive burns served as controls.

Of the 75 burned animals, 25 were not fluid resuscitated and served as untreated burn controls, 20 were resuscitated with lactated Ringer's (LR) solution for 24 hours, and the remaining 30 animals were treated with an initial bolus of HSD, followed by 1 mL, 2 mL, or 4 mL of LR per kg per percent burn. The animals were decapitated and the hearts rapidly removed and perfused. The effects of LR and HSD resuscitation were assessed in isolated coronary perfused hearts.

Cardiac function in animals were untreated burns was significantly impaired compared with findings in unburned controls. Hearts from burned animals treated with LR alone showed no significant improvement in cardiac function compared with hearts from untreated burn animals. However, hearts from burned animals treated with HSD plus LR had significantly improved cardiac function compared with hearts from untreated burn controls. At 24 hours after burn injury, the mortality was 29% for untreated burns, 0% for unburned controls, 0% for burned animals treated with HSD plus LR in volumes of 1 or 2 mL/kg per percent burn, and 17% for animals treated with HSD plus 4 mL/kg per percent-burn

LR. Further, HSD plus 1 mL/kg per percent burn LR was the optimal fluid therapy for maintaining normal cardiac function after burn injury. The enhanced cardiac contractile function after hypertonic resuscitation appeared to be related to an increase in cellular calcium in the myocardium. An initial HSD bolus prevents myocardial dysfunction after major burn injury and decreases the subsequent volume of isotonic crystalloid resuscitation.

▶ The important thing to realize about this preliminary experimental paper is that the senior author (Dr. Baxter) is the father of pure isotonic fluid resuscitation of burns. The fact that he and his co-authors now show that HSD resuscitation prevents myocardial dysfunction and decreases the amount of fluid resuscitation required is notable. We hope that they will be able to repeat these cardiac studies in humans and report to us an improvement on the "Parkland Formula."—M.C. Robson, M.D.

Early Burn Wound Excision Significantly Reduces Blood Loss
Desai MH, Herndon DN, Broemeling L, Barrow RE, Nichols RJ Jr, Rutan RL
(Univ of Texas, Galveston)
Ann Surg 211:753–762, 1990   7–6

Recent developments in the intraoperative monitoring of blood volume have improved mortality rates associated with early near-total burn wound excision compared with those reported after delayed excisional procedures. To determine whether children with large burn wounds can safely undergo early near-total burn wound excision during the resuscita-

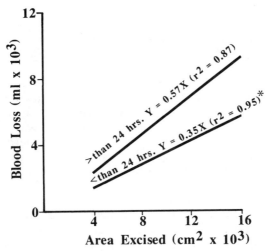

Fig 7–1.—Regression slopes and equations for patients with 30% or greater TBSA burn excised within 24 hours of injury (n = 15) and those excised after 24 hours (n = 299). *Asterisk* indicates significantly lower slope at $P < .001$. (Courtesy of Desai MH, Herndon DN, Broemeling L, et al: *Ann Surg* 211:753–762, 1990.)

tion period, studies were made in 1,662 children who were treated in 1982–1989 for acute burn injuries; 594 of these had cutaneous flame or scald burn injuries requiring excision and grafting.

All 594 children underwent near-total excison in a single procedure, including 318 with burns over more than 30% of the total body surface area (TBSA). Of the latter group, 15 underwent excision within the first 24 hours after injury, 262 had burn wound excision on postburn days 2–16, and 41 underwent excision more than 16 days after the burn injury.

There were no intraoperative deaths. Surgery took less than 3 hours in all patients. Blood loss in those with more than 30% TBSA was significantly less when surgical burn excision was performed either within the first 24 hours after burn injury or after postburn day 16 compared with that in patients operated on between days 2 and 16 after burn injury (Fig 7–1). The mortality rate after early excision was not increased when compared with rates at later burn excision times.

Children with large burn wounds can safely undergo near-total primary burn wound excision during the resuscitative phase after burn injury. Early excision results in less blood replacement without adversely affecting hemodynamic stability or mortality.

▶ Total burn excision within 24 hours is a goal that few have attempted. In adult patients the blood loss was exorbitant. However, these authors have demonstrated their success in achieving this goal in children. Blood loss was least when the excision was performed within the first 24 hours. In the patients having excision in the first 24 hours, the TBSA was 64% ± 6% and the survival rate was 93%. These figures speak for themselves to support the early excision technique.—M.C. Robson, M.D.

The Continuing Challenge of Burn Care in the Elderly
Saffle JR, Larson CM, Sullivan J, Shelby J (Univ of Utah)
Surgery 108:534–543, 1990   7–7

Recent advances in the treatment of burn injuries have resulted in greatly improved survival rates; however, problems remain, especially in the treatment of elderly burn patients. An attempt was made to determine the likelihood of survival of older patients with thermal injuries and to define the factors affecting survival. Also studied were the costs of care for these patients and the impact of treatment of elderly burn patients on available resources and public funding.

A review was made of the records of all patients at least 45 years old who had sustained acute thermal, chemical, or electrical burns between 1978 and 1987. Data collected included age, sex, cause and size of burns, numbers and types of preexisting medical problems, complications during care, volume of fluid required for resuscitation, surgical procedures performed, and outcome. Hospital billing records were reviewed to determine total charges for each patient's care.

There were 278 older burn patients treated during the 10-year period. Overall, the survival rate was 80%; for those older than age 75 years the survival rate was 67%. Mortality rates correlated with age, burn size, presence of inhalation injury, fluid resuscitation requirements, and number of complications of care. Mortality rates did not correlate with the number of preexisting medical problems. Burn wounds were often excised and treated with grafting; these procedures were well tolerated.

During the study period there was a fourfold increase in hospital charges. Daily charges for nonsurvivors were significantly greater than those for survivors, but nonsurvivors had a slightly shorter mean length of stay than survivors. Daily charges for those who died early did not differ significantly from daily charges for those who died later, but total charges for those who died late were more than twice the charges for survivors despite a similar length of stay. As patients aged, funding sources shifted from industrial and private insurance to Medicare-Medicaid programs. These latter programs accounted for 87% of funding in patients over the age of 75 years. Hospital charges exceeded diagnosis related group-based reimbursement by a mean of more than $18,000 per patient, for a total of more than $1.2 million. For patients with extensive burns, the mean loss per patient was more than $41,000.

Aggressive care for elderly burn patients would appear justified by the improved outcomes found in these patients. However, the high nonreimbursable cost of treatment poses a dilemma in terms of allotment of resources.

▶ The management of burns in the elderly has been the subject of many recent reports. Unfortunately, authors cannot agree on the definition. Certainly, age 45 cannot be considered elderly. Despite this problem the authors do report on 39 patients older than age 75. In these patients, they achieved a remarkable 67% survival rate, which is much better than that reported in other series. In this group of patients, the diagnosis related group reimbursement fell short by $18,000 per patient. As burn patient survival continues to increase, this financial burden is something with which society will have to deal.— M.C. Robson, M.D.

Tissue Expansion in the Correction of Burn Alopecia: Classification and Methods of Correction
McCauley RL, Oliphant JR, Robson MC (Shriners Burns Inst, Galveston, Texas)
Ann Plast Surg 25:103–115, 1990   7–8

Burn deformities of the head and neck are difficult to correct. The use of tissue expanders in the correction of burn alopecia has greatly facilitated treatment because the technique has virtually eliminated the need for complex staged operations. However, the technical approach currently is based on trial and error. A protocol and classification were developed for tissue expansion in the treatment of burn alopecia.

During a 4-year study period, 102 children aged 3–17 years (mean, 9

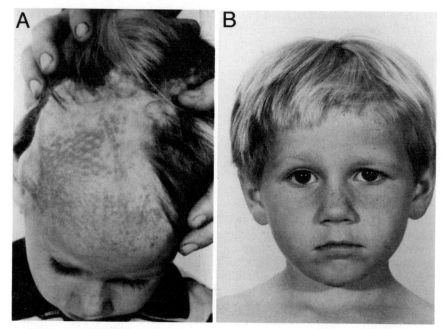

Fig 7–2.—**A,** preoperative view of a 5-year-old boy with type 1B burn alopecia. Full expansion with 2 tissue expanders totaling 950 mL was performed. **B,** postoperative appearance 6 months after wound closure. (Courtesy of McCauley RL, Oliphant JR, Robson MC: *Ann Plast Surg* 23:103–115, 1990.)

years) underwent tissue expansion. All procedures were performed with the use of general anesthesia. Forty-three patients had previously undergone partial excision or rotation of scalp flaps. A total of 222 tissue expanders were placed during 178 operations. Patterns of burn alopecia were classified as type I through type IV, reflecting primarily the depth of the injury. In this classification, type I represents uniform alopecia (Fig 7–2); type II, segmental alopecia; type III, patchy alopecia; and type IV, total alopecia. The extent of alopecia within each pattern is further stratified into subtypes A through D, reflecting the extent of the burn alopecia.

Seventeen patients (17%) required early expander removal because of exposure, infection, or traumatic extrusion, resulting in a loss of 24 (10.8%) of the expanders. At the time of the report, total coverage had been attained in 78 patients (76.5%). Treated areas in the remaining patients were still in various stages of expansion.

Reconstruction for patients with burn alopecia should be a well-thought-out, planned procedure. Proper classification of burn alopecia provides a basis for comparison and description and identifies those who are not candidates for tissue expansion. On the basis of the proposed classification, patients with type III and type IV alopecia are usually not suitable candidates.

▶ This paper represents the largest series of tissue expansions performed for burn alopecia and the first attempt to classify the patterns of alopecia. Classifying the patterns of burn alopecia allows division of cases into homogeneous subgroups so that indications, results, and complications can be refined.—M.C. Robson, M.D.

Intestinal Permeability Is Increased in Burn Patients Shortly After Injury
Deitch EA (Louisiana State Univ, Shreveport)
Br J Surg 77:587–592, 1990   7–9

Attention has been focused on the role of the gastrointestinal tract as a promotor or potentiator of organ dysfunction and sepsis in high-risk surgical patients. Data from Wilmore's laboratory have shown that a single dose of endotoxin increases intestinal permeability in healthy human volunteers. Another study found that intestinal permeability is increased in burn patients with sepsis.

To determine whether a major thermal injury is associated with increased intestinal permeability shortly after injury in the absence of infection, intestine permeability was measured within 24 hours of injury in 15 hemodynamically stable, aseptic patients with burns over more than 20% of their total body surface area. Two nonmetabolizable sugars, lactulose and mannitol, were used as permeability markers. Eight healthy volunteers served as controls.

Patients had increased intestinal absorption of lactulose, but not of mannitol, after thermal injury. The mean amount of lactulose excreted in the urine during 6-hour timed urine collection was almost 4 times greater in patients than in controls. Because absorption of mannitol is primarily transcellular and absorption of lactulose is paracellular, these findings suggest that only paracellular permeability is increased after thermal injury.

In this study intestinal permeability was increased within 24 hours after thermal injury in the absence of infection. Although others have found early elevations of plasma levels of endotoxin after burn injury, plasma levels of endotoxins in these patients were not significantly different from those in controls.

▶ Dr. Deitch has presented many elegant studies in experimental animals documenting bacterial translocation and elucidating its mechanism. In this study he conclusively demonstrates that this phenomenon occurs in man after uncomplicated thermal injury. The problem with the study is that the techniques require the patient to be in the fasting state. Early enteral feeding protects against bacterial translocation, but such feeding was prohibited by the methodology of the study. Therefore, an article that appears to provide an answer is not quite definitive.—M.C. Robson, M.D.

8 Transplantation

Renal Transplant Rejection: Transient Immunodominance of HLA Mismatches
Gilks WR, Gore SM, Bradley BA (Med Research Council, Cambridge; United Kingdom Transplant Service, Bristol, England)
Transplantation 50:141–146, 1990   8–1

Long-term benefit from HLA matching in renal transplantation has been confirmed. Rates of graft loss were evaluated in consecutive post-transplant intervals, using data from the United Kingdom Transplant Service; analysis included 3,991 first and 848 second cadaver kidney transplantations done in 1983–1987.

The long-term benefit of HLA matching was based on a reduction in graft failures within 5 months of transplantation. After that period, HLA-A, B, DR matching appeared to have little influence on rates of graft loss. The transition to lack of effect of HLA matching was fairly abrupt. Beneficial matching was most advantageous when 2 distinct DR antigens were distinguished.

Renal graft losses occurring more than 5 months after transplantation may be secondary to non-HLA targets. Alternatively, some HLA mismatches may be more immunopotent than others.

▶ Nearly 5,000 cadaver kidney transplant recipients were included in this study from England, and the results are quite interesting. Failure because of rejection in the first 5 months after transplant was half as great in patients with little or no HLA incompatibility (0 DR mismatch, no more than 1 A,B mismatch) as that in any other group. The powerful antigenic effect of HLA seems to make or break the graft early; late failures because of rejection may represent cumulative effects of other stimuli. To detect this effect it is important to use strict criteria, as was done here, to classify patients into good match categories.— O. Jonasson, M.D.

Evidence That Zero Antigen-Matched Cyclosporine-Treated Renal Transplant Recipients Have Graft Survival Equal to That of Matched Recipients: Reevaluation of Points
Greenstein SM, Schechner RS, Louis P, Senitzer D, Matas A, Veith FJ, Tellis VA (Montefiore Med Ctr/Albert Einstein College of Medicine, Bronx)
Transplantation 49:332–336, 1990   8–2

Controversy still surrounds the value of HLA matching in cadaver renal transplantation (CRT). It has been suggested that greater importance be given to HLA matching for the distribution of cadaver kidneys. How-

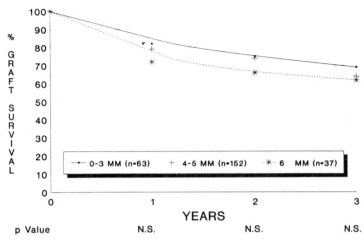

Fig 8−1.—Actuarial graft survival of adult cyclosporine-treated cadaver kidney recipients based upon mismatching. (Courtesy of Greenstein SM, Schechner RS, Louis P, et al: *Transplantation* 49:332– 336, 1900.)

ever, this policy would increase the delay and expense of CRT, increases that are justifiable only if results are significantly improved.

The results of CRT in 252 cyclosporine-treated adults undergoing transplantation between 1984 and 1989 were reviewed. Initially, kidneys were transplanted to cross-match-negative recipients on the basis of waiting time, regardless of match. At the end of 1987 a points system based on United Network for Organ Sharing (UNOS) criteria was implemented. Eighty-four patients with 0 antigen match with their donors were compared with 168 sharing 1−6 antigens. The cumulative life-table method was used to determine actuarial graft and patient survival (Fig 8−1). Better matching or mismatching had no significant effect on graft survival.

There is no significant difference in graft survival in cyclosporine-treated adult cadaver kidney recipients on the basis of matching, mismatching, or the UNOS point system, except for 6 antigen-matched kidneys. Therefore, a point system heavily weighted toward HLA matching should not be instituted in the United States. To do so is both unjustified and contrary to the principle of equal access for all.

▶ Patients in this series received transplants based on how long they had waited, not on HLA matching. It is no surprise then, that in this and other series in which this policy applies, very few patients have received HLA-matched organs. If more emphasis were placed on bringing well-matched (0 DR mismatches, no more than 1 A or B mismatch) organs to recipients, the group of matched recipients would be much larger and the data more convincing. It is a circular argument to say that, because the well-matched group is so small, the good results in this category can be ignored, especially as the poorly matched group of recipients are "doing well" (enough). Greenstein's group has lumped together up to 3 mismatches, including the important DR antigens, into the "good match" group. This is unacceptable, because we have much data showing that both DR and at least 3 of 4 A and B antigens must be matched to achieve behefit. In fact, the data in this study speak more for a change in the institution's policy toward selecting for matched organ than for abandonment of all matching attempts. After all, their 3-year graft survival was only 50% to 70%, whereas the well-matched recipients in England (see Abstract 8–1) had a 72% to 90% graft survival during the same period.— O. Jonasson, M.D.

The Transfusion Effect in Cadaver Kidney Transplants—Yes or No
Iwaki Y, Cecka JM, Terasaki PI (Univ of California, Los Angeles)
Transplantation 49:56–59, 1990   8–3

Blood transfusions are considered one of the strongest means of improving the outcome of renal transplantation, but many kidney recipients fail to receive transfusions. In a series of first cadaver kidney recipients followed for at least a year, graft survival rates were 71% for nontransfused patients at 1 year and 75% in those given a single transfusion. Two transfusions conferred a graft survival rate of 77%, and 3 or 4 transfusions a rate of 78%. Further transfusions did not improve the outcome. No transfusion effect was apparent in patients lacking HLA-DR mismatches, whereas transfusions improved the 1-year graft survival by 10% in those with 2 DR-mismatched grafts (Fig 8–2).

Two or 3 random transfusions probably are optimal before cadaver kidney transplantation. Patients are a relatively high risk of sensitization, such as multiparous women, may be matched for HLA-DR as an alterna-

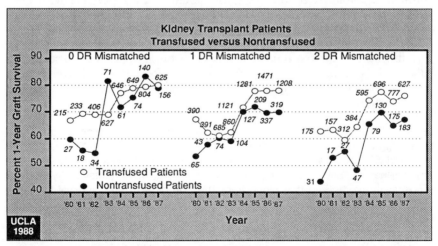

Fig 8–2.—The influence of HLA-DR matching on transfusion effect yearly since 1980. (Courtesy of Iwaki Y, Cecka JM, Terasaki PI: *Transplantation* 49:56–59, 1990.)

tive. Previously transfused patients may not require further transfusion before transplantation.

▶ There are many reasons to avoid blood transfusion in any patient, although with improved viral testing the risks are now minimal. Sensitization to HLA antigens occurs in a small number of heavily transfused patients, but the risk of sensitization is small with few transfusions. A clear benefit is demonstrated after transfusion of at least 2 units of blood to recipients of kidneys mismatched for at least 1 DR antigen, even if cyclosporine A is given. The transfusion effect is seen only in mismatched recipients (see Abstracts 8–4 and 8–5).—O. Jonasson, M.D.

Evidence That HLA Class II Disparity Is Required for the Induction of Renal Allograft Enhancement by Donor-Specific Blood Transfusions in Man
Lazda VA, Pollak R, Mozes MF, Barber PL, Jonasson O (Univ of Illinois, Chicago)
Transplantation 49:1084–1087, 1990   8–4

Many mechanisms that potentially underlie the efficacy of donor-specific transfusion in renal allograft recipients may require some degree of major histocompatibility complex mismatch. Forty-six living-related primary renal allograft recipients were matched for a single HLA haplotype but differed at various HLA loci on the unshared haplotype. Patients received 200 mL of donor-specific blood, either 3 times at 2-week intervals, or once 3–4 weeks before transplantation, along with oral azathioprine. Patients were followed for at least a year.

Incompatibility for class II determinants on the unshared haplotype promoted stable, rejection-free graft function. Of 7 patients with graft loss 6 were HLA class II compatible with the blood/kidney donor. Mismatching for HLA class I determinants did not influence the outcome.

Induction of tolerance by donor-specific transfusion appears to be grounded in factors within the major histocompatibility complex, particularly class II disparity. Improved HLA matching in cadaver kidney transplantation may help to explain the declining prominence of the "transfusion effect."

▶ It is the HLA-DR or class II antigens that appear to be most important in matching to achieve improvement in graft survival. In the preceding papers, recipients with no class II mismatch (and no more than 1 class I or HLA-A,B mismatch) had superior graft survival, without regard for transfusion. In Abstract 8–3, analysis showed that blood transfusion improved graft survival by nearly 10%, but only if there was a class II mismatch. In the present study, Lazda et al. found that donor-specific transfusions were effective only when the mismatched allele had an incompatible class II antigen. The transfusion effect thus appears to be an active immunologic event, initiated by a blood transfusion and carried over to the transplanted organ.—O. Jonasson, M.D.

Suppressed Antidonor MLC Responses in Renal Transplant Candidates Conditioned With Donor-Specific Transfusions That Carry the Recipient's Noninherited Maternal HLA Haplotype

Bean MA, Mickelson E, Yanagida J, Ishioka S, Brannen GE, Hansen JA (Virginia Mason Research Ctr and Clinic; Puget Sound Blood Ctr; Pacific Northwest Research Found, Seattle)
Transplantation 49:382–386, 1990   8–5

Renal graft survival is substantially improved in high-risk patients who are preconditioned with donor-specific blood transfusions. The mechanisms involved were examined in 47 patients with end-stage renal disease who received 3 whole-blood infusions of 250 mL every 2 weeks before transplantation. Fourteen patients became sensitized; 31 others received a transplant from the transfusion donor.

The 31 transplant recipients had an estimated 2-year graft survival rate of 97%, a 3-year rate of 88%, and a 4-year rate of 69%. Eleven recipients exhibited a reduced antidonor mixed lymphocyte cytotoxicity (MLC) response after completion of transfusion therapy. Deletion of CD8$^+$ lymphocytes from suppressed MLCs restored antidonor MLC reactivity in 4 of 6 instances. Decreased MLC reactivity after transfusions correlated with expression of noninherited maternal HLA antigens by cells of the transfusion donor.

Specific antidonor T suppressor cells appear as a result of donor-specific transfusion in renal transplant recipients. It may be that transplant recipients who are mismatched for 2 haplotypes but nevertheless have a good outcome are given grafts that express the noninherited maternal HLA haplotype to which the immune system was exposed in utero.

▶ One third of the recipients of donor-specific transfusions had marked decreases in in vitro proliferation of lymphocytes after exposure to donor's cells after transfusion (MLC response). Most of these were restored to normal by depleting the responding cells of the suppressor T cells (CD8$^+$). Of even more interest is the observation that it was usually the mismatched maternal, rather than paternal, haplotype involved in this response. Exposure of the fetus in utero to its noninherited maternal HLA antigens may make it tolerant to those antigens in later life.— O. Jonasson, M.D.

Analysis of the Donor-Specific Cytotoxic T Lymphocyte Repertoire in a Patient With a Long Term Surviving Allograft: Frequency, Specificity, and Phenotype of Donor-Reactive T Cell Receptor (TCR)-$\alpha\beta^+$ and TCR-$\gamma\delta^+$ Clones

Vandekerckhove BAE, Datema G, Koning F, Goulmy E, Persijn GG, Van Rood JJ, Claas FHJ, De Vries JE (Univ Hosp of Leiden, The Netherlands; UNICET Labs for Immunological Research, Dardilly, France)
J Immunol 144:1288–1294, 1990   8–6

The induction of transplantation tolerance in man is not well understood, although there is some evidence that a suppressor mechanism is involved. In-depth studies were conducted in a patient in apparent good health 9 years after she received a poorly HLA-matched renal graft. Cell-mediated lympholysis nonresponsiveness developed after transplantation.

A series of TCR-αβ$^+$ and TCR-γδ$^+$ clones specific for donor class I or class II antigen were isolated. Transplant-specific cytotoxic T lymphocytic (CTL) clones were generated in high frequency from T cell bulk cut lures activated by phytohemagglutinin in the absence of any sensitization by donor antigen in vitro. The patient did not generate specific cytolytic activity against donor-derived blasts in the mixed lymphocyte cytotoxicity test, using donor spleen cells or B lymphoblastoid cells as stimulators. Precursor frequencies of CTL against donor alloantigens were low.

Clones of CTI specific for donor HLA antigens were isolated in relatively high frequency from this patient. The CTL clones apparently are not operational in vivo, possibly because of ongoing immunosuppressive therapy. Alternatively, specific suppressor mechanisms not affecting normal immune responses may explain the absence of transplant-specific activity in vivo.

▶ More information about rejection may be found in patients with successful grafts than in those whose grafts have failed. In this study clones of T cells with cytolytic potential against the graft were found but seemed not to be operational. Because all other cell-mediated responses were normal, the authors suggest that donor-specific suppressor activity may be present. Rejection results when this activity is absent.— O. Jonasson M.D.

Induction of Antibody-Dependent Cellular Cytotoxicity Against Endothelial Cells by Renal Transplantation

Miltenburg AMM, Meijer-Paape ME, Weening JJ, Daha MR, van Es LA, van der Woude FJ (Univ Hosp of Leiden, The Netherlands)
Transplantation 48:681–688, 1989   8–7

Endothelial cells are the most accessible target for graft injury, because they form the primary interface between a vascularized organ graft and its recipient circulation. Antibodies reactive with endothelial cells of umbilical veins are present in renal transplant recipients, and their presence correlates with clinical rejection. Severe rejection developed in a patient with extensive lymphocytic infiltration of vessel walls after she received an HLA-identical family transplant.

Antibody-inducing antibody-dependent cellular cytotoxicity (ADCC) of umbilical vein endothelial cells were detected using the patient's serum. No such reactivity was found before transplantation. Studies using endothelial cells from various donors confirmed the specificity of the antibody. Sera from 2 of 9 other renal transplant recipients were positive in the ADCC assay; 20 normal serum donors were negative. Antibody-dependent cellular cytotoxicity was not secondary to classic antiendothelialmonocyte antibodies. Endothelial cell lysis was shown to be caused by natural killer/killer (NK/K) cells present in the peripheral blood mononuclear cell population.

Renal allotransplantation can induce IgG1 antibodies directed against non-HLA antigens on endothelial cells. These antibodies can, by interacting with NK/K cells, be responsible for ADCC against endothelial cells. The antibodies may activate Fc receptor-positive lymphocytes infiltrating the renal graft.

▶ Early and severe vascular rejections that occur even when HLA-identical donors are involved seem to be related to donor endothelial cell antigen–recipient antibody reactions. This study documents that the damage is done by recipient's NK cells, which are not specifically immunologically targeted to the endothelial cells but, rather, are fixed to the cells by the Fc portion of antibody. The antibody is directed specifically not against traditional transplant antigens but against an endothelial cell antigen system. The importance of this type of vascular rejection event is not entirely clear, and it is infrequent.—O. Jonasson, M.D.

Characterization of High Endothelial-Like Properties of Peritubular Capillary Endothelium During Acute Renal Allograft Rejection
Renkonen R, Turunen JP, Rapola J, Häyry P (Univ of Helsinki)
Am J Pathol 137:643–651, 1990   8–8

It has been suggested that lymphocytes enter rejecting renal allografts via the peritubular, but not other capillary, endothelium. This has been confirmed using a frozen section ex vivo binding assay. Cells present during acute renal allograft rejection in rats were characterized by immunofluorescence staining and by light and electron microscopy.

Increased lymphocyte binding to peritubular capillaries preceded peak leukocyte accumulation in the graft. Pretreatment of lymphocytes against CD11a and CD18 (LFA-1α and β chains) reduced lymphocyte binding, but ICAM-1 pretreatment was ineffective. Marked activation of peritubular capillary endothelial cells was noted in the allografts but not in syngeneic controls or normal kidneys. An antibody that stains rat lymph node high endothelial venules failed to react with peritubular capillaries of the allograft.

The peritubular capillaries become morphologically and functionally similar to lymph node high endothelial venules during acute renal allograft rejection in the rat. The phenomenon appears to be locally induced and organ specific. A new immunosuppressive approach may lie in blocking the entry of white blood cells into the allograft at the level of the microvascular endothelium.

▶ The endothelial cells of the vascular structures of an organ allograft are the first site of donor and host interaction. Lymphocyte attachment and penetration of venules has been localized to peritubular capillaries. The endothelial cells of the capillaries develop an appearance much like the high, plump endothelial cells of the postcapillary venules of lymph nodes where recirculating lymphocytes enter the node. The attachment of lymphocytes to the high endothelium is the first event in rejection, thus agents that block lymphocyte binding to high endothelial cells may be useful in preventing the lymphocyte invasion characteristic of rejection.—O. Jonasson, M.D.

Accelerated Arteriosclerosis in Heart Transplant Recipients Is Associated With a T-Lymphocyte–Mediated Endothelialitis
Hruban RH, Beschorner WE, Baumgartner WA, Augustine SM, Ren H, Reitz BA, Hutchins GM (Johns Hopkins Med Inst)
Am J Pathol 137:871–882, 1990   8–9

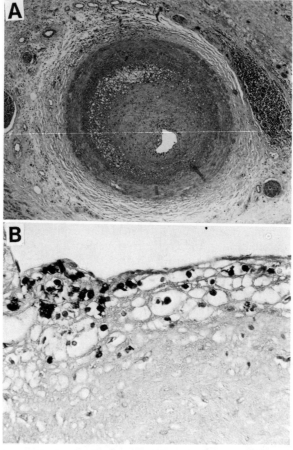

Fig 8–3.—The accelerated arteriosclerosis in this heart transplant case was characterized by a concentric luminal narrowing (**A**). Intimal thickening was associated with a T lymphocyte endothelialitis (**B**). **A:** hematoxylin and eosin; original magnification, ×60. **B:** immunohistochemical staining for CD45RO; original magnification, ×400. (Courtesy of Hruban RH, Beschorner WE, Baumgartner WA, et al: *Am J Pathol* 137:871–882, 1990.)

Graft arteriosclerosis can occur in pediatric and adult heart transplant recipients as soon as 3 months after transplantation. Its pathogenesis is not clearly understood. Arteriosclerotic lesions in 2 surgically explanted hearts and 23 transplants obtained at autopsy were examined immuno-histochemically. Of 117 patients given 119 heart transplants in 1983–1990, 32 died and 24 were autopsied.

Marked endothelialitis was seen in the coronary arteries of the 2 explanted hearts. Both patients had marked transplant-related accelerated arteriosclerosis. In all, 10 of 11 recipients with accelerated arteriosclerosis and 3 of the other 14 had moderate to marked lymphocytic endothelialitis (Fig 8–3). Most lymphocytes in the subendothelial space of affected vessels were T cells. Macrophages accumulated in conjunction with the infiltrate, and smooth muscle cells proliferated in the vascular intima. Analysis in 1 case showed the T cells to be chiefly cytotoxic T lymphocytes. Thrombosis was present in 3 cases in association with lymphocytic endothelialitis. The accelerated arteriosclerosis seen in some heart transplant recipients may represent, in part, a cytotoxic T lymphocyte-directed endothelialitis that is a manifestation of rejection.

Major Histocompatibility Complex Antigen Expression on Parenchymal Cells of Thyroid Allografts Is Not by Itself Sufficient to Induce Rejection
La Rosa FG, Talmage DW (Univ of Colorado)
Transplantation 49:605–609, 1990   8–10

Organ culture in hyperbaric oxygen may be effective in removing passenger leukocytes and eliminating tissue antigenicity. To determine whether hyperexpression of allo-major histocompatibility complex (MHC) antigens on the parenchymal cells of transplanted tissue can enhance rejection, fresh H-2^d mouse thyroid lobes were cultured in oxygen and normal atmospheric pressure, representing a suboptimal culture, and grafted into H-2^b mice. In some of these tissues, culture was done with recombinant mouse γ-interferon; before grafting, these tissues had high antigen levels.

After 3 weeks no difference was noted between the rejection rates of MHC-induced grafts and uninduced tissues—50% in each group. When fresh, uncultured grafts were placed, all were rejected within less than 2 weeks. Also grafted into normal H-2^b mice were H-2^d thyroids that were freed of donor leukocytes by preculture in hyperbaric oxygen and more than 1 year parking in normal H-2^b recipients and incubated with or without recombinant mouse γ-interferon. In both groups there was 100% acceptance, regardless of the expression of allo-MHC molecules on thyroid cells.

Grafts with a single antigenic difference at the MHC locus were inserted in a second series of experiments. Only when the recipients were immunized with donor spleen cells and fresh tissues were implanted did rejection occur. Generally, rejection did not occur in the same immune recipients when cultured and MHC-induced thyroids were grafted in the opposite kidney.

By itself, expression of allo-MHC molecules on graft cells appears to be insufficient to engender tissue immunogenicity. This finding supports the hypothesis that tissue culture's main effect is to inactivate passenger leukocytes. Only when they are properly presented by these cells do MHC antigens appear to be immunogenic.

▶ Even hyperexpression of transplant antigens on parenchymal cells of an allograft is insufficient to initiate rejection. Equally interesting is the finding that dendritic cells, the passanger cells thought to be essential for presenting antigen to the host, must be assisted by other factors, presumably cytokines, to be effective. These were clever experiments in which allografts were manipulated in several ways to affect the passenger cell population. Again, the critical importance of functional passenger cells in initiating rejection, was demonstrated.—O. Jonasson, M.D.

Induction of Donor-Specific Unresponsiveness by Intrathymic Islet Transplantation

Posselt AM, Barker CF, Tomaszewski JE, Markmann JF, Choti MA, Naji A (Univ of Pennsylvania)
Science 249:1293–1295, 1990   8–11

The most specific therapy for insulin-dependent diabetes mellitus is isolated pancreatic islet transplantation; however, its applicability is hampered by the vulnerability of allografts to immunologic rejection. To assess whether the thymus might be an immunologically privileged site, islets were taken from rat donors and transplanted into major histocompatibility complex incompatible rats in which diabetes had been induced. Islets were inoculated into conventional transplant sites; into the testicle, which is known to be a privileged site; and into the thymus. Some islets were fresh and others were cultured before transplantation. Some recipients had a single injection of rabbit antiserum to rat lymphocytes.

All islet allografts into the thymus in recipients who received antilymphocyte serum survived indefinitely. Survival of a second donor strain islet allograft was permitted by a state of donor-specific unresponsiveness. This state may have been induced by maturation of T cell precursors in a thymic microenvironment that was harboring foreign alloantigen.

Pancreatic islet allografts transplanted into the thymus survive indefinitely and can induce donor-specific unresponsiveness. This model may offer a method for successful pancreatic islet transplantation and information on the development of tolerance.

▶ These are elegant experiments. By giving a dose of antilymphocyte serum at the time of transplantation of islet cells into the thymus, peripheral mature circulating T cells are depleted and prothymocyte traffic to the thymus is increased. The new T cells matured in the thymus in the presence of the allografted pancreatic islet cells and were tolerant. Even a new dose of islet cells from the original donor strain implanted in an ordinary site was protected. Extension of this work to large adult animals is eagerly awaited.—O. Jonasson, M.D.

Causes of Graft Loss Beyond Two Years in the Cyclosporine Era
Dunn J, Golden D, Van Buren CT, Lewis RM, Lawen J, Kahan BD (Univ of Texas, Houston)
Transplantation 49:349–353, 1990   8–12

Two-year renal transplant survival has improved since cyclosporine A (CsA) came into use in preference to azathioprine (Aza). However, one study found no difference in long-term graft survival between patients treated with CsA-prednisolone and those treated with Aza-prednisolone. Long-term graft survival rates in 343 patients treated with CsA at a single center were investigated, including the causes of graft loss. All had received renal transplants over a 6-year period, and the grafts had functioned for at least 2 years. Almost all patients had CsA-prednisolone immunosuppression.

The 6-year primary and cadaveric graft survival rate was 59%, and the graft half-life, 10 years. This result was better than the 40% survival rate and 7.7-year half-life in primary cadaveric kidney recipients treated with Aza-prednisolone in the multicenter study of Terasaki et al. in 1987; it was also better than the 41% survival and 5.5-year half-life reported in a multicenter study. Primary living related donor (LRD) grafts had a 6-year survival of 77% and a half-life of 23.4 years, which was close to that of HLA-identical LRD grafts in patients treated with Aza. Cyclosporine A was thought to mitigate the effects of HLA incompatibility to reduce graft survival.

After 2 years, chronic rejection caused 36.2% of graft losses and noncompliance, 27.6% (table). Of 58 patients with graft loss, 13 died, most of cardiovascular diseases. Two patients died of sepsis and 1 of viral hepatitis; these were the only deaths that could be attributed to CsA immu-

Causes of Graft Loss Beyond 2 Years in 343 Renal Transplant Recipients

Cause	N	Percent
Chronic rejection	21	36.2
Noncompliance	16	27.6
Death[a]	13	22.4
Acute rejection	6	10.3
Congestive heart failure	1	1.7
Recurrent of original disease	1	1.7

[a]Causes of death included myocardial infarction (4), liver failure (2), stroke (2), sepsis (2), ruptured abdominal aortic aneurysm (1), complications secondary to AIDS (1) and suicide (1).
(Courtesy of Dunn J, Golden D, Van Buren CT, et al: *Transplantation* 49:349–353, 1990.)

nosuppression. During continuous CsA therapy, acute rejection caused 8.6% of graft losses. A higher proportion of retransplant patients were in the graft-loss group than in the graft-survival group; previous transplantation seemed to carry a higher risk of long-term as well as acute rejection. Patients undergoing a second transplantation were significantly less prone to graft loss because of noncompliance; male patients were significantly more noncompliant.

Better long-term primary cadaveric renal graft survival is reported in patients who receive CsA-prednisolone than in those who receive Aza-prednisolone. After 2 years the major causes of graft loss are chronic rejection, noncompliance, and retransplantation. The improved results in single-center studies may be explained by increased experience with the use of CsA-prednisolone.

▶ Late graft losses of nearly 20% during a 5–10 year period diminish the effectiveness of organ transplantation. Although approximately 20% of the loss is attributable to the patient's death, predominantly from cardiovascular events, nearly two thirds of late losses are caused by rejection. Regrettably, almost half of this is because of noncompliance with the immunosuppressive regimen. Establishment of specific unresponsiveness (tolerance) of the allograft without the need for long-term immunosuppression, such as was achieved in rodents by the intrathymic inoculation of islet cells cited in Abstract 8–11, is the ultimate goal in organ transplantation.— O. Jonasson, M.D.

Results of Single-Lung Transplantation for Bilateral Pulmonary Fibrosis

Grossman RF, Frost A, Zamel N, Patterson GA, Cooper JD, Myron PR, Dear CL, Maurer J, and the Toronto Lung Transplant Group (Toronto Gen Hosp; Mt. Sinai: Hosp, Toronto)
N Engl J Med 322:727–733, 1990   8–13

Single-lung transplantation may be useful in patients with severe pulmonary fibrosis. During a 6-year period, single-lung transplantation was done in 20 patients with end-stage pulmonary fibrosis, evidenced by progressive interstitial lung disease with relentless deterioration and increasing oxygen requirements despite corticosteroid therapy. All were younger than 60 years. Patients were weaned from steroids, had adequate nutrition, were ambulatory and motivated, had no major psychiatric or drug abuse problem, and had adequate psychosocial support. Four patients died in the perioperative period, 3 died of chronic rejection complications, 1 of Epstein-Barr virus lymphoma, and 1 of viral pneumonia.

Nine patients survived for more than 1 year. Preoperatively, the mean vital capacity was 43%; it increased to 65% of predicted after 3 months and then stabilized, reaching 69% after 12 months. There was an increase in relative perfusion to the transplanted lung from 63% within 3 days after surgery to 73% after 1 month. Perfusion in the transplanted

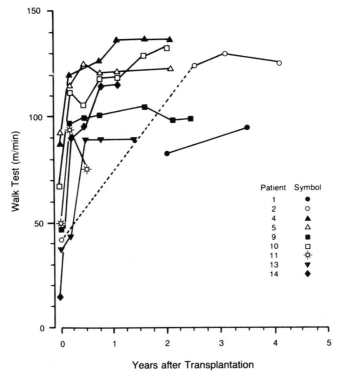

Years after Transplantation

Fig 8–4.—Results of the 6-minute walk test. Patient 1 was not tested before surgery. Rapid improvement in exercise tolerance was apparent within 3–6 months, and tolerance stabilized thereafter. In patient 11 exercise tolerance declined in conjunction with the appearance of chronic rejection. (Courtesy of Grossman RF, Frost A, Zamel N, et al: *N Engl J Med* 322:727–733, 1990.)

lung was either stable or progressively increased in all 9 patients; final measurements ranged from 76% to 99%. Rapid improvement in exercise tolerance occurred for a few months after surgery and then became relatively stable (Fig 8–4). The forced expiratory volume in 1 second, diffusing capacity for carbon monoxide, and arterial oxygen tension all improved, and no patient needed supplemental oxygen.

Single-lung transplantation is effective in carefully selected patients with end-stage pulmonary fibrosis. Results compare favorably to those of heart-lung transplantation. Improved organ preservation, rapid diagnosis of rejection, and a larger donor pool are needed.

► Although 20% of this group of 20 patients died in the perioperative period (of complications related to the donor and recipient procedures), only one third of the survivors failed to achieve long-term benefit. Especially in recipients who are not infected, single-lung transplantation has provided an excellent quality of life and deserves wider application.—O. Jonasson, M.D.

Heart-Lung Transplantation for Cystic Fibrosis and Subsequent Domino Heart Transplantation

Yacoub MH, Banner NR, Khaghani A, Fitzgerald M, Madden B, Tsang V, Radley-Smith R, Hodson M

J Heart Transplant 9:459–467, 1990
8–14

One feature of cystic fibrosis includes recurrent pulmonary infections that lead to progressive deterioration in respiratory function. Twenty-seven patients received combined heart-lung transplantation for end-stage respiratory disease. Survival was 78% after 1 year and 72% at 2 years. Bacterial respiratory infections were frequent shortly after surgery. More cyclosporine was needed than in other transplant recipients. Lung function improved greatly, and survivors had an excellent quality of life. Lymphoproliferative disease developed in 2 patients but resolved after immunosuppressive therapy was reduced. Two patients required retransplantation, 1 because of obliterative bronchiolitis and the other because of respiratory failure after recurrent infections related to tracheal stenosis. A modified technique permitted subsequent ("domino") heart transplantation in 20 instances. These recipients had a survival rate of 75% at 1 year. At 1 year, in none of the 12 patients was coronary artery disease observed on angiography.

Heart-lung transplantation has yielded very encouraging clinical results in patients with end-stage respiratory disease caused by cystic fibrosis. Nevertheless, improvement may be less marked than in patients with other parenchymal lung disorders because of the effects of repeated respiratory infections.

▶ The patients are infected and require bilateral pneumonectomy. Although others have successfully applied double-lung transplants, Yacoub et al. elected instead to use the recipient's good heart for another recipient and to transplant heart and lungs en bloc. Surprisingly good results were achieved in both groups, but the difficulties of cyclosporine administration and absorption were evident in that the domino group seemed to be overimmunosuppressed—a troublesome incidence of Epstein-Barr-virus–related lymphoproliferative disorders were seen. Although gene therapy for cystic fibrosis seems to be at hand, there are many patients now living with this disease who may benefit from transplantation as they reach adulthood and a terminal stage.—O. Jonasson, M.D.

Application of Reduced-Size Liver Transplants as Split Grafts, Auxiliary Orthotopic Grafts, and Living Related Segmental Transplants

Broelsch CE, Emond JC, Whitington PF, Thistlethwaite JR, Baker AL, Lichtor JL (Univ of Chicago)

Ann Surg 212:368–377, 1990
8–15

Apart from a limited supply of pediatric liver donors, the need for sufficiently small grafts is an important problem. Use of a liver lobe as a graft could overcome size disparity and shift available organs from older

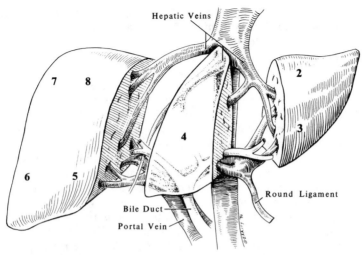

Fig 8–5.—Simplified schema of the intrahepatic anatomy is depicted (For clarity, the arterial structures have been omitted.) Most important is the location of the junction of the bile ducts to segments *2*, *3*, and *4*. If the liver is transected to the left of the round ligament, 2 separate biliary orifices (segments *2* and *3*) will be encountered. This has technical implications for both split-liver transplantation and transplantation using a living related donor. (Courtesy of Broelsch CE, Emond JC, Whitington PF, et al: *Ann Surg* 212:368–377, 1990.)

donors to younger recipients. Between 1986 and 1990, 26 reduced-size liver transplant procedures were performed. In addition, 25 children and 5 adults underwent split-liver transplantation using the technique shown in Figure 8–5. An additional 5 patients received a transplant from a living related donor, and 1 patient underwent orthotopic auxiliary liver grafting. Sixty-two percent of all pediatric transplant procedures involved the use of a liver lobe as a graft.

Split-liver transplantation is associated with the highest mortality and complication rates. Living related liver transplantation also has caused complications, both in donors and recipients, but all patients have survived. Orthotopic auxiliary liver transplantation was effective in a patient with ornithine transcarbamylase deficiency. The overall results are comparable to those achieved using full-size grafts. Pretransplantation mortality has been lower than 2%. Reduced-size liver transplants of various types are more complex and produce more complications, but global mortality is lowered in children with end-stage liver disease.

▶ Both Broelsch and Bismuth successfully pioneered the precise anatomical techniques that make it possible to transplant a large liver to a small patient. Broelsch has pointed out that at the age and size when pediatric recipients most need liver transplantation, the accidental or sudden death rate of children is lowest and the donor pool smallest. Extending this technique to parental donors for small children is highly controversial, but this group has done their homework and have embarked on the procedure with appropriate safeguards and caution.—O. Jonasson, M.D.

Optimal Therapy for Patients With Biliary Atresia: Portoenterostomy ("Kasai" Procedures) Versus Primary Transplantation

Wood RP, Langnas AN, Stratta RJ, Pillen TJ, WIlliams L, Lindsay S, Meiergerd D, Shaw BW Jr (Univ of Nebraska)
J Pediatr Surg 25:153–162, 1990   8–16

The relative merits of portoenterostomy and liver transplantation in infants with biliary atresia remain uncertain, as does the effect of portoenterostomy on a subsequent transplant procedure. The results of transplantation in 48 children with biliary atresia were compared with those obtained in 35 children given transplants for other liver diseases, including metabolic disorders, neonatal hepatitis, and acute liver failure.

Preoperative laboratory values were comparable in the 2 groups, and there were no differences in operating time. The survival rate was significantly greater in patients with biliary atresia, but there were no differences in hospital time or rate of retransplantation. Reoperation for bowel complications was equally frequent in the 2 groups. The posttransplantation course generally was less smooth in patients who had a stoma made as part of their portoenterostomy surgery.

Portoenterostomy is the preferred primary treatment for jaundiced infants with biliary atresia who have favorable characteristics. If obvious cirrhosis, portal hypertension, or unfavorable histologic findings are present, the chances of achieving adequate biliary decompression are very low and referral for transplantation is appropriate. Because most patients eventually undergo transplantation, a stoma is best avoided.

▶ Although the Kasai portoenterostomy is successful in some patients, most infants with biliary atresia are not cured and their disease progresses to end-stage biliary cirrhosis. The intent is to reserve transplantation for those in whom portoenterostomy is certain to fail and to avoid compromising their chances with repeated right upper quadrant operations. This seems to make good sense.— O. Jonasson, M.D.

Liver Transplantation in Patients With Alcoholic Cirrhosis: Selection Criteria and Rates of Survival and Relapse

Bird GLA, O'Grady JG, Harvey FAH, Calne RY, Williams R (King's College Hosp, London; King's College School of Medicine and Dentistry; Addenbrooke's Hosp, Cambridge, England)
Br Med J 301:15–17, 1990   8–17

A 9-year retrospective study was done to assess the outcome of liver transplantation in patients with alcoholic cirrhosis. In 3 women and 21 men with alcoholic cirrhosis who received liver transplants, the main outcome measures were survival, rehabilitation, and clinical and laboratory signs of a return to harmful drinking after surgery. Of the 24 patients, 15 were selected to undergo liver transplantation because of repeated admission for complications of advanced portal hypertension despite abstinence; 6 were selected because they had hepatocellular carcinoma superimposed on alcoholic cirrhosis, and 3 were given transplants but were not abstinent.

Sixty-six percent of the patients were still alive at 1 year. Of the 18 patients, 17 who survived for at least 3 months were rehabilitated. Laboratory and histologic assessment of the liver suggested a return to drinking, although they denied it, in 3 patients who were not abstinent before transplantation.

The survival and rehabilitation of patients receiving transplants for alcoholic cirrhosis compare favorably with the outcome in transplant recipients with cirrhosis of other causes. The criteria for selecting transplant recipients with alcoholic cirrhosis should include recurrent complications related to severe portal hypertension despite maximal medical treatment and a minimum 6 months' abstinence.

▶ Liver transplantation for alcoholic cirrhosis is highly controversial, mainly because the number of patients with end-stage alcoholic liver disease is vastly larger than any other group. Donor organs, already in short supply, would go to the alcoholic liver disease population in overwhelming numbers, and the issue of fairness can be raised, especially because small children with biliary atresia who now have access to a reduced-size liver (and who have the best long-term success rates) would again face restricted access to a donor organ. Those who favor offering liver transplants to patients with alcoholic cirrhosis point out that a 6-month trial of abstinence before eligibility is arbitrary and unnecessary because other psychological indicators appear to be accurate predictors of future abstinence. At present, the number of patients receiving transplants for alcoholic liver disease is steadily increasing. Long-term follow-up is not yet available.— O. Jonasson, M.D.

Hepatocyte Transplantation for the Low-Density Lipoprotein Receptor-Deficient State: A Study in the Watanabe Rabbit

Wiederkehr JC, Kondos GT, Pollak R (Univ of Illinois, Chicago)
Transplantation 50:466–471, 1990   8–18

The Watanabe heritable hyperlipidemic (WHHL) rabbit simulates human familial hypercholesterolemia because of a congenital deficiency of low-density lipoprotein (LDL) receptor. Affected animals have increased serum levels of LDL cholesterol and early atherosclerosis.

Isolated normal hepatocytes were transplanted into WHHL rabbits to augment the number of LDL receptors and thereby lower the serum level of LDL cholesterol level. Pure hepatocyte preparations were derived from the collagenase-digested liver. Both hepatocytes and nonparenchymal cells were incubated with fluorescein-labeled monoclonal antirabbit class I, anti-class II, and anti-T cell antibodies. The cells also served as stimulators in one-way mixed lymphocyte-hepatocyte cultures before and after exposure to ultraviolet light B. Allogeneic hepatocytes were injected intraportally and intrasplenically in homozygous WHHL rabbits. For intraperitoneal injection, hepatocytes were attached to collagen-coated dextran microcarriers. Recipients were given a single dose of cyclosporine.

No marked changes in lipid profiles followed either the intrasplenic or intraportal injection of hepatocytes, but intraperitoneal injections significantly lowered serum LDL cholesterol levels to 50% to 60% of baseline for 3–4 weeks. Total serum cholesterol levels changed similarly, but serum triglyceride, high-density lipoprotein cholesterol, and very-low-density lipoprotein cholesterol levels did not change significantly. Ongoing studies will show whether WHHL rabbits given hepatocytes by transplantation are less apt to have atherosclerosis.

▶ This is a clever approach to replacing a genetic deficiency in lipid metabolism. Starzl's group has performed whole-organ transplantation for this particular disorder in several patients. Although single-cell transplants are highly susceptible to rejection, if modification of the cells and immunosuppression can be applied successfully—as in these studies in Watanabe rabbits—it appears that this serious congenital disorder of LDL receptor deficiency could be repaired.— O. Jonasson, M.D.

Prevention of Acute Graft Rejection by the Prostaglandin E₁ Analogue Misoprostol in Renal-Transplant Recipients Treated With Cyclosporine and Prednisone

Moran M, Mozes MF, Maddux MS, Veremis S, Bartkus C, Ketel B, Pollak R, Wallemark C, Jonasson O (Univ of Illinois, Chicago; GD Searle and Co, Skokie, Ill)

N Engl J Med 322:1183–1188, 1990   8–19

Prostaglandins of the E series have immunosuppressive effects. It was hypothesized that prophylactic treatment with misoprostol, a prostaglandin E₁ analogue, would improve renal function and reduce graft rejection in recipients of renal allografts. In a randomized, double-blind, placebo-controlled trial, 77 renal allograft recipients received standard immunosuppression with cyclosporine and prednisone; 38 of the 77 patients received misoprostol, 200 μg, 4 times daily by mouth and 39 received placebo for the first 12 weeks after transplantation. All patients were observed for an additional 4 weeks after misoprostol or placebo was discontinued.

Serum creatinine concentrations were significantly lower and creatinine clearances were significantly higher in patients given misoprostol, compared with the placebo group. Furthermore, the incidence of acute graft rejection was significantly reduced in the misoprostol group (Fig 8–6). This reduced incidence of acute graft rejection was not related to cyclosporine blood levels, although cyclosporine blood levels and the incidence of acute nephrotoxicity caused by cyclosporine tended to be higher in the misoprostol group. Infectious complications were fewer in the misoprostol group, and there was less need for rehospitalization.

The data indicate that the prostaglandin E₁ analogue misoprostol sig-

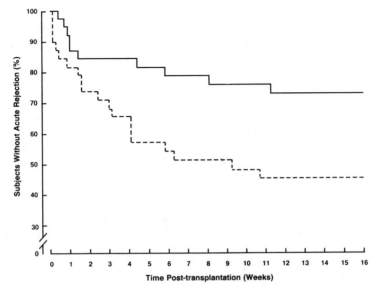

Fig 8–6.—Kaplan-Meier survival curve (time to first event) for acute graft rejection. Treatment with misoprostol is associated with a significant reduction in acute rejection ($P = .02$ by log-rank test). (Courtesy of Moran M, Mozes MF, Maddux MS, et al: *N Engl J Med* 322:1183–1188, 1990.)

nificantly improves renal function in recipients of renal allografts. Furthermore, it reduces the incidence of acute graft rejection in recipients treated with cyclosporine and prednisone without increasing the risk of posttransplantation complications.

▶ Prostaglandins of the E series are clearly potent adjuncts to conventional immunosuppression and appear to exert this effect without added risk. Although the original premise of this study was that prostaglandin E_1 might alleviate cyclosporine nephrotoxicity, this was not the case. The striking reduction in rejection activity was independent of cyclosporine levels.—O. Jonasson, M.D.

Prolonged Survival of Nonhuman Primate Renal Allograft Recipients Treated Only With Anti-CD4 Monoclonal Antibody
Cosimi AB, Delmonico FL, Wright JK, Wee S-L, Preffer FI, Jolliffe LK, Colvin RB (Massachusetts Gen Hosp, Boston; Ortho Pharmaceutical Corp, Raritan, NJ)
Surgery 108:406–414, 1990   8–20

The CD4 lymphocyte population may play a major role in allograft rejection. The immunosuppressive effectiveness of OKT4A reactive with human and monkey CD4 cells was evaluated in cynomolgus monkeys who underwent heterotopic renal transplantation. Recipient-donor pairs were selected for classes I and II histocompatibility antigen mismatching. Ten recipients received intact monoclonal antibodies and 2 received F(ab')2 fragments; dosage was .1–.3 mg/kg/day for 12 days. Five animals received OKT4A, 10 mg/kg, on the day of transplantation as their only immunosuppressive treatment. Controls were 4 animals that had either no treatment or treatment with OKT3 monoclonal antibody, which was nonreactive with monkey cells.

Controls and animals who received F(ab')2 survived for a maximum of 11 days. In animals that received low-dose OKT4A, the mean survival was 25.4 days, compared to 39 days for animals that received high-dose OKT4A. Immunologic monitoring showed "coating" and CD4 modulation in all OKT4A recipients. Recipients of F(ab')2 showed no modulation. At biopsy nearly complete reduction in lymphocyte infiltration was seen in animals treated with high-dose OKT4A. Those that received low-dose OKT4A showed regular generation of donor-reactive cytotoxic T cell lines during periods of stable function; high-dose OKT4A recipients did not have this finding. An immunoglobulin G antimurine humoral response developed in all animals that received monoclonal antibodies.

Even when administered in a single bolus, OKT4A provides potent immunosuppression, and this effect does not require depletion of CD4 cells. It may be useful clinically to prevent early rejection; a limited number of higher-dose injections may be all that is necessary.

▶ Inactivation (modulation) of the helper T cell population, CD4$^+$ T cells, at the time the transplant is placed is a novel approach to immunosuppression. One high dose of the monoclonal antibody OKT4A prevented entry of the CD4$^+$ cells into the graft. This type of approach, wherein the immune response is blunted only at the moment of transplantation, may be the means by which tolerance of the allograft can eventually be achieved. The major problem of the rapid development of an immune response to monoclonal antibodies of mouse origin still limits their usefulness.— O. Jonasson, M.D.

Randomized Controlled Trial of a Monoclonal Antibody Against the Interleukin-2 Receptor (33B3.1) as Compared With Rabbit Antithymocyte Globulin for Prophylaxis Against Rejection of Renal Allografts
Soulillou J-P, Cantarovich D, Le Mauff B, Giral M, Robillard N, Hourmant M, Hirn M, Jacques Y (Centre Hospitalier Régional Univ, Nantes; Inst National de la Santé et de la Recherche Medicale, Nantes; Immunotech et Faculté de Sciences, Marseille, France)
N Engl J Med 322:1175–1182, 1990   8–21

A monoclonal antibody that targets a specific molecule involved in activating the growth signal for T lymphocytes offers a more specific means of immunosuppression than the polyclonal antilymphocyte globulin in prophylaxis against graft rejection. The Tac chain component of the interleukin-2 receptor is expressed only on a small fraction of activated lymphocytes, and antibodies directed at this Tac chain component have been shown to prevent allograft rejection in animals. A rat monoclonal antibody against the human Tac chain, 33B3.1, has potent interleukin-2-receptor-binding inhibitory activity.

In a randomized controlled trial, the immunosuppressive effect of 33B3.1 was compared with that of a rabbit polyclonal antithymocyte globulin in 100 recipients of first cadaveric renal transplants. In addition to prednisone and azathioprine, 50 patients received 33B3.1, 10 mg/day, and 50 received antithymocyte globulin during a 14-day period after transplantation.

Injections of 33B3.1 were well tolerated, whereas 32% of patients receiving antithymocyte globulin experienced major side effects that necessitated discontinuation of treatment. The incidence of acute rejection did not differ significantly between treatment groups at 1, 2, and 3 months after transplantation. Six acute rejection episodes occurred in the 33B3.1 group during the first 14 days of treatment, but all were reversible after discontinuation of monoclonal antibody and rescue treatment. Similar graft function and similar actuarial survival of patients and grafts were observed during a mean 12 months of follow-up in the 33B3.1 and anti-lymphocyte-globulin groups. The drop in peripheral blood lymphocyte concentrations was significantly greater in patients treated with antithymocyte globulin. The level of circulating Tac chain-bearing lymphocytes remained below 1% during 33B3.1 treatment, compared with 4% to 5% during antithymocyte-globulin treatment. Fewer episodes of infection were observed in the 33B3.1 group. Induction treatment with 33B3.1 is as effective as antithymocyte globulin in preventing acute rejection in recipients of first cadaveric renal allografts, with fewer infections and side effects.

▶ This is a different approach to specific blockade of the immune response: interaction of a rat monoclonal antibody with the receptor for interleukin-2 on the lymphocytes actively participating in the rejection. This antibody proved as effective as the pan-T cell antibody customarily used, with the benefit that normal host defenses were less reduced. Antibodies to the agent developed in more than 80% of the patients, and effectiveness appeared to be reduced.—O. Jonasson, M.D.

Platelet-Activating Factor and Hyperacute Rejection: The Effect of a Platelet-Activating Factor Antagonist, SRI 63–441, On Rejection of Xenografts and Allografts in Sensitized Hosts
Makowka L, Chapman FA, Cramer DV, Qian S, Sun H, Starzl TE (Cedars-Sinai Med Ctr, Los Angeles; Univ of Pittsburgh; VA Med Ctr, Pittsburgh)
Transplantation 50:359–365, 1990   8–22

Hyperacute transplantation reactions begin with a cascade of nonspecific inflammatory reactions and result in destruction of the target organ. Platelet-activating factor (PAF) is an important part of these reactions. Therefore, the influence of a specific PAF receptor antagonist, SRI 63–441, in inhibiting hyperacute rejection was studied in animal allografts and xenografts.

Two experimental models were used: rat cardiac allografts in presensitized recipients, and guinea pig-to-rat and mouse-to-rat cardiac xenografts. Four minutes before revascularization of the donor heart, SRI 63–441 was given in a single intravenous bolus injection.

In sensitized Brown-Norway rats that received ACI rat cardiac allografts, SRI 63–441 did not prolong graft survival, either alone or with cyclosporine A (CsA), FK 506, or prostaglandin E_2. In sensitized Lewis rats that received ACI rat cardiac allografts, SRI 63–441 did prolong graft survival, and the effect was synergistic when SRI 63–441 was combined with CsA. Administration of FK 506 prolonged survival still further.

In concordant mouse-to-rat xenografts, there is relative resistance to graft survival after treatment with SRI 63–441, either alone or in combination with CsA or FK 506. Therefore, SRI 63–441's inhibition of PAF function had a variable effect on the survival of cardiac allografts. Survival of guinea pig-to-rat xenografts was significantly prolonged when either the donor or recipient was given SRI 63–441, either alone or in combination with CsA or FK 506. Earlier results had shown the same effect in preventing rejection of cat-to-rabbit kidney grafts.

The use of SRI 63–441 to interfere with PAF function prolongs graft survival in systems in which preformed antibody or complement activation play an important role in hyperacute reaction. This substance, one of a family of compounds that can be modified to balance their therapeutic and toxic qualities, may prove to be very important in the control of graft rejection.

▶ This approach ignores the immune response and is directed to the cascade of events that follow injury to endothelial cells and subsequent vascular thrombosis. The experiments were most successful when the anticipated reaction was most intense, such as in discordant xenografts. Even hyperacute rejection is a multifactorial event, and inhibition of the effect of PAF is only partially effective.—O. Jonasson, M.D.

Liver, Kidney, and Thoracic Organ Transplantation Under FK 506
Todo S, Fung JJ, Starzl TE, Tzakis A, Demetris AJ, Kormos R, Jain A, Alessiani M, Takaya S, Shapiro R (Univ of Pittsburgh; VA Med Ctr, Pittsburgh)
Ann Surg 212:295–307, 1990   8–23

An immunosuppressive drug—FK 506—was introduced to replace cyclosporine for liver recipients with intractable rejection or drug toxicity. Results of FK 506 use were reported in 140 liver recipients, 120 receiving a primary transplantation and 20 undergoing retransplantation; 11 heart transplant patients (8 adults and 3 children); 2 double-lung recipients; 1 heart-lung recipient; and 36 kidney recipients, two thirds of whom had other transplantations or complications that would normally have precluded kidney transplantation.

The initial FK 506 dose was .075 mg/kg by intravenous infusion over a

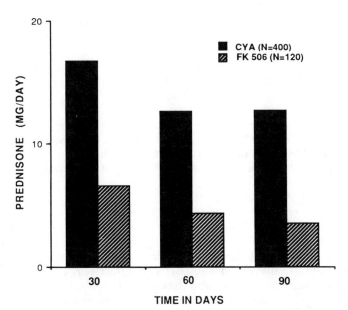

Fig 8–7.—Daily prednisone after 1, 2, and 3 months in the primary liver recipients treated with FK 506 vs. historical controls. *CYA,* cyclosporine. (Courtesy of Todo S, Fung JJ, Starzl TE, et al: *Ann Surg* 212:295–307, 1990.)

4-hour period, beginning in the operating room and repeated every 4 hours, followed by oral doses of .15 mg/kg every 12 hours. Intravenous and oral doses were usually overlapped for 1 day. Variations in this approach were made later; liver recipients had reduced doses if graft function was substandard, and doses were kept as high as possible in thoracic organ recipients. All except the lung and heart-lung recipients also received methylprednisolone, 1 g, intravenously during the operation and a 200-mg burst on the first day, reduced daily in 40-mg increments, less for children.

Among primary liver transplant patients, the 2-month to 8-month survival rate was 93.3%, with original graft survival of 87.5%. For liver retransplant patients, 85% were still alive. Almost all surviving liver transplant patients had good liver function. All 14 thoracic organ recipients survived and were unusually free from the hypertension seen in historical controls. Results in the kidney recipients were reported elsewhere. Overall, rejection was usually controlled without other drugs and with reduced steroid dosages (Fig 8–7). Some nephrotoxicity was observed. Serum cholesterol levels were reduced, but it cannot be proved that this was an effect of FK 506 treatment. The adverse reactions and immunosuppressive mechanisms of the drug were similar to those of cyclosporine.

Preliminary observations suggest that FK 506 has a better therapeutic index than cyclosporine. Good patient and graft survival rates have been attained, and liver function is generally good. Future randomized trials are needed, but FK 506 appears to have a major role in transplantation practice.

▶ The initial excitement over FK 506 appears to have been justified, at least in part. This immunosuppressive drug is very effective and appears to be better tolerated than cyclosporine.— O. Jonasson, M.D.

Suppression of Allograft Rejection With FK 506: I. Prolonged Cardiac and Liver Survival in Rats Following Short-Course Therapy
Murase N, Kim D-G, Todo S, Cramer DV, Fung JJ, Starzl TE (Univ of Pittsburgh; VA Med Ctr, Pittsburgh)
Transplantation 50:186–189, 1990   8–24

Lymphocyte proliferation appears to be inhibited by FK 506 during the recognition and induction phase of allograft reaction and not during production and binding of lymphokines. Brief courses of treatment have prolonged allograft survival in animals. This effect was examined in more detail in the survival of heart and liver allografts in rats. The donors were ACI rats and the recipients were Lewis rats; heterotopic heart and orthotopic liver grafts were done. Recipient animals had a 3- or 4-day course of intramuscular FK 506 beginning on postoperative day 0, 2, 3, 4, 5, or 6. Most groups received a dose of 1.28 mg/kg on each treatment day. Controls in both transplant groups were untreated.

The trial drug prolonged survival of heart grafts from a median of 6 days in controls to 91 days in animals who received FK 506 beginning on day 4. When treatment began before or after day 4, results were inferior; however, animals that did not receive FK 506 until day 5 still survived for a median of 50 days. Rats treated on days 0 to 3 had a median graft survival of only 36 days. Similar results were achieved in liver grafts; the median time to rejection was 10 days in controls, whereas animals who had treatment starting on day 0, 2, 3, and 4 usually survived permanently. Liver recipients first treated on day 6 had no improvement in survival.

A short course of FK 506 treatment, begun as late as 4 days after transplantation, appears to prolong graft survival in rats. This agent has an extraordinary ability to switch off the destructive immune process, practically on the eve of destruction. Its mechanism is unclear.

▶ These data came from an experimental model, but, to quote the authors, "The ability of FK 506 to switch off the destructive immune process, practically on the eve of rejection, was extraordinary." Even after waiting until the fourth posttransplant day to begin treatment, 3 days of therapy was sufficient to greatly prolong strongly incompatible heart allografts and to allow permanent acceptance of liver allografts. Data such as these question the commonly held concepts of rejection mechanisms.— O. Jonasson, M.D.

Increased Incidence of Lymphoproliferative Disorder After Immunosuppression With the Monoclonal Antibody OKT3 in Cardiac-Transplant recipients

Swinnen LJ, Costanzo-Nordin MR, Fisher SG, O'Sullivan EJ, Johnson MR, Heroux AL, Dizikes GJ, Pifarre R, Fisher RI (Loyola Univ Med Ctr, Maywood, Ill; Hines VA Hosp, Hines, Ill)

N Engl J Med 323:1723–1728, 1990   8–25

A sharp increase in incidence of posttransplantation lymphoproliferative disorder was noted in heart transplantation patients in association with the monoclonal antibody OKT3. Heart transplantation patients at one institution were reviewed to identify factors that predict the development of this disorder.

The study sample comprised 154 patients who received cardiac transplants during a 6-year period. Of these, 79 received OKT3 prophylactically or for treatment of rejection and 86 received prophylaxis with antithymocyte globulin. All patients received methylprednisolone, azathioprine, prednisone, and cyclosporine. Statistical analysis of the results included univariate analyses and multivariate analysis by logistic regression.

Posttransplantation lymphoproliferative disorder occurred in 1 of 75 patients who did not receive OKT3, a rate of 1.3%, compared to 11.4% of patients who did receive OKT3. The OKT3-treated group was 9 times more likely to have the disorder. The use of OKT3 was shown by multivariate analysis to be the only factor having a significant association with development of the disorder. Increasing doses of this agent significantly increased the risk; the disorder developed in only 4 of 65 patients whose overall dose was 75 mg or less but in 5 of 14 patients who received more than 75 mg. Seven deaths were attributed to posttransplant lymphoproliferative disorder.

Apparently, OKT3 increases the incidence of posttransplantation lymphoproliferative disorder in heart transplant patients, especially those given cumulative doses of more than 75 mg. The use of prophylactic OKT3 should be reassessed, particularly as the value of prophylactic immunotherapy is yet to be firmly established. All patients who have received OKT3 should be monitored closely for signs of posttransplantation lymphoproliferative disorder.

▶ It is very tempting to pull out all of the stops when immunosuppressing heart transplant recipients because the stakes are so high. The grim observation that lymphomas occurred in a third of the recipients receiving prolonged OKT3 treatment certainly raises the question of the risk-benefit ratio of the prophylactic use of a pan-T cell agent in all patients when only a fraction of them will need this treatment.—O. Jonasson, M.D.

Immunohistology of Epstein-Barr Virus–Associated Antigens in B Cell Disorders from Immunocompromised Individuals

Thomas JA, Hotchin NA, Allday MJ, Amlot P, Rose M, Yacoub M, Crawford DH (Imperial Cancer Research Fund; Royal Postgrad Med School; Royal Free Hosp, London; Harefield Hosp, Middlesex, England)
Transplantation 49:944–953, 1990   8–26

Epstein-Barr virus (EBV) is associated with various B cell tumors in immunodeficient patients. Lymphoproliferative lesions from organ allograft recipients and patients having acute, rapidly fatal infectious mononucleosis were analyzed for EBV-coded antigens, cell adhesion molecules, and B cell markers implicated in EBV-induced proliferation. Eight patients given kidney, heart, or heart-lung transplants were studied, along with 2 children in whom rapidly fatal mononucleosis-like disorders developed.

All of the lesions examined expressed EBV gene products, but no lytic cycle antigens associated with productive viral infection were detected. The pattern resembled the viral gene expression seen in normal B cells immortalized by EBV in vitro. The findings support a primary role for EBV in the development of posttransplant and X-linked proliferative syndrome B cell disorders. This contrasts with the subsidiary role played by EBV in the development of Burkitt's lymphoma.

▶ These are careful and complete studies contrasting Burkitt's lymphoma and EBV-induced lymphomas in immunosuppressed patients. The EBV-infected tumor cells of the transplant patients express viral antigens, but T cell surveillance responses are suppressed. Once T cell responsiveness is restored through withdrawal of immunosuppression, the infected cells are attacked and the tumor often regresses. In Burkitt's lymphoma, the viral and cellular adhesion molecules required to incite T cell activity are missing. Immunosuppression that is broad and nonspecific suppresses tumor surveillance.—O. Jonasson, M.D.

The Influence of Immunosuppression on Peptic Ulceration Following Renal Transplantation and the Role of Endoscopy

Steger AC, Timoney ASA, Griffen S, Salem RR, Williams G (Royal Postgrad Med School, London)
Nephrol Dial Transplant 5:289–292, 1990   8–27

Peptic ulcers often develop in renal transplant patients. A prospective study was done to determine whether a change in routine immunosuppressive therapy could result in less peptic ulceration.

Group 1 consisted of 90 patients who had renal transplantation over a 3-year period and received azathioprine and prednisolone. Group 2 consisted of 44 patients who received transplants over a subsequent 2-year period and were given cyclosporine and low-dose azathioprine and prednisolone. At 7–14 days after surgery, all patients had endoscopy to as-

Endoscopic Findings in Relation to Receipt of Methylprednisolone

Endoscopy findings	Azathioprine/ prednisolone (n = 75)	A/P plus methylprednisolone (n = 15)	Triple therapy/ cyclosporin (n = 9)	Triple/cyclosporin plus methylprednisolone (n = 35)
Normal	29 (39%)	5 (33%)	5 (56%)	11 (31%)
Duodenal ulcer	14 (19%)	2 (13%)	1 (11%)	9 (26%)
Gastric ulcer	5 (7%)	1 (7%)	0 (0%)	3 (9%)
Oesophagitis	19	4	2	12
Gastritis	17	2	3	5
Duodenitis	11	2	2	6

(Courtesy of Steger AC, Timoney ASA, Griffen S, et al: *Nephrol Dial Transplant* 5:289–292, 1990.)

certain whether they had any peptic ulcers, esophagitis, gastritis, or duodenitis. Patients in group 2 received significantly more methylprednisolone for rejection.

The 2 groups were not different in incidence of peptic ulceration or inflammatory lesions. Patients in both groups who received 2 g or more of methylprednisolone by the time of endoscopy were more likely to have ulcers or inflammatory lesions (table). Thus any reduction in the incidence of ulcers was outweighed by the use of high-dose methylprednisolone.

There continues to be a high incidence of peptic ulcers and inflammatory lesions in renal transplant patients. The incidence of such changes after transplantation is much higher than if investigation begins with presenting symptoms. Regular postoperative endoscopy allows prompt diagnosis and treatment, thereby achieving low mortality from peptic ulceration of .75% overall or 4% in those with ulcers.

▶ Even with modern immunosuppression using reduced maintenance steroids, two thirds of transplant recipients have peptic ulcer disease—usually duodenal or pyloric channel ulcers. Perhaps prostaglandin E_1 analogues, which are cytoprotective for gastric mucosal cells suppress acid production, and also appear to be useful adjuncts to immunosuppression (see Abstract 8–19), should be tested in both contexts.—O. Jonasson, M.D.

9 Oncology and Tumor Immunology

Tumor Immunization: Improved Results After Vaccine Modified With Recombinant Interferon Gamma
Sigal RK, Lieberman MD, Reynolds JV, Williams N, Ziegler MM, Daly JM (Univ of Pennsylvania; Childrens' Hosp of Philadelphia)
Arch Surg 125:308–312, 1990   9–1

Studies have shown that adding recombinant murine interferon-γ to cultured murine neuroblastoma explants augments tumor immunogenicity. The ability of interferon-modified tumor cells to serve as a vaccine against unmodified tumor was assessed by culturing the murine neuroblastoma C1300 for 3 days with recombinant interferon-γ, 500 units per mL. Mice received either irradiated tumor cells or cells incubated in interferon intradermally and were rechallenged a week later with viable tumor cells.

Animals immunized with tumor cells incubated with interferon-γ had delayed development of tumors and also a survival advantage compared with mice given irradiated tumor cells. Administration of tumor cells incubated with interferon significantly increased the level of nonspecific systemic immunity. The addition of bacille Calmette-Guerin to cultures reduced the efficacy of each of the vaccines.

Vaccination of mice with interferon-modified neuroblastoma cells enhances host cytotoxicity and leads to better survival after rechallenge with tumor. These findings may have clinical application. Vaccination may be most effective at the time of operation when the tumor burden is low but the risk of metastasis is relatively high.

▶ Although the results of these experiments were less than dramatic, the approach of modifying the tumor cells in a vaccine to enhance their antigenicity is logical. Tumor-associated antigens have been regularly identified elsewhere, but these appear to be weak and ineffective stimulators of a meaningful immune response. Upregulation of the antigens by interferon-γ is a logical approach.—O. Jonasson, M.D.

Lymphocyte Subset Alterations in Nodes Regional to Human Melanoma
Farzad Z, Cochran AJ, McBride WH, Gray JD, Wong V, Morton DL (Univ of California, Los Angeles; Univ of Southern California)
Cancer Res 50:3585–3588, 1990   9–2

Lymphocyte subsets involved in immune responses to tumors reflect the nature of the response and may help to determine the outcome of the tumor-host interaction. Two-color flow cytometry was used to delineate lymphocyte subpopulations in tumor-draining lymph nodes of 24 patients with malignant melanoma. Axillary nodes were removed from 14 patients with clinical stage I melanoma and from 10 with clinical stage II disease.

Uninvolved nodes from patients with stage II disease (nodal metastasis) had significantly reduced helper/inducer T cells and an increased number of cytotoxic/suppressor cells compared with nodes from stage I patients. The presence of tumor in a node sometimes was associated with a substantial reduction in total T cells. Natural killer cells were increased in nodes closest to the tumor and were more numerous in uninvolved nodes from stage II cases.

The findings support a critical role for altered subsets of immunocompetent cells in the process of melanoma progression as metastasis. Studies of lymphocyte subpopulations may help to identify those immunocompromised patients who are at the highest risk of recurrent disease and who would be most likely to benefit from adjuvant treatment.

▶ The findings that lymph node lymphocyte populations are deranged in uninvolved nodes in stage I melanoma patients is interesting, as are the findings that the population of helper T cells (CD4[+]) as reduced in patients with larger or more invasive tumors. The implication is that products of the tumor are immunosuppressive and facilitate metastases.— O. Jonasson, M.D.

Human Natural Killer Cell Adhesion Molecules: Differential Expression After Activation and Participation in Cytolysis

Robertson MJ, Caligiuri MA, Manley TJ, Levine H, Ritz J (Dana-Farber Cancer Inst, Boston; Harvard Med School)
J Immunol 145:3194–3201, 1990   9–3

Cell adhesion molecules (CAMs) help to regulate interactions between lymphocytes, accessory cells, and target cells involved in immune responses. The expression of several CAMs by isolated human natural killer (NK) cells and by NK cells activated in vitro by interleukin-2 (IL-2) was compared with CAM expression by T lymphocytes.

Freshly isolated human NK cells were positive for LFA-3 (CD58), a target cell ligand, and expressed two- to threefold more LFA-1 (CD11a/CD18), an adhesion molecule, than resting T lymphocytes did. In addition, more NK than T cells expressed the intercellular adhesion molecule-1 (CD54). Natural killer cells incubated with IL-2 had four- to sixfold increases in surface levels of CAM CD11a/CD18, CD2, CD54, CD58, and CD56. Essentially all NK cells became CD54 positive within 3 days of exposure to IL-2. In contrast, T cells did not exhibit comparable upregulation of CAM when incubated with IL-2. Increased CAM expression in NK cells correlated with enhanced killing of NK-sensitive targets and induction of cytotoxicity for previously NK-resistant targets.

Cell adhesion molecules have an important role in regulating NK cytolysis. Altered expression of CAM may change the target cell specificity of activated NK effectors, and CAM might be involved in both initial conjugate formation and triggering of the cytolytic process.

▶ The importance of various CAMs in mediating many physiologic events is becoming evident. In this study, the mechanism by which NK cells become activated by IL-2 to exert an antitumor effect seems to be through upregulation of the CAMs that permit NK and target cell interaction.— O. Jonasson, M.D.

LFA-3, CD44, CD45: Physiologic Triggers of Human Monocyte TNF and IL-1 Release

Webb DSA, Shimizu Y, Van Seventer GA, Shaw S, Gerrard TL (Food and Drug Administration, Bethesda, Md; Natl Cancer Inst, Bethesda, Md)
Science 249:1295– 1297, 1990   9– 4

The monocyte-derived cytokines, tumor necrosis factor-α (TNF-α) and interleukin-1β (IL-1β) are important factors regulating immune responses, but the physiologic basis for their release is not well understood. Monoclonal antibodies to 8 monocyte surface receptors were surveyed for their ability to induce TNF-α and IL-1β release by monocytes.

Monoclonal antibodies specific for CD44, CD45, and lymphocyte function-associated antigen-3 (LFA-3) induced release of TNF-α and

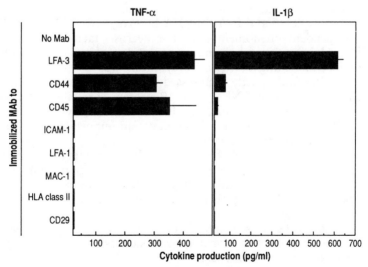

Fig 9– 1.—Antibodies to LFA-3, CD44, and CD45 stimulate tumor necrosis factor-α (TNF-α) and interleukin-1β (IL-lβ) production by human monocytes. The lowest detectable concentration of TNF-α or IL-1β was 25 pg/ml. Results are the mean of triplicates ± SRM. Endotoxin (500 ng/ml) was used as a positive control and induced the release of 1285 pg of TNF-α and 6400 pg of IL-lβ per milliliter. (Courtesy of Webb DSA, Shimizu Y, Van Seventer GA, et al: *Science* 249:1295– 1297, 1990.)

IL-1β from monocytes (Fig 9–1). Tumor necrosis factor-α was released when monocytic LFA-3 bound immobilized, purified CD2—its physiologic receptor. None of the antibodies induced monokine release when not bound to plastic, indicating that they act by cross-linking the respective antigens. The findings show that a receptor-ligand interaction that mediates cell-to-cell adhesion can trasmit signals promoting the release of monokines.

▶ Cell-cell contact may be an important physiologic stimulus for the release of important cytokines. For instance, when a monocyte contacts a tumor cell, TNF-α is released. In these experiments, an adhesion event (binding to plastic surfaces) is used to mimic cell-cell contact, and cytokine release is demonstrated.—O. Jonasson, M.D.

Coordinated Induction of Autocrine Tumor Necrosis Factor and Interleukin 1 in Normal Human Monocytes and the Implications for Monocyte-Mediated Cytotoxicity
Smith DM, Lackides GA, Epstein LB (Univ of California, San Francisco)
Cancer Res 50:3146–3153, 1990   9–5

Cytokine production and cytotoxicity are important monocyte functions. Normal human monocytes were examined for autocrine tumor necrosis factor (TNF) and interleukin-1β (IL-1β) induction using cells from murine fibrosarcoma WEHI-164 as a tumor target. Accumulation of mRNA was measured by Northern blot analysis, and protein synthesis by specific enzyme-linked immunosorbent assays.

Induction of TNF and IL-1β mRNA by exogenous TNF or IL-1β was a time-dependent phenomenon. Tumor necrosis factor mRNA was induced first by each stimulus, and its accumulation was enhanced by cycloheximide, indicating that protein synthesis was not required. In contrast, cycloheximide partly suppressed the later accumulation of IL-1β mRNA. Production of TNF and IL-1β protein correlated well with induction of the respective mRNAs. Interleukin-1β downregulates autocrine TNF function. Autocrine TNF playes an important role in mediating tumor cell lysis by monocytes.

The findings affirm a role for TNF and IL-1β in regulating monocyte-mediated antitumor cytotoxic effects. The broad range of biologic activities induced by these cytokines helps to explain why regulatory mechanisms have evolved to keep their production in check.

▶ Tumor necrosis factor is an important product of macrophages and does enhance cytotoxicity. In these experiments, regulation of TNF production also was demonstrated.—O. Jonasson, M.D.

Adoptive Immunotherapy of Human Cancer: The Cytokine Cascade and Monocyte Activation Following High-Dose Interleukin 2 Bolus Treatment

Boccoli G, Masciulli R, Ruggeri EM, Carlini P, Giannella G, Montesoro E, Mastroberardino G, Isacchi G, Testa U, Calabresi F, Peschle C (Istituto Superiore di Sanita; Blood Transfusion Ctr; Istituto di Patologia Medica; Univ "La Sapienta"; Istituto Regina Elena, Rome)
Cancer Res 50:5795–5800, 1990   9–6

Adoptive immunotherapy for cancer involves the in vitro activation of lymphokine-activated killer (LAK) cells by recombinant interleukin-2 (rIL-2) and their subsequent administration. Serum levels of interferon-γ neopterin, 2'-5'A synthetase, and tumor necrosis factor (TNF-α) were monitored in 5 cancer patients given adoptive immunotherapy with high-dose IL-2 plus LAK cells. Three patients had melanoma, 1 had colon cancer, and 1 had carcinoma of the adrenal cortex.

The markers increased significantly after IL-2 administration in all cases. The increase in neopterin was delayed compared with that of interferon-γ, implying that macrophages (the source of neopterin) were activated by interferon after IL-2–mediated lymphocyte induction. The antitumor effect of high-dose IL-2 may be mediated in part by activation of endogenous cytokines, including interferon-γ and TNF-α. Macrophages may participate in this antitumor effect.

▶ Activation has been demonstrated through measurement of the macrophage products TNF-α and neopterin. The macrophages, themselves activated by products of LAK cells, especially interferon-γ, may significantly participate in antitumor activity during IL-2 therapy, and the cytokines they secrete may also play an important independent role.— O. Jonasson, M.D.

Immunohistochemical Correlates of Response to Recombinant Interleukin-2-Based Immunotherapy in Humans

Rubin JT, Elwood LJ, Rosenberg SA, Lotze MT (Natl Cancer Inst, Bethesda, Md)
Cancer Res 49:7086–7092, 1989   9–7

The immunologic mechanisms underlying immunotherapy remain incompletely understood. The immunohistochemical characteristics of the tumors were examined in 48 patients with advanced malignancy who received immunotherapy based on recombinant interleukin-2 (rIL-2). Some patients received cyclophosphamide, tumor necrosis factor, interferon α, or antimelanoma antibody in conjunction with rIL-2. Adoptively transferred tumor infiltrating lymphocytes and lymphokine-activated killer cells also were used in some cases. Metastatic melanoma and renal cell carcinoma were the most frequent malignancies.

About half of the melanomas and nearly 60% of renal cell cancers expressed class II antigen before treatment, but this did not predict the clinical response to immunotherapy. After treatment, all 7 biopsied regressing metastases expressed DR antigen intensely in more than half of the cells (Fig 9–2). Unresponsive lesions, in contrast, usually did not express

62x   250x

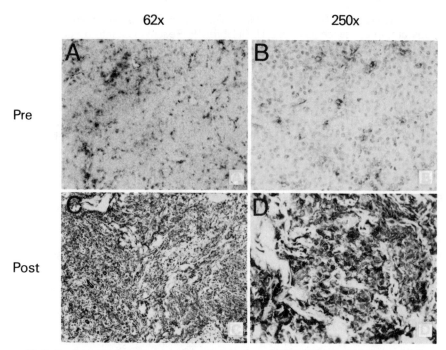

Pre

Post

Fig 9–2.—Regressing lesions express DR antigen on most of their cells. These 2 subcutaneous lesions were excisionally biopsied from a woman with disseminated melanoma before and during therapy. Her pretreatment biopsy (**A,B**) is nearly devoid of tumor associated staining with anti HLA-DR antibody. A regressing lesion (**C,D**) obtained after 5 days of therapy, however, is intensely stained. (Courtesy of Rubin JT, Elwood LJ, Rosenberg SA, et al: *Cancer Res* 49:7086–7092, 1989.)

DR antigen to this extent. Regressing lesions exhibited macrophages and both CD4 and CD8 T cells.

Both T cells and macrophages are involved in the response to rIL-2–based immunotherapy, given for advanced malignancy. The biologic role of DR antigen expression remains uncertain.

▶ These are interesting analyses of metastatic tumors during rIL-2 and combination immunotherapy. It appears that the cytokines have induced transplantation antigen expression on the tumor cells and, perhaps, a subsequent rejection reaction.— O. Jonasson, M.D.

Successful Combination Immunotherapy for the Generation In Vivo of Antitumor Activity With Anti-CD3, Interleukin 2, and Tumor Necrosis Factorα
Yang SC, Fry KD, Grimm EA, Roth JA (Univ of Texas, Houston)
Arch Surg 125:220–225, 1990   9–8

An alternative to adoptive immunotherapy, which may cause severe toxicity, is the activation of endogenous immune responses using combinations of biologic agents. An attempt was made to generate lymphokine-activated killer (LAK) cells using a murine anti-CD3 analogue combined with low-dose interleukin-2 (IL-2) and tumor necrosis factor-α (TNF-α). Low doses of anti-CD3 induce T cell functions and are mitogenic for T cells. Treatment was evaluated against pulmonary metastasis from various mouse tumor cell lines.

A single dose of anti-CD3, followed by low-dose IL-2 and TNF-α, potentiated a reduction in metastases compared with either a higher dose of IL-2 or combined IL-2 plus TNF-α. The addition of anti-CD3 prolonged survival and allowed long-term survival in 60% of treated mice. No animal given other combinations or single agents survived. The LAK activity and natural killer activity of murine splenocytes increased after treatment with anti-CD3 combined with IL-2 and TNF-α.

Effective immunotherapy appears to be feasible using appropriate combinations of biologic agents. This approach can lower the dose of IL-2 required and thereby reduce toxicity from IL-2. In addition, selective activation of the endogenous lymphocyte populations needed for lytic activity should be possible.

► A cocktail of cytokines combined with an antibody to the T cell receptor anti-CD3 has been shown to reduce experimental metastases. Tumor necrosis factor probably also increases adhesion molecule expression and may activate macrophages to participate in the response. The benefit of the combination approach is the ability to markedly reduce doses of IL-2, which has severe systemic toxicity.— O. Jonasson, M.D.

Anti-Tac-H, a Humanized Antibody to the Interleukin 2 Receptor With New Features for Immunotherapy in Malignant and Immune Disorders
Junghans RP, Waldmann TA, Landolfi NF, Avdalovic NM, Schneider WP, Queen C (Natl Cancer Inst, Bethesda, Md; Protein Design Labs, Palo Alto)
Cancer Res 50:1495–1502, 1990   9–9

The interleukin-2 receptor peptide Tac (CD25) is markedly upregulated in adult T cell leukemia and other malignancies, and in T cells activated in autoimmunity or allografts. Past attempts to use anti-Tac, a murine monoclonal antibody directed against Tac peptide, were limited by weak recruitment of effector functions and by neutralization by antimouse immunoglobulin (Ig) antibodies.

Chimeric "humanized" anti-Tac antibodies were prepared through genetic engineering. In the "hyperchimeric" antibody anti-Tac-H, the molecule is totally human except for small hypervariable segments of the complementarity-determining regions retained from the murine antibody (Fig 9–3). The chimeric constructs maintained high affinity for antigen and the ability to block T cell activation. In addition, they exhibited a capability for antibody-dependent cell-mediated cytotoxicity, which is not a feature of mouse anti-Tac. Anti-Tac monoclonal antibody was able to block antigen-induced T cell proliferation.

Antibody-dependent cell-mediated cytotoxicity is an important feature

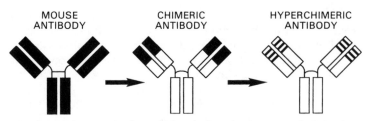

MOUSE ANTIBODY   CHIMERIC ANTIBODY   HYPERCHIMERIC ANTIBODY

Fig 9–3.—Strategy for preparing humanized antibodies. The chimeric antibody has human heavy and light chain constant regions and mouse heavy and light chain variable regions, whereas the hyperchimeric antibody is human except for the complementarity-determining regions (CDRs), which are retained from the mouse antibody. *Filled square,* sequences of mouse origin; *open square,* sequences of human origin. (Courtesy of Junghans RP, Waldmann TA, Landolfi NF, et al: *Cancer Res* 50:1495–1502, 1990.)

of human–mouse chimeric and hyperchimeric antibodies to the Tac T cell activation antigen. Anti-Tac-H may have applications in treating adult T cell leukemia and other malignancies and also in the allograft and autoimmune settings.

▶ This beautifully written paper describes new technology used to eliminate the major disadvantages of the usual mouse-derived monoclonal antibodies to the CD25, T cell receptor for IL-2. The mouse monoclonal antibody has been "humanized" by replacement of 90% of the antibody with human IgG1 sequences, thus possibly reducing its immunogenicity and early immune elimination. The second effect is that the humanized antibody, although as effective as the mouse in blocking the T cell IL-2 receptor, also recruited natural killer cells to perform cell-mediated cytotoxicity. The potential of these humanized antibodies for killing T cell leukemic cells is obvious; the possibility of using the antibody not only to block antigen-specific T cell activation in transplant recipients, but even to eliminate these specifically activated cells, is truly exciting.— O. Jonasson, M.D.

Gene Transfer Into Humans: Immunotherapy of Patients With Advanced Melanoma, Using Tumor-Infiltrating Lymphocytes Modified by Retroviral Gene Transduction
Rosenberg SA, Aerbersold P, Cornetta K, Kasid A, Morgan RA, Moen R, Karson EM, Lotze MT, Yang JC, Topalian SL, Merino MJ, Culver K, Miller AD, Blaese RM, Anderson WF (Natl Cancer Inst, Bethesda, Md; Natl Heart, Lung, and Blood Inst, Bethesda, Md; Genetic Therapy, Rockville, Md; Fred Hutchinson Cancer Ctr, Seattle)
N Engl J Med 323:570–578, 1990   9–10

Therapy using tumor-infiltrating lymphocytes (TILs) along with interleukin-2 mediates substantial regression of advanced malignant melanoma in about 50% of cases. Retroviral-mediated gene transduction of TIL before infusion was studied. The new gene provided a genetic marker for the infused cells.

The gene-modified TILs were given to 5 patients with metastatic melanoma, who also received standard treatment to manage the side effects of cell infusion and interleukin-2 therapy. Genomic DNA from the peripheral blood mononuclear cells and, when available, tumor biopsy specimens and lymphocytes grown from those specimens were tested by polymerase chain reaction assay for the presence of the transduced neomycin resistance (NeoR) gene.

All patients had the new gene, as shown by Southern blot analysis. In 4 of the 5 patients, TILs were also cultured from cells in the neomycin analogue G418, in which the nontransduced cells died in concentrations of greater than 300 μg/mL. In all patients the NeoR gene was present for at least 19–22 days. One patient had the gene for 51 days and another for 60 days. There were no toxic effects beyond those that would be expected with cell infusion and interleukin-2 treatment, and no evidence of infectious virus.

This study was the first clinical protocol in which foreign genes were approved for introduction into humans. Retroviral-mediated gene transduction appears to be feasible and safe. It may have important implications for the therapeutic effectiveness of TILs for cancer. The finding that these lymphocytes remain in circulation and tissue for long periods after infusion may also have implications for therapy of inherited genetic defects.

▶ This exciting study is the first in which gene transfer techniques were used to modify cells infused into patients. Although the cells were used only as a marker in these studies, the safety of the technology was demonstrated, and the possibility is opened of inserting genes into defective cells to repair diseases such as hemophilia.— O. Jonasson, M.D.

Elimination of Small Cell Carcinoma of the Lung From Human Bone Marrow by Monoclonal Antibodies and Immunomagnetic Beads

Vredenburgh JJ, Ball ED (Dartmouth Med School)
Cancer Res 50:7216–7220, 1990   9–11

Up to half of the patients with limited small cell carcinoma of the lung (SCCL) and a large majority of those with extensive disease have malignant cells in the bone marrow. To achieve a good outcome with high-dose chemotherapy and autologous marrow transplantation it may be necessary to purge the marrow of contaminating tumor cells.

A panel of monoclonal antibodies reactive with SCCL was used in conjunction with immunomagnetic beads in an attempt to eliminate SCCL cells from a mixture of 90% normal marrow cells and 10% malignant cells. Immunomagnetic separation removed 4–5 log of SCCL cells in this model system without adversely affecting normal hematopoietic progenitor cells, as assessed by counts of marrow colony-forming units.

The use of immunomagnetic beads with monoclonal antibodies against SCCL cells can effectively and safely remove such cells from the bone marrow. The procedure is expected to facilitate autologous marrow transplantation after high-dose chemotherapy in patients with SCCL.

▶ This and the next 3 abstracts (9–12, 9–13, and 9–14) describe new techniques for super-high-dose chemotherapy with rescue by autologous bone marrow in patients with advanced metastatic malignances. The approach described in Abstract 9–11 is incredibly simple in concept and seems to sweep the marrow of tumor cells with great efficiency.— O. Jonasson, M.D.

Selective Elimination of Breast Cancer Cells From Human Bone Marrow Using an Antibody-*Pseudomonas* Exotoxin A Conjugate

Bjorn MJ, Manger R, Sivam G, Morgan AC Jr, Torok-Storb B (NeoRx Corp, Seattle; Fred Hutchinson Cancer Research Ctr, Seattle)
Cancer Res 50:5992–5996, 1990   9–12

The presence of malignant cells in the bone marrow impedes marrow transplantation, and agents used to purge the marrow may not eliminate all residual tumor cells. In addition, prolonged hematopoietic depression may increase the risk of infection. A pancarcinoma monoclonal antibody, NR-LU-10, which reacts homogeneously with human breast cancer cells, was used to eliminate tumor cells from the marrow without compromising hematopoietic potential. The antibody was conjugated to *Pseudomonas* exotoxin A. Marrow samples were contaminated by MCF-7 breast cancer cells.

The immunotoxin did not react with normal marrow. Immunofluorescence microscopy readily detected 1% contamination by cancer cells. The immunotoxin was highly cytotoxic to both the MCF-7 and ALAB human breast cancer cell lines. The colony-forming ability of hematopoietic progenitor cells was not significantly inhibited by the immunotoxin.

An immunotoxin can effectively deplete breast cancer cells from human bone marrow while preserving the proliferative capacity of progenitor cells. Apart from breast tumors, this approach might be applicable to small cell lung cancer, colon cancer, and other malignancies in which marrow metastases are relatively common.

▶ In these experiments, a monoclonal antibody directed to tumor determinants was used to carry an exotoxin to the tumor cells contaminating bone marrow. The specificity was so great that normal marrow stem cells were not affected.— O. Jonasson, M.D.

Phase I Study of Intravenously Administered Bacterially Synthesized Granulocyte-Macrophage Colony-Stimulating Factor and Comparison With Subcutaneous Administration

Lieschke GJ, Maher D, O'Connor M, Green M, Sheridan W, Rallings M, Bonnem E, Burgess AW, McGrath K, Fox RM, Morstyn G (Ludwig Inst for Cancer

Research; Royal Melbourne Hosp, Victoria; Schering-Plough Corp, Kenilworth, NJ)
Cancer Res 50:606–614, 1990   9–13

Monocytes stimulated by granulocyte-macrophage colony-stimulating factor (GM-CSF) appear to exhibit tumoricidal properties in vitro. A phase I study was done to assess the effects of subcutaneous recombinant human GM-CSF (rhGM-CSF), and an additional phase I study was done to determine whether intravenous rhGM-CSF could avoid the rashes caused by subcutaneous administration.

Subjects were 21 patients with advanced malignancy or neutropenia for whom no other treatment was appropriate. A 10-day course of rhGM-CSF was administered, either .3 to 3 µg/kg/day by intravenous bolus injection or 3–20 µg/kg/day by 2-hour intravenous infusion. At all doses, the intravenous administration of rhGM-CSF resulted in an immediate but transient decrease in circulating neutrophils, eosinophils, and monocytes; leukocyte levels were restored within 6 hours. Except in 1 neutropenic patient, bolus dosing did not elevate leukocyte levels. A dose-dependent leukocytosis was seen with a 2-hour infusion, with neutrophils increased up to 4.3 times, eosinophils up to 18 times, and mono-

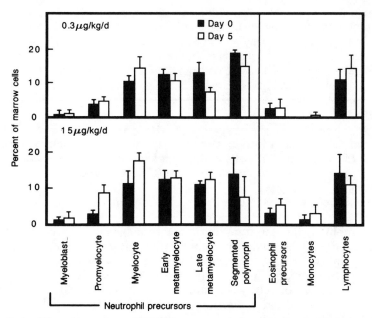

Fig 9–4.—Effect of intravenous rhGM-CSF on marrow leukopoiesis. Results for the lowest dose level (.3 µg/kg/day by intravenous bolus) and maximal tolerated dose level (15 µg/kg/day by intravenous 2-hour infusion) are shown. *Columns,* mean of groups of 3 patients at each dose level; *bars,* SE. The patient with chronic lymphocytic leukemia treated with 15 µg/kg/day was not included in this analysis, because lymphocytes comprised 59.3% of nucleated marrow cells. (Courtesy of Lieschke GJ, Maher D, O'Connor M, et al: *Cancer Res* 50:606–614, 1990.)

cytes up to 3.5 times. Increased proportions of promyelocytes and my-elocytes were noted in marrow aspirates (Fig 9–4).

After 10 days without rhGM-CSF, retreatment at doses of 10 µg/kg/day, or more, caused more pronounced leukocytosis. There was a decrease in platelet levels during the first 3 days, followed by an increase during the first course of treatment. Transient reduction of lymphocytosis was noted in 2 chronic lymphocytic leukemia patients. Treatment decreased serum cholesterol and albumin levels but increased vitamin B_{12} levels. The agent was relatively well tolerated, but bone pain, fever, rash, and weight gain were noted. At doses of 1 µg/kg, or more, there was a first-dose reaction characterized by hypoxia and hypotension. Intravenous dosing induced less leukocytosis than equivalent subcutaneous doses and resulted in a more frequent incidence of rash and first-dose reactions. The maximum tolerated intravenous dose was 15/µg/kg/day.

When given as an intravenous bolus, rhGM-CSF is an ineffective stimulant of leukopoiesis. When given by short intravenous infusion, however, it is effective. Subcutaneous or continuous intravenous infusions are more potent and generally preferable to short intravenous infusions. In phase II studies that seek to raise leukocyte levels, doses of 3–15 µg/kg/day should be used.

▶ These were toxicity studies of intravenous infusions of rhGM-CSF reported by a group that has pioneered studies of these agents. This material is clearly toxic and causes some early reactions such as hypoxia, hypotension, and capillary leak. But the advantages of colony stimulation and substantial increases in granulocyte count in leukopenic patients would be considerable. Whether leukemic patients will also have increases in leukemic activity is not yet clear.— O. Jonasson, M.D.

Effect of Recombinant Human Granulocyte-Macrophage Colony Stimulating Factor on Progenitor Cells in Patients With Advanced Malignancies
Villeval J-L, Dührsen U, Morstyn G, Metcalf D (Royal Melbourne Hosp, Victoria, Australia)
Br J Haematol 74:36–44, 1990   9–14

Recombinant human granulocyte-macrophage colony-stimulating factor (rhGM-CSF) stimulates the proliferation of hematopoietic progenitor cells lacking self-renewal capacity. Concern exists over the possibility of stem cell depletion, but a rise in circulating progenitor cell levels has been reported. Progenitor cells were estimated in the blood and marrow of 37 patients with advanced malignancy who received rhGM-CSF, .3–30 µg/kg/day for 10 days.

A biphasic increase in peripheral blood progenitor cells was associated with administration of rhGM-CSF (Fig 9–5). A slight bias toward granulocyte-macrophage progenitors was evident. When 20 µg/kg was given there was a mean eightfold increase in the GM-CFC and a threefold increase in the BFU-E levels. Patients with malignant lymphoma had a rel-

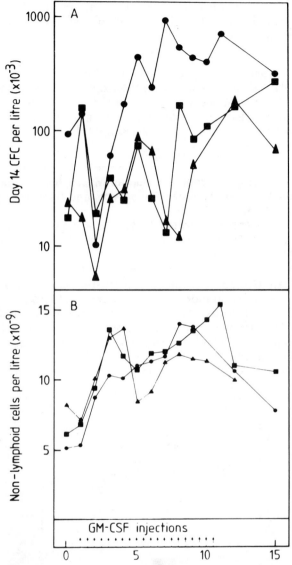

Fig 9–5.—Variation of day 14 colony-forming cell frequencies *(A)* and granulocyte plus monocyte counts *(B)* in peripheral blood of 3 patients treated with rGM-CSF. Day 14 CFC frequencies are mean counts of duplicate agar cultures stimulated by a combination of rGM-CSF plus rG-CSF. *Filled circles* represent patient 29, *filled triangles* represent patient 30, and *filled squares* represent patient 30. *Arrows* indicate time of injection (Courtesy of Villeval J-L, Dührsen U, Morstyn G, et al: *Br J Haematol* 74:36– 44, 1990.)

atively marked response to a given dose of rhGM-CSF. Parallel increases in CFU-E and hematocrit were noted. Progenitor cells in the bone marrow changed variably during treatment.

It appears that rGM-CSF may have value in raising circulating levels of hematopoietic progenitor cells in patients with advanced malignancy. In this way, it may be feasible to harvest peripheral blood cells to reconstitute the bone marrow.

▶ There are exciting possibilities for the use of these CSFs. In this study, all progenitor cells, including erythrocyte precursors, were stimulated to proliferate. Protocols to using CSFs to increase bone marrow progenitor cells before harvest, followed by lethal chemotherapy and reinfusion of the autologous marrow, are now being developed.—O. Jonasson, M.D.

Effects of Parenteral Recombinant Human Macrophage Colony-Stimulating Factor on Monocyte Number, Phenotype, and Antitumor Cytotoxicity in Nonhuman Primates

Munn DH, Garnick MB, Cheung N-KV (Mem Sloan-Kettering Cancer Ctr, New York; Genetics Inst, Cambridge, Mass)
Blood 75:2042–2048, 1990   9–15

Recombinant human macrophage colony-stimulating factor (rhM-CSF) induces peripheral blood monocytes to differentiate into macrophage-like cells that mediate cytotoxicity against human melanoma and neuroblastoma cells. The effects of exogenous rhM-CSF on white cells and on in vitro antitumor antibody-dependent cell-mediated cytotoxicity (ADCC) were evaluated in cynomolgus monkeys.

Circulating monocytes began to increase within 48 hours of rhM-CSF

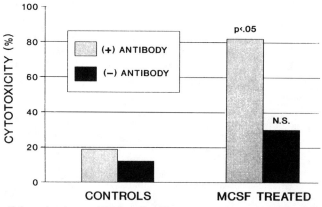

Fig 9–6.—Enhanced antitumor ADCC mediated by monocytes from rhM-CSF-treated monkeys. Peripheral blood monocytes from rhM-CSF-treated animals and control animals were purified and then precultured for 3 days in medium containing 10% monkey serum and 100 μm/ml rhM-CSF. Target cells (human melanoma) with or without antitumor antibody (3F8) were added on day 3, and co-incubated for 72 hours. Cytotoxicity was determined by enzyme-linked immunoabsorbant assay. For incubations with antibody, there was significantly higher ADCC in the animals receiving rhM-CSF ($P < .05$, average of 8 experiments) than in control. For antibody-independent killing, there was no significant difference between the 2 groups (average of 7 experiments). The E:T ratio was 4:1 in all experiments. (Courtesy of Munn DH, Garnick MB, Cheung N-KV: *Blood* 75:2042–2048, 1990.)

administration. Many cells were large, granular, and very vacuolated. The expanded cell population expressed HLA-DR, LFA-3, CD11b, and CD14. It was 77% positive for CD16. After 3 days of in vitro culture in rhM-CSF, monocytes of treated animals mediated efficient ADCC against human melanoma cells (Fig 9–6). Monocytes from control animals exhibited little ADCC.

Parenterally administered rhM-CSF is well tolerated by monkeys and produces marked monocytosis and enhanced monocyte antitumor cytotoxicity in the presence of tumor-specific antibody. The factor might also be helpful in treating chemotherapy-induced neutropenia.

▶ These are clearly preclinical studies with immediate relevance. Melanoma is often chosen as the target tumor because tumor-associated antigens are readily identified and monoclonal antibodies are available. The side effects were minimal, so application of this technique to humans seems appropriate.—O. Jonasson, M.D.

Relationship Between Epidermal Growth Factor Receptor Status and Various Prognostic Factors in Human Breast Cancer

Toi M, Nakamura T, Mukaida H, Wada T, Osaki A, Yamada H, Toge T, Niimoto M, Hattori T (Hiroshima Univ, Japan)
Cancer 65:1980–1984, 1990   9–16

An inverse relationship has been reported between epidermal growth factor receptor (EGFR) and estrogen receptor (ER) in human breast cancer tissue. Expression of EGFR may be important, not only for the hormone-independent tumor growth, but also for predicting poor prognoses. Patients with EGFR-positive tumors have a higher recurrence rate than those with EGFR-negative tumors.

The relationship between EGFR status and various clinical and histologic features shown to be of prognostic importance was investigated in 91 human breast cancer tissue specimens. Epidermal growth factor receptor was assessed using biochemical competitive binding assay with iodine-125-labeled epidermal growth factor.

Status of EGFR did not correlate with axillary lymph node involvement, tumor size, stage, or histologic type. However, it was significantly correlated with histologic grading and lymphatic invasion. The EGFR status and the ER status were clearly inversely related. The Ki-67-positive stained cell rate, which shows the proportion of cycling cells, was significantly higher in EGFR-positive tumor tissues than in EGFR-negative cases. A preliminary postoperative survey showed a high tendency of recurrence rate for patients with EGFR-positive tumors compared with patients with EGFR-negative tumors.

Status of EGFR may be an important predictor of biologically high malignant potential. Multidrug chemotherapy should be considered for patients who are EGFR positive with high growth factors, even if the tumors are in an early stage.

▶ The presence of EGFRs on breast cancer cells, indicating tumor growth stimulation by the cytokine, EGF, is clearly correlated with a poor prognosis. This study demonstrates that EGFR-positive tumors are poorly differentiated and likely to demonstrate lymphatic invasion. As the authors suggest, demonstration of EGFR-positive cells in a tumor might be used to choose the patients who would benefit from adjuvant chemotherapy.—O. Jonasson, M.D.

The Epidermal Growth Factor Receptor and the Prognosis of Bladder Cancer

Neal DE, Sharples L, Smith K, Fennelly J, Hall RR, Harris AL (Univ of Newcastle Upon Tyne; Freeman Hosp, Newcastle Upon Tyne, England)
Cancer 65:1619–1625, 1990   9–17

Epidermal growth factor (EGF) is present in high concentration in urine, and its receptor (EGFr) is present in certain high-grade bladder tumors. Retrospective evaluations were made to correlate EGFr positivity with the prognosis in 101 patients with newly diagnosed primary bladder

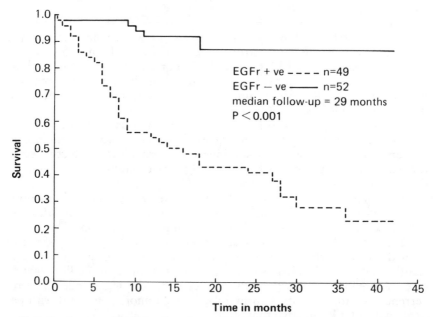

EGFr + ve ---- n=49
EGFr − ve ——— n=52
median follow-up = 29 months
P < 0.001

Fig 9–7.—Cancer-specific death rates and survival for all 101 patients plotted out for EGFr-positive patients (**lower curve**) and EGFr-negative patients (**upper curve**). A significant difference in survival was found ($P < 0.001$). (Courtesy of Neal DE, Sharples L, Smith K, et al: *Cancer* 65:1619–1625, 1990.)

cancer, usually transitional cell carcinoma. In addition to resection, patients with muscle-invasive tumors received systemic chemotherapy or radiotherapy.

Nearly half of the tumors stained strongly for EGFr, and a significant association with high-grade tumor was evident, as well as with tumor size. Among patients with non—muscle-invasive tumors, those whose tumors stained for EGFr were more likely to have multiple lesions. Both tumor stage and EGFr status significantly influenced cancer-specific mortality (Fig 9—7). The presence of EGFr correlated with both a higher risk of recurrence and future progression of disease.

An association was confirmed between the aggressiveness of bladder cancer and the presence of EGFr. Mechanisms by which a high receptor level could influence tumor behavior include facilitation of enzymes such as plasminogen activator. Drug targeting is a possibility.

▶ Epidermal growth factor, a potent mitogen, is found in urine and in many tissues. Tumor cells of many types may express receptors for this growth factor and be responsive to growth stimulation by EGF. As in breast cancer, bladder cancer grade and invasiveness are correlated with the presence of the receptor. Immunotherapy using antibodies to the receptor conjugated with immunotoxins may be feasible.—O. Jonasson, M.D.

Detection of Somatostatin Receptors in Surgical and Percutaneous Needle Biopsy Samples of Carcinoids and Islet Cell Carcinomas

Reubi JC, Kvols LK, Waser B, Nagorney DM, Heitz PU, Charboneau JW, Reading CC, Moertel C (Sandoz Research Inst, Berne, Switzerland; Mayo Clinic and Found, Rochester, Minn; Univ of Zurich)
Cancer Res 50:5969–5977, 1990   9–18

Octreotide, a somatostatin (SS) analogue, helps reduce symptoms of both islet cell carcinoma and carcinoid in ways that are not clear. Somatostatin receptor status was determined in 62 cases of carcinoid tumor and 15 of islet cell carcinoma. Receptor autoradiography was carried out using 2 iodinated SS analogues as radioligands. Both primary and metastatic carcinoid tumors were examined.

Somatostatin receptor-positive tumors were present in 87% of patients with carcinoid tumor and all those with islet cell carcinoma. The wide range of islet cell tumors included vipomas, insulinomas, glucagonomas, and nonfunctioning tumors. High-affinity binding sites pharmacologically specific for bioactive analogues were identified. Receptor was densely distributed in a majority of tumors, including hepatic metastases. Many negative carcinoids were poorly differentiated bronchial lesions; receptor-positive tumors were never anaplastic. All but 1 of the tumors from patients given octreotide were SS receptor-positive.

In islet cell cancers and carcinoid tumors, SS receptors may be the molecular basis for octreotide action. A test for SS receptor content accordingly may predict the effectiveness of octreotide therapy.

▶ Demonstration of SS receptors on these octreotide-responsive tumors suggests that SS suppresses hormone secretion and tumor cell growth by mechanisms similar to those of other neuroendocrine systems. Targeting these tumors by radiolabeling the octreotide analogue of SS is now under investigation.— O. Jonasson, M.D.

Immunohistochemical Demonstration of Human Papilloma Virus Antigen in Human Colon Neoplasms

Kirgan D, Manalo P, McGregor B (Univ of Nevada; VA Med Ctr, Reno)
J Surg Res 48:397–402, 1990   9–19

Human papillomavirus (HPV) has been found in benign and malignant neoplasms of the colon, but the frequency with which it is found in normal colon mucosa and in malignant tumors of the mucosa is unknown. Both types of mucosa were studied by immunohistochemical techniques for the presence of HPV antigen.

Pathologic specimens were obtained for study: 30 normal colon samples, 30 single tubulovillous adenomas, and 30 invasive carcinomas. Samples were fixed in formalin, embedded in paraffin, and prepared for examination by immunohistochemical techniques. Slides were read in a blinded fashion by a pathologist, who rated them as either positive or negative for HPV antigen.

The 3 groups varied dramatically in the presence of HPV antigen (table). The antigen was present in 23% of normal colon specimens, 60% of benign tubulovillous adenomas, and 97% of invasive carcinomas. Antigen was distributed uniformly throughout the colon. The protocol was repeated several times on separate sections and with several blind readings, each time with the same results.

Demonstration of Human Papillomavirus (HPV) Antigen by Immunohistochemistry

Tissue type	Positive for HPV	Statistical significance compared to normal colon
Normal colon (N = 30)	7/30 (23%)	
Benign TVA (N = 30)	18/30 (60%)	$P < 0.001$
Carcinoma (N = 30)	29/30 (97%)	$P < 0.001$

Note: Immunohistochemical demonstration of HPV antigen comparing normal colon mucosa, benign tubulovillous adenomas, and invasive carcinomas of the colon. Significant difference by chi-square analysis ($P < .001$).
(Courtesy of Kirgan D, Manalo P, McGregor B: J Surg Res 48:397–402, 1990.)

There is an association between colon neoplasms and the presence of HPV antigen. Human papillomavirus may have a causative role in the development of colon cancer.

▶ Demonstration of papillomavirus in nearly all colon cancers and in most polyps is interesting, but by no means do these observations prove cause and effect. Although papillomavirus is strongly associated with urologic and airway cancers, and may well have an important role in the pathogenesis of these lesions, it is ubiquitous. Koch's postulates must be more definitely fulfilled before a role in etiology of colon cancer can be defined.— O. Jonasson, M.D.

Utility and Cost of Carcinoembryonic Antigen Monitoring in Colon Cancer Follow-Up Evaluation: A Markov Analysis
Kievit J, van de Velde CJH (State Univ of Leiden, The Netherlands)
Cancer 65:2580–2587, 1990   9–20

Monitoring of carcinoembryonic antigen (CEA) after resection of colon cancer can improve life expectancy through the early detection of recurrences. Nevertheless, falsely positive findings are a disadvantage, as is the fear of an incurable recurrence being detected in an asymptomatic patient. The effects of CEA monitoring on life expectancy and quality of life were studied using Markov analysis, defining variables on the basis of reported data. The analysis simulated an oncologic follow-up of 2 years.

Any effect of CEA monitoring on quality-adjusted life expectancy appeared to be modest. Adverse effects of monitoring were most prominent in older patients having a favorable Duke's stage of the primary tumor. Total costs of monitoring, including the diagnostic and therapeutic measures necessitated by a true or false positive rise in CEA, were considerable. Both high cost and a low return account for a high marginal cost-effectiveness ratio.

Monitoring the CEA level would not appear to be appropriate in the routine follow-up of colon cancer patients. A controlled trial of CEA monitoring is needed to demonstrate its true value.

▶ Dogma demands that postoperative follow-up in colon cancer patients include periodic CEA measurements. When confronted with a rise in the CEA level, evaluation and probable reexploration are logical. In this elegant statistical analysis, a decision tree approach was taken. Disappointingly, no overall benefit of detection of recurrence based on the CEA level could be demonstrated. The mortality associated with reexploration, especially considering the possibility of a falsely positive CEA result, outweighs the occasional benefit.— O. Jonasson, M.D.

N-*myc* Oncogene Expression and Amplification in Metastatic Lesions of Stage IV-S Neuroblastoma

Garvin J Jr, Bendit I, Nisen PD (Columbia Univ; Long Island Jewish Med Ctr, New Hyde Park, NY; Univ of Texas, Dallas)
Cancer 65:2572–2575, 1990
9–21

Amplification of the N-*myc* oncogene often is found in primary tumors from patients with stages III and IV neuroblastoma. The role of N-*myc* in neuroblastoma was investigated by determining levels of oncogene amplification and RNA expression in 3 infants with metastatic neuroblastoma. Two patients had stage IV-S disease, a stage with limited metastatic potential and a generally favorable prognosis. The remaining patient had stage IV disease.

Southern blot studies showed a normal N-*myc* copy number in the primary tumor from one of the patients with stage IV-S disease and extensive gene amplification in the other. Intermediate gene amplification was found in the primary and metastatic lesions of the patient with stage IV disease. All of the primary and metastatic lesions tested expressed N-*myc* RNA; overexpression was found in the stage IV-S patient without gene amplification. The latter patient did well, but the other 2 died of progressive disease.

Amplification of the N-*myc* oncogene is characteristic of advanced neuroblastoma. It is important to assess gene amplification when a diagnosis of stage IV-S disease is under consideration.

▶ These are interesting studies of a fascinating disease. Neuroblastoma, stage IV-S, which has such a good prognosis despite extensive tumor burden, is shown to be very different from other extensive forms of the disease in degree of amplification of the N-*myc* oncogene.— O. Jonasson, M.D.

An Immunohistochemical Analysis of *ras* Oncogene Expression in Epithelial Neoplasms of the Colon

Jansson DS, Radosevich JA, Carney WP, Rosen ST, Schlom J, Staren ED, Hyser MJ, Gould VE (Rush Med College, Chicago; Swedish Univ of Agricultural Sciences, Uppsala; Northwestern Univ; Du Pont, Billerica, Mass; Natl Cancer Inst, Bethesda)
Cancer 65:1329–1337, 1990
9–22

Monoclonal antibodies were used in immunohistochemical studies for *ras* oncogene products in 101 colonic epithelial tumors of several types. Villoglandular adenomas, carcinomas in situ, adenocarcinomas, and neuroendocrine carcinomas were included. Samples of multiple polyposis ranging from adenoma without dysplasia to invasive carcinoma also were examined.

Enhanced staining was found in mucosa near tumors or sites of inflammation, but the degree of staining did not correlate with depth of invasion or with clinical stage of disease. Some metastases stained positively for *ras* oncogene products. Staining was strongest and most extensive in the villoglandular adenomas, dysplastic adenomas, and carcinomas in situ. It was not uncommon for immunostaining to be unevenly distributed in carcinomas.

These findings suggest that *ras* expression is an early event in tumorigenesis in the colon. Enhanced *ras* expression in colon cancers does not appear to correlate with advanced tumor stage.

▶ The interesting finding in this report is the intense expression of *ras* proteins in premalignant colon neoplasms, suggesting that *ras* expression is an early event in tumorigenesis.— O. Jonasson, M.D.

K-*ras* Oncogene Activation as a Prognostic Marker in Adenocarcinoma of the Lung
Slebos RJC, Kibbelaar RE, Dalesio O, Kooistra A, Stam J, Meijer CJLM, Wagenaar SS, Vanderschueren RGJRA, van Zandwijk N, Mooi WJ, Bos JL, Rodenhuis S (Netherlands Cancer Inst, Amesterdam; Free Univ of Amsterdam; St Antonius Hosp, Nieuwegein; Univ of Leiden, The Netherlands)
N Engl J Med 323:561–565, 1990   9–23

Activated oncogenes can induce malignant transformation of immortalized cells in vitro; they may play a similar role in the development of human tumors. To determine whether the presence of the K-*ras* oncogene, which occurs in about one third of lung adenocarcinomas, has prognostic significance, studies were done in 69 adults with adenocarcinoma whose tumors could be completely resected.

By means of the polymerase chain reaction, *ras*-specific DNA sequences were isolated from frozen tumor samples in 35 patients and from formalin-fixed, paraffin-embedded tumor material from 34 patients. Subsequently, mutation-specific oligonucleotide probes were used to detect and classify *ras* point mutations. Clinical data were then gathered and analyzed for each patient.

A point mutation in codon 12 of the K-*ras* oncogene was present in 19 tumors. Age at diagnosis, sex, and presence of previous or concurrent neoplasm were not associated with K-*ras* point mutation. The K-*ras*-positive tumors were generally smaller and less differentiated. Of the 19 patients with K-*ras*-positive tumors, 12 died during the median 36-month follow-up; of the 50 patients with K-*ras*-negative tumors, only 16 died. Duration of disease-free survival and number of deaths from cancer also suggested that the K-*ras* codon-12 point mutation was a strong, unfavorable prognostic factor (Fig 9–8).

In lung adenocarcinoma K-*ras* point mutation is associated with a poor prognosis and short disease-free survival despite radical resection and small tumor size. There is also evidence to suggest that these tumors may

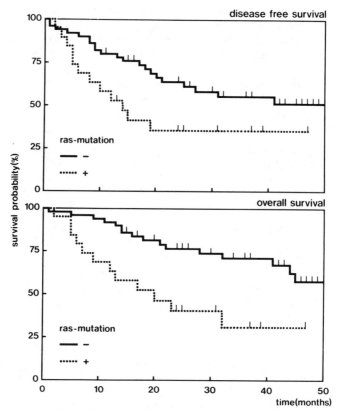

Fig 9–8.—Survival of 69 patients after radical surgery for adenocarcinoma of the lung. In analysis of disease-free survival, 12 of the 19 patients with K-*ras* point-mutation-positive tumors relapsed or died during the follow-up period, as compared with 22 of the 50 patients with no mutation in K-*ras* (*P* = .038 by log-rank test). In the analysis of overall survival, 12 of the 19 patients with K-*ras* point-mutation-positive tumors died during the follow-up period, as compared with 16 of the 50 patients without the mutation (*P* = .002 by log-rank test). (Courtesy of Slebos RJC, Kibbelaar RE, Dalesio O, et al: *N Engl J Med* 323:561–565, 1990.)

become resistant to radiation and to many chemotherapeutic agents. These findings should be studied further in clinical investigations.

▶ A striking difference in outcome after curative surgical resection was found in this study of patients with adenocarcinoma of the lung, with or without the oncogene point mutation. Those with no mutation had quite good outcomes and should be selected for curative surgical treatment.—O. Jonasson, M.D.

Increased Expression of Mutant Forms of p53 Oncogene in Primary Lung Cancer
Iggo R, Gatter K, Bartek J, Lane D, Harris AL (ICRF Molecular Immunochemistry Laboratory, Potter's Bar, Hertfordshire; John Radcliffe Hosp, Oxford, En-

gland; Research Inst of Clinical and Experimental Oncology, Brno, Czechoslovakia)
Lancet 335:675– 679, 1990   9– 24

The human gene p53 may be the tumor suppressor gene responsible for allele loss in common human cancers, including lung cancers. With the use of cell staining with highly specific antibodies to p53, primary lung cancer samples were examined for expression of this gene. Samples were frozen and sectioned for light microscopic study and immunocytochemical staining with the mouse monoclonal antibody PAb240 and the high-titer rabbit antiserum JG8.

Of 40 carcinomas studied, abnormalities of p53 expression were found in 28. Of 17 squamous tumors studied, 14 had abnormal p53 expression. There was no expression of p53 in 7 carcinoid tumor samples or in 10 normal lung samples. An asymmetric polymerase chain reaction mRNA sequencing strategy was used to provide direct evidence of homozygous expression of mutant p53 mRNA in representative carcinomas; this procedure allowed sequencing without any cloning step. All of the mutations observed were G to T transversions, which resulted in mis-sense mutations in amino acids that are highly conserved in evolution.

Simple immunohistologic methods can provide strong evidence of genetic change in human lung cancer, of which mutation of the p53 gene is the most common. Its interaction with other oncogenes and prognostic significance remain to be determined, but new therapeutic approaches may be based on restoring normal p53 activity or inducing a specific cell-mediated immune response.

▶ Not only are transforming oncogenes abnormally expressed in many cancers, but the normal control or suppressor genes are abnormal as well and probably dysfunctional. Identification of these defects may lead to innovative therapeutic techniques, such as gene therapy.— O. Jonasson, M.D.

HER-2/Neu Oncogene Expression and DNA Ploidy Analysis in Breast Cancer
Bacus SS, Bacus JW, Slamon DJ, Press MF (Cell Analysis Systems, Inc, Lombard, Ill; Univ of Southern California Med Ctr; Univ of California, Los Angeles)
Arch Pathol Lab Med 114:164– 169, 1990   9– 25

Biological parameters such as tumor ploidy are becoming increasingly important as prognostic adjuncts to histologic grading in breast cancer. Other major research efforts are aimed at assessing the correlation between gene alteration and the clinical behavior of cancers. Proto-oncogenes, such as the HER-2/neu oncogene, are a family of normal cellular genes involved in cell growth and differentiation. Evidence suggests that alterations in gene structure, gene copy, or overexpression may play a role in the pathogenesis of some cancers. The correlation between HER-

2/neu gene expression and DNA ploidy patterns was evaluated in 45 patients with breast cancer.

Twenty-two cases were scored visually to be positive for HER-2/neu protein overexpression. These cases also contained more than 10% HER-2/neu protein compared with the standard control cell line. All 22 of these patients had near-tetraploid DNA content. Cells from the 23 women who did not have HER-2/neu protein overexpression contained DNA amounts ranging from euploid to various degrees of aneuploid.

Tumors with HER-2/neu protein overexpression have tetraploid or near-tetraploid DNA content. This pattern may be associated with the biological behavior of breast cancer.

▶ Demonstration of this oncogene in large amounts was correlated with a poor prognostic characteristic—polyploidy of the tumor cells. Like the epidermal growth factor receptor (see Abstracts 9–16 and 9–17), a variety of cell membrane characteristics that can be readily measured can be used to target the patients with a poor prognosis and, perhaps, to select them for additional treatment.—O. Jonasson, M.D.

10 Skin, Subcutaneous Tissue, and the Hand

Correlation of Tissue Constituents With the Acoustic Properties of Skin and Wound
Olerud JE, O'Brien WD Jr, Riederer-Henderson MA, Steiger DL, Debel JR, Odland GF (Univ of Washington; Univ of Illinois, Urbana)
Ultrasound Med Biol 16:55–64, 1990   10–1

Ultrasound may be useful in assessing skin and healing wounds if the measurements obtained correlate with the tensile strength and morphological and biological characteristics of wounds. To investigate the potential usefulness of ultrasound, tissue water, total collagen, and acetic-acid-soluble collagen concentrations were correlated with acoustic speed and attenuation coefficient in wounds created in dogs.

A scanning laser acoustic microscope was used to examine the tissue specimens. Ultrasonic speed and attenuation coefficient measurements were obtained for skin 2–3 cm from the wound, which served as a control; for skin within .3 mm of the wound; and for wound tissue. Wound tissue had the lowest ultrasonic speed and attenuation coefficient values, followed by adjacent tissue and then control tissue. Both speed and attenuation values increased as wound healing progressed, but the changes varied among individual animals. The values began increasing and continued to increase at different times. For control skin, a duplicate sample measurement of wave speed was precise within 1.7%; the measurement of attenuation was precise within 16%. Both values correlated directly with the tissue collagen concentration and had an inverse correlation with the tissue water concentration. The acetic-acid-soluble collagen concentration, which reflects collagen changes during healing, showed the best correlation with attenuation coefficient. Attenuation measurements made with the scanning laser acoustic microscope at 100 MHz were compared with backscatter acoustic techniques made at 10–40 MHz. Each technique used tissue samples obtained from adjacent locations on the animals.

Both ultrasonic speed and attenuation coefficient appear to be directly correlated with tissue collagen concentration and inversely correlated with tissue water concentration. In the long term, objective, noninvasive clinical measurements of surgical wounds may be possible by acoustic methods. Careful, expert definition of the acoustic properties of connective tissue is needed.

▶ Noninvasive techniques are necessary if one is going to gain further information about wound healing in humans. In 1987 these same authors suggested that ultrasonic measurements made with a scanning laser acoustic microscope might provide such a technique (1). They have now extended those observations and correlated the noninvasive findings with edema, collagen, and tensile strength. Combining this technique with nuclear magnetic resonance spectroscopy may begin to allow one to "sample" a healing wound both during normal healing and in the event of proliferative scar formation.—M.C. Robson, M.D.

Reference

1. Olerud JE, et al: *J Invest Dermatol* 88:615, 1987.

Effects of Electrical Nerve Stimulation (ENS) in Ischemic Tissue
Kjartansson J, Lundeberg T (St Joseps Hosp, Hafnarfjördur, Iceland; Karolinska Inst, Stockholm)
Scand J Plast Reconstr Hand Surg 24:129–134, 1990   10–2

At present, there is no effective means of reversing established tissue ischemia if it develops after reconstructive surgery. However, electrical nerve stimulation and acupuncture may increase the peripheral blood flow. The effects of electrical nerve stimulation (ENS) were examined in ischemic skin flaps.

Fifteen women and 5 men underwent surgery with cutaneous or fasciocutaneous skin flaps. All flaps had slow capillary refill, edema, and stasis. Patients were treated according to a randomized crossover scheme with either ENS or placebo-ENS. Patients underwent 1 or the other treatment for an hour, then had a rest period of 6–10 hours, after which the alternate treatment method was given. After the initial crossover trial, pa-

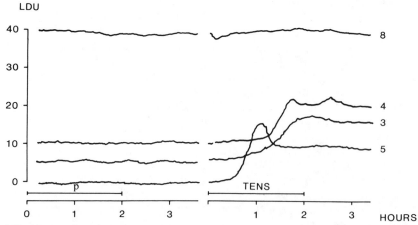

Fig 10–1.—Effect of placebo-ENS *(p)* and electrical nerve stimulation (ENS) on peripheral blood flow as assessed with laser Doppler flowmetry on the distal part of the flap in the patients undergoing reconstructive surgery. *LDU,* laser Doppler arbitrary units. (Courtesy of Kjartansson J, Lundeberg T: *Scand J Plast Reconstr Hand Surg* 24:129–134, 1990.)

tients began a therapeutic course of ENS for 2 hours twice daily until there was significant improvement in signs of ischemia.

Before the crossover trial, there was no significant difference in blood flow. Treatment with ENS resulted in a significant increase in blood flow, whereas placebo-ENS had no significant effect (Fig 10–1). Repeated ENS treatment significantly reduced both stasis and edema. Capillary refill was also improved significantly. The only side effect was allergic dermatitis caused by the adhesive tape used to hold the electrodes in position. Erythema developed in 2 of the 5 patients who had this reaction.

In this series, the postoperative ENS treatment of ischemic flaps increased peripheral blood flow and may have prevented necrosis. The treatment is easy to apply, and it causes no major side effects. Treatment with ENS is contraindicated in patients with pacemakers or other implanted electrical devices.

▶ The use of ENS may well be a way to increase perfusion in an ischemic flap. Unfortunately, this paper is not convincing. The crossover methodology severely limits the conclusions, although one can understand the difficulty in persisting with a placebo when ischemia persists. Time alone will increase perfusion, as ischemia-provoking mediators such as thromboxane and prostaglandin $F_{2\alpha}$ decrease after the insult (1). Possibly, a well-controlled animal trial would allow the placebo-ENS group to proceed and determine whether those flaps go on to necrosis or improve with time. There is good theoretical evidence to support this technique, and if it can be substantiated, it would be a significant contribution.—M.C. Robson, M.D.

Reference

1. Murphy RC, et al: *Br J Plast Surg* 38:272, 1985.

Stretching Skin: Undermining Is More Important Than Intraoperative Expansion
Mackay DR, Saggers GC, Kotwal N, Manders EK (Milton S Hershey Med Ctr; Pennsylvania State Univ, Hershey, Penn)
Plast Reconstr Surg 86:722–730, 1990   10–3

Conventional soft tissue expansion has been used for closure of surgical defects, but this takes time and creates temporary deformities. Active stretching of soft tissue with intraoperative expansion has been attempted. The force required to close a wound before and after its edges were undermined and after intraoperative expansion were compared.

The young piglet was chosen as the experimental animal, because of the close similarity of the elasticity of its skin to that encountered in abdominoplasty and mammaplasty in humans. The series comprised 10 young pigs (average weight, 11.5 kg). Defects were created on the animals' back, belly, and midflank cephalad and caudally, for a total of 80

Wound Closure Tensions: Direct Closure, Undermining, and after Acute Expansion

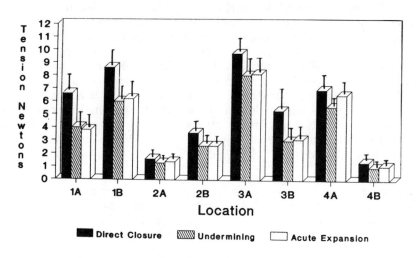

T Represents 1 Standard Error

Fig 10–2.—Graphic representation of tension measurements clearly illustrating no additional advantage of intraoperative expansion over that of undermining alone at the 8 flap sites. (Courtesy of Mackay DR, Saggers GC, Kotwal N, et al: *Plast Reconstr Surg* 86:722–730, 1990.)

flaps. One set of animals had intraoperative expansion, and another set had graded amounts of undermining.

Undermining of the wound significantly decreased the tension required to close wounds (Figs 10–2 and 10–3). Intraoperative expansion showed no significant effect toward decreasing tension. There was little difference between the reduction in force achieved by undermining and that produced by intraoperative expansion. Advancement of the undermined flaps was not aided significantly by intraoperative expansion. The sequential increase in the amount of undermining progressively decreased the force required to advance the edge of the wound.

Undermining appears to be of primary importance in skin stretching. Intraoperative expansion did not additionally reduce the tension required to approximate the edges of the wounds. The location of the wound has much to do with the tension required to close it. Tests of intraoperative human skin expansion are underway in appropriately selected patients.

▶ Dr. Manders and his group have studied tissue responses for years. Therefore, special attention should be paid to this negative report. The rationale for intraoperative sustained limited expansion as reported by Sasaki (1) has always eluded me. Now the authors of this paper demonstrate convincingly that un-

Tension vs. Undermining at Different Locations

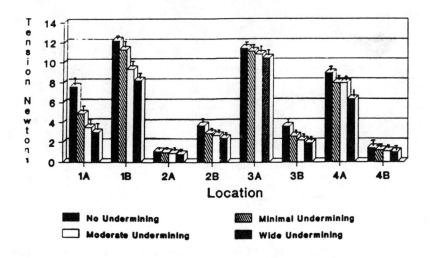

No Undermining **Minimal Undermining**
Moderate Undermining **Wide Undermining**

T Represents 1 Standard Error

Fig 10–3.—Graph shows progressive decrease in tension with progressive undermining. Importance of location is also evident with tension measurements of back skin (1A, 1B, 3A, 4A) being significantly higher than those of abdominal skin (2A, 2B, 3B, 4B). (Courtesy of Mackay DR, Saggers GC, Kotwal N, et al: *Plast Reconstr Surg* 86:722–730, 1990.)

dermining is more useful in reducing wound tension and advancing skin flaps than intraoperative tissue expansion.—M.C. Robson, M.D.

Reference

1. Sasaki GH: *Clin Plast Surg* 14:563, 1987.

Cultured Keratinocyte Sheets Enhance Spontaneous Re-Epithelialization in a Dermal Explant Model of Partial-Thickness Wound Healing

Regauer S, Compton CC (Massachusetts Gen Hosp, Boston; Shriners Burn Inst of Boston)
J Invest Dermatol 95:341–346, 1990   10–4

A model of epidermal wound healing was developed in which porcine sheets of mid-dermis reepithelialize by means of keratinocyte outgrowth from hair follicle infundibula. This model was used to assess the growth-promoting effects of cultured human keratinocyte sheets and the effects of topically applied growth factors on epidermal regeneration. Explants .02-in. thick are used. Growth factors were assessed in a serum-free setting.

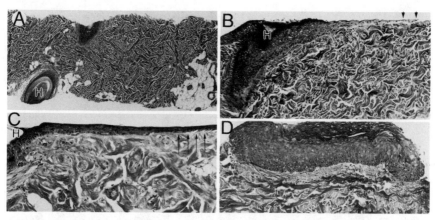

Fig 10-4.—**A,** mid-dermal explant, 20/1000-in. thick, after harvest (magnification, ×75). **B,** at 3 days in culture, keratinocytes have migrated outward from the root sheath of the follicular infundibulum (magnification, ×150, *arrows* at migrating edge). **C,** at 12 days, the regenerating epithelium at the edge of perifollicular collar appears attenuated (magnification, ×150, *arrows*). **D,** Regenerated island in a cholera toxin-treated explant shows marked mitotic activity (magnification, ×75). *H,* hair. (Courtesy of Regauer S, Compton CC: *J Invest Dermatol* 95:341–346, 1990.)

Centrifugal migration of keratinocytes was followed by bridging of adjacent perifollicular epithelial collars. Regenerated epidermis was slightly thinner and somewhat less well organized than normal skin (Fig 10–4). Application of cultured keratinocyte sheets to the explant surface markedly enhanced epithelial outgrowth (Fig 10–5). Cholera toxin, alone and combined with insulin-like growth factor, promoted epithelial outgrowth. Epidermal growth factor and bombesin were relatively inactive. No growth factor induced complete reepithelization during the 8-day study period.

These findings support clinical observations that cultured human keratinocyte grafts enhance wound healing. An example is the use of cultured allografts to heal chronic ulcers that are resistant to conventional measures.

▶ Reports of long-term viability of sheets of cultured autologous keratinocytes have been contradictory. This work goes a long way toward explaining the confusion. If the cultured keratinocytes act by stimulating the remaining dermis to regenerate lost epidermis, then possibly the applied keratinocytes do not have to survive to be useful. This experiment needs to be repeated in explants of human dermis instead of porcine dermis to determine whether the conclusions are applicable to the clinical situation.—M.C. Robson, M.D.

In Vitro Effects of Matrix Peptides on a Cultured Dermal-Epidermal Skin Substitute

Cooper ML, Hansbrough JF, Foreman TJ (Univ of California, San Diego)
J Surg Res 48:528–533, 1990   10–5

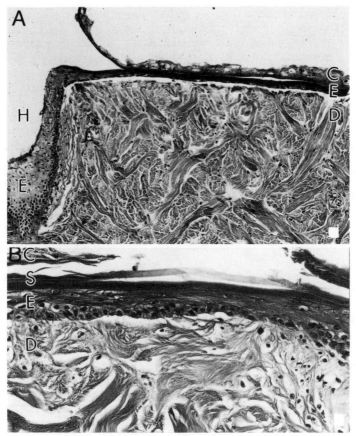

Fig 10–5.—A, 4 days after topical application of second-passage cultured keratinocyte sheets (magnification, ×70). Note the outgrowth of keratinocytes from the hair follicle and the degenerating cell sheet on top of the regenerating epithelium. **B,** mid-dermal explant, 7 d (magnification, × 150). C, cell debris from degenerating cultured xenograft; D, dermis; E, epidermis; H, hair follicle; S, stratum corneum. (Courtesy of Regauer S, Compton CC: *J Invest Dermatol* 95:341–346, 1990.)

Composite dermal-epidermal skin substitutes cultured from autologous cells are used in the treatment of burn wounds that are too large to be covered with dermal autografts. The technique involves obtaining a skin biopsy specimen from the burn patient shortly after admission. Human keratinocytes from the epidermis and human fibroblasts from the dermis are cultured and attached to a collagen-chondroitin 6-sulfate (GAG) membrane. An in vitro study was conducted to determine whether the addition of matrix peptides to the dermal substrate would increase epithelial thickness.

Human keratinocytes and fibroblasts were isolated from surgical discard. Cultured grafts were made by attaching the keratinocytes to the external surface of a GAG membrane and inoculating fibroblasts internally. Synthetic peptides containing the arginine-glycine-aspartic acid (RGD) sequence were used as the matrix peptide. The effect of the matrix peptide was tested under 3 in vitro conditions, including a standard human keratinocyte and fibroblast graft without RGD peptide; a graft of keratinocytes, fibroblasts, and RGD peptide; and a keratinocyte graft with RGD peptide without fibroblasts. The thicknesses of the resulting epithelial layers were measured after a standard 4-day culture period.

The addition of RGD peptide to the collagen-GAG membrane before placement of the keratinocytes and fibroblasts resulted in a significantly thicker epithelial layer at the end of the 4-day culture period compared with the keratinocyte-fibroblast graft without RGD. Subjectively, the fibroblast content on the RGD peptide-treated grafts also was greater. When fibroblasts were not placed on the cultured graft and only RGD peptide, keratinocytes, and the collagen-GAG substrate were used, the resultant epithelial thickness was even greater. The addition of matrix peptides appears to increase cell attachment to the dermal substrate, which should improve the effectiveness of cultured composite dermal-epidermal skin substitutes in the treatment of large burn wounds.

▶ The use of synthetic and biological dressings for wound closure is a rapidly expanding area of burn care. These authors have pioneered a composite membrane populated by human fibroblasts and keratinocytes. This paper suggests the use of a matrix peptide, RGD, for increasing adherence of the "artificial skin" and increasing the thickness of the epithelial layer. The authors, however, fail to convince the reader of the importance of a thicker epithelium, nor does the paper address the durability or water vapor properties of the thicker epithelium. However, these attempts at improving on wound closure from other than pure autologous sources must be continued and closely followed by the practicing surgeon.—M.C. Robson, M.D.

Inferior Epigastric Artery Skin Flaps Without Rectus Abdominis Muscle
Koshima I, Soeda S (Univ of Tsukuba, Ibaraki, Japan)
Br J Plast Surg 42:645–648, 1989   10–6

The use of the rectus abdominis musculocutaneous flap was first reported in 1977 by Mathes and Bostwick and by Dever in 1979. Its clinical usefulness as an island flap and a free flap has been stressed by other surgeons. However, this musculocutaneous flap is bulky because of the thickness of the muscle involved, which may present problems in some situations, and the removal of the rectus abdominis muscle can result in postoperative abdominal herniation.

Inferior epigastric artery skin flaps without rectus abdominis muscle were used successfully in 2 patients.

Case 1.—Man, 64, had a malignant lymphoma in the left groin. Despite chemotherapy, the tumor increased in size, and palliative resection of the involved tissues became necessary. After resection of the tumor and overlying skin, the large defect in the groin was repaired with an inferior epigastric artery flap without the rectus abdominis muscle. A skin flap measuring 28 × 17 cm was outlined on the right side of the abdominal wall. The first incision was made through the lateral border of the flap and then extended medially, superficial to the fascia of both the external oblique and rectus abdominis muscles. The dissection continued/ toward the umbilicus until the main perforator was seen. The fibers of the rectus abdominis muscle were separated from around the perforator with a pair of retractors, and the small muscle branches of the perforator were divided. The perforator was then dissected, cutting deeply through the muscle to its origin from the inferior deep epigastric artery, the distal end of which was divided. The inferior deep epigastric artery and venae comitantes were freed from the muscle until the flap, without the rectus abdominis muscle, could be transferred to the prepared groin defect as an island flap. The secondary defect was covered with a meshed skin graft. No postoperative problems were encountered. No herniation of the lower abdominal wall occurred. A small area of partial necrosis of the most inferior section of the flap needed minor repair with a split-skin graft.

Case 2.—Man, 44, had a squamous cell carcinoma on the lateral aspect of the tongue. A free inferior epigastric artery skin flap was used to reconstruct the oral floor. In this patient also, the postoperative course was smooth and without complications.

A possible disadvantage of the flap described is that the location and size of the perforator may vary. Also, there is the technical difficulty of dissecting the perforator within the muscle because there are many small muscle branches originating from it; however, careful ligation of these branches and dissection of the perforator with retractors assist in the safe elevation of the flap.

▶ If success with this flap can be duplicated by others, this will be a significant advance. Large amounts of skin can presently be transferred only by incorporating the underlying fascia or muscle, or by using multistaged procedures keeping the flap pedicle intact. Isolation of the perforating vessel requires meticulous dissection. In the cases reported, the end appears to justify the means.—M.C. Robson, M.D.

Reconstruction of the Upper Extremity With Multiple Microvascular Transplants: Analysis of Method, Cost, and Complications
Whitney TM, Buncke HJ, Lineaweaver WC, Alpert BS (Davies Med Ctr, San Francisco; Univ of California, San Francisco)
Ann Plast Surg 23:396–400, 1989   10–7

Upper extremity reconstruction with free microsurgical transplants can now achieve success rates of more than 90%. Multiple microvascular transplants, the simultaneous transfer of 2 or more microvascular transplants during the same operation to reconstruct complex injuries, can result in cost savings and reduction in hospitalization time. The records of 62 patients who underwent multiple microvascular transplants were reviewed to determine the costs and complications of this method.

The patients all had severe upper extremity defects. Group I (35 patients) underwent reconstruction with 70 flaps transferred in simultaneous pairs during 35 operations. The 27 patients in group II had reconstruction with sequential transplantation of 61 individual flaps transplanted in 2 or more procedures.

Both groups had excellent results. Despite salvage attempts, 2 flaps were lost in each group. Patients in group I required significantly more reexplorations ("take-backs") than patients in group II. The most common clinical reason for reexploration was arterial insufficiency (70%). The overall occurrence of complications, the frequency of infection, and the incidence of partial flap necrosis or hematoma were similar in the 2 groups.

Rehospitalization in patients receiving sequential reconstruction resulted in significantly elevated costs. Surgical fees were 25% lower for the 2 simultaneous flaps than for the 2 separate sequential flaps. Simultaneous multiple microvascular transplants, particularly in patients admitted with acute injuries, can be performed without an increase in complications or flap failure.

▶ Simultaneous reconstruction with free tissue transfer is feasible and, as shown by these authors, cost effective. The cost savings may be much greater than reported, because not all of the data were available to the authors. Sequential repeated free flaps spread out over several operations and/or hospitalizations are not rational from a wound healing prospective. Fibrosis, contracture, and perivascular inflammation make repeated exploration of potential recipient vessels difficult. What is not discussed in this article is the number of surgeons used when multiple flaps are performed in a single procedure. This may be a limitation when only a single surgeon with microsurgical capabilities is available, or may suggest the need for regional centers to treat this type of injury.—M.C. Robson, M.D.

The Value of Current Staging Systems for Melanoma of the Extremities
Ghussen F, Krüger I, Groth W (Univ of Cologne, Germany)
Cancer 66:396–401, 1990   10–8

The many classifications available for staging melanoma have made it difficult to compare treatment results in a reliable manner. A prospective study was conducted to assess the validity of current staging systems for malignant melanoma of the extremities.

During an 8-year study period, 62 men and 158 women (mean age, 48 years) in whom malignant melanoma of the extremities was diagnosed underwent wide excision of the primary lesion, dissection of regional lymph nodes, and cytostatic extremity perfusion. None of the patients had previously undergone radiation, chemotherapy, or lymphadenectomy. Lymph node dissection was performed during perfusion.

Of the 220 patients, 46.6% had nodular melanoma, 25.8% had superficial spreading melanoma, and 18.6% had acral lentiginous melanoma. The remaining patients could not be classified; 54 patients had ulceration of the primary lesion. Patients were classified according to the original 3-stage system, the M.D. Anderson staging system, the classification system of the American Joint Committee of Cancer Staging and End Results Reporting (AJCC), and the current International Union Against Cancer (UICC) classification system.

The original 3-stage system yielded a statistically significant differentiation of the patients with a distinct preference for stage I. The M.D. Anderson staging system did not divide the patients into prognostically significant different tumor stages. The AJCC classification provided the best differentiation into tumor stages that were evenly distributed and significant for prognoses. The UICC staging system yielded a numerical preference of stages II and III, but the differentiation of stages I and II was not significant. The staging system of the AJCC provides the best differentiation of patients with melanoma of the extremities into stages of prognostic relevance.

▶ Although most surgeons now believe that a combination of tumor thickness as popularized by Breslow (1) and depth of tumor invasion as popularized by Clark et al. (2) is the best prognosticator for malignant melanoma, it is nice to have that demonstrated in a series of patients. The AJCC staging system, which proved to be the best in this series of patients, is derived from a combination of thickness and depth of invasion. If more series would apply all of the different staging systems to the same data set, possibly some of the systems would disappear, making it easier for the practicing surgeon.—M.C. Robson, M.D.

References

1. Breslow A: *Ann Surg* 172:902, 1970.
2. Clark WH, et al: *Cancer Res* 29:705, 1969.

Defect Coverage in Malignant Melanoma: A Retrospective Analysis of 422 Cases
Germann G, Doertenbach J, Inglis R, Encke A (Klinikum Merheim, Köln, Germany; JW Goethe Univ, Frankfurt, Germany)
Eur J Plast Surg 13:52–54, 1990   10–9

Despite intensive clinical research for many decades, the surgical treatment of cutaneous melanoma continues to be debated. Acceptable excision margins, elective lymph node dissection, or regional extremity perfusion in high-risk melanomas are still under investigation. In a retrospective study of 422 patients seen from 1977 through 1986, the tendency toward a more conservative surgical approach was examined and the patterns of defect coverage studied.

Development of Mean Safety
Margins

Tumor diameter	1977	1986
< 10 mm	33 mm	13 mm
> 10 mm	36 mm	26 mm

(Courtesy of Germann G, Doertenbach J,
Inglis R, et al: *Eur J Plast Surg* 13:52–54,
1990.)

The table demonstrates the extent of safety margins throughout the study period. The mean excision margins decreased in thin melanomas (thickness less than 1 mm) from 33 mm to 13 mm. In tumors of maximal thickness (more than 1 mm), margins were reduced from 36 mm to 26 mm on average. During the 10-year study period there was a steady increase in the use of local flaps or primary closure. This correlates well with the changing theory that margins can safely be decreased in size. Local recurrence did not increase during the 10-year period and was noted to be 4% to 6.5% in all primary melanomas not treated previously.

The prognosis of malignant melanoma has improved markedly since the first half of this century. Because death from melanoma is generally caused by systemic dissemination of the disease, improvement in survival is probably the result of earlier diagnosis rather than therapeutic progress. The prognosis is further improved by a steady increase of the spherically growing superficial spreading melanoma.

For almost 7 decades, excision with a 5-cm margin of normal skin has been the customary procedure of local treatment in malignant melanoma. This procedure was based on observation of a single case by Handley in 1907 and a misinterpretation of his proposals. However, several studies have revealed that conventional "safety margins" fail to affect patient survival favorably.

The present findings are consistent with other reports in the literature. The excision margins for thin melanomas have decreased continuously during the past decade. A wider margin seems reasonable in intermediate (thickness 1–1.5 mm, level II-III) or high-risk melanomas (thickness greater than 1.5 mm, level IV-V, and all nodular melanomas).

The results of this analysis demonstrate that the surgical strategy was influenced largely by the worldwide trend to reduce excision margins. Concurrently, the use of local flaps or primary closure increased. Tumor type and stage-adapted surgical procedure apparently do not adversely affect the local recurrence rate or survival.

▶ All data available suggest that margins for malignant melanoma resection can be markedly less than originally thought. Despite this, many surgeons persist with wide margins. Recently, closure of the resultant defects has been shown to be safe. Cuono and Ariyan (1) showed the safety of primary flap coverage, as have the authors of this article. If local flaps are safe, the size of the defect becomes important. The data in this article should be scrutinized closely by those who still believe that "wide" margins and skin grafts are necessary to treat malignant melanoma successfully.—M.C. Robson, M.D.

Reference

1. Cuono CB, Ariyan S: *Plast Reconstr Surg* 76:281, 1985.

11 The Breast

Management of Nipple Discharge

Leis HP Jr (Univ of South Carolina, Columbia)
World J Surg 13:736–742, 1989   11–1

Nipple discharge, which is an important presenting feature in patients with breast disease, is more often associated with benign than with malignant lesions in all settings. Discharge was the presenting symptom in 7.4% of 8,703 women who had breast surgery. These patients were operated on because of a clear, serous, serosanguineous, or bloody discharge.

Intraductal papillomas were found in 48% of 586 patients who had surgery, and there were fibrocystic changes in 33%. Cancer was present in 14% of the group, and precancerous mastopathy was found in 7%. Among 84 patients with cancer, results of mammography were false negative in 9.5%; results of cytology were false negative in 18%. The risk of cancer increased when the discharge was bloody or watery, when a lump was present, or when discharge occurred unilaterally and was from a single duct. Age older than 50 years also was a risk factor for malignancy.

Apart from near-term patients without a mass or cytologic abnormality, patients with surgically significant nipple discharge must undergo biopsy. In women younger than age 35 years and those who wish to have children, only the clinically involved duct need be removed with a wedge of surrounding breast tissue. In other patients complete excision of the central ducts (Fig 11–1) will help to prevent recurrence and will ensure the removal of all intraductal papillomas.

▶ The article serves as a keystone in the management of patients with nipple discharge. The false negative and false positive indices for both mammography and cytology are of particular importance. The importance of a pure watery discharge and its likelihood of cancer association is generally not appreciated. The technique described provides excellent cosmetic results.— S.I. Schwartz, M.D.

Fibroadenoma

Dent DM, Cant PJ (Univ of Cape Town; Groote Schuur Hosp, Cape Town)
World J Surg 13:706–710, 1989   11–2

Breast fibroadenomas are usually single breast masses that are found during the early reproductive years. Such masses are considered to be abnormalities of normal development and involution rather than neoplasms. The frequency of fibroadenomas identified at breast clinics has been reported to range from 7% to 12%. Between one third and one half

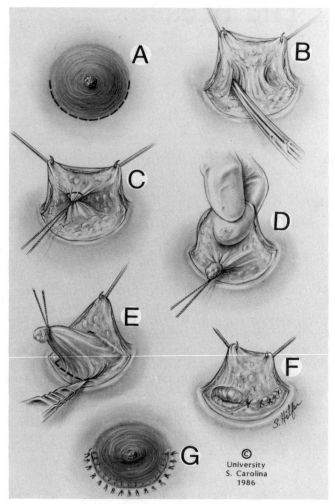

Fig 11–1.—Seven basic steps of complete central duct excision. **a,** circumareolar incision; **b,** elevation of aerolar flap; **c,** encircling and ligating central ducts; **d,** coning out of nipple; **e,** diamond-shaped incision and removal of central ducts; **f,** meticulous hemostatis and only limited deep closure; **g,** skin closure. (Courtesy of Leis HP Jr: *World J Surg* 13:736–742, 1989.)

of the biopsy specimens for benign breast disease yield fibroadenomas, a proportion that increases to over more than three fourths in teenagers. Although fibroadenomas are thought to be more prevalent among darker skinned populations, this assumption was not confirmed in a recent study.

The biologic behavior of fibroadenomas is variable. Short-term follow-up of 63 young women with 201 clinically and cytologically confirmed fibroadenomas showed that 31% of the masses resolved, 12% became smaller, 25% did not change in size, and 32% increased in size.

The tendency to regression was slightly greater with single lesions. Long-term follow-up data are not available.

It is widely believed that fibroadenoma is not a risk factor for breast cancer, but greater than expected frequencies of breast carcinoma in women with fibroadenomas have been reported. The occurrence of carcinoma within a fibroadenoma is rare; only 96 such cases have been reported in the literature. Because these tumors are totally benign and do not predispose to future malignancy, excision is not required. However, excision remains the principal management because most women want to get rid of any breast growths, even if benign, because of an inherent fear of breast cancer. Only 19 of 70 women younger than age 25 years who had a conclusive diagnosis of fibroadenoma chose not to undergo excision. Cytologic confirmation of benign disease and routine monitoring in women who opt for the conservative approach are essential.

▶ This excellent review of a subject that has rarely been discussed in depth addresses several interesting points. The fact that the lesion may not represent a neoplasm is a new concept. The suggestion that masses thought to be fibroadenomas on clinical and cytologic grounds resolve in a significant number of cases is also contrary to common opinion. It is generally believed that a skilled examiner can probably detect a fibroadenoma with an accuracy of about 80%, but biopsy is regarded as mandatory. It is my opinion that the lesion should always be removed, and the procedure generally can be carried out in an outpatient setting.—S.I. Schwartz, M.D.

Treatment Options and Recurrence Potential for Cystosarcoma Phyllodes
Palmer ML, De Risi DC, Pelikan A, Patel J, Nemoto T, Rosner D, Dao TL (Roswell Park Mem Inst, Buffalo, NY; Kunz Regional Hosp, Banska Bystrica, Czechoslovakia)
Surg Gynecol Obstet 170:193–196, 1990   11–3

Cystosarcoma phyllodes, a rare tumor of the breast, is usually benign; however, local recurrence and systemic spread can be fatal. The surgical treatment and outcomes were reviewed in 31 women (mean age, 50 years) treated between 1955 and 1988.

The average tumor size, documented in 29 patients, was 9 cm; 16 lesions were no more than 5 cm in diameter. Surgical treatment included total mastectomy in 7 patients, radical mastectomy in 2, and modified radical mastectomy in 2. The remaining 20 patients initially underwent local excision. Tumors removed by mastectomy were larger, averaging 15 cm in diameter.

Local recurrences were histologically confirmed in 6 women 2–18 months after initial surgery; 3 had excision of the recurrent tumor and 3 underwent mastectomy. Of the women who had mastectomy because of recurrence, 1 subsequently died of distant disease, but the remaining 5 women were disease free. No patient younger than 30 years had a recurrence. Metastatic cystosarcoma phyllodes developed in 4 women whose average age was 57 years.

The histologic appearance or size of the tumor cannot predict the clinical behavior of cystosarcoma phyllodes. Wide surgical treatment, rather than mastectomy, should be the initial treatment. Of 20 patients treated by excision, 15 had no further local recurrence. Nodal dissection appears necessary only when axillary nodes are clinically suspicious. Although cystosarcoma can be benign, 4 patients in this group died of malignant spread.

▶ As the authors point out, only 1 lesion in 10 is truly malignant, and many regard the majority as a benign variant of fibroadenoma. In those cases, the synonyms of giant intracanalicular or pericanalicular fibroadenoma have been used. The issue of the applicability of axillary dissection is controversial. Many think that axillary metastases are so uncommon that simple mastectomy is an adequate procedure for both the benign and the malignant forms. The malignant variant metastasizes most commonly to the lungs, bones, and subcutaneous tissue.—S.I. Schwartz, M.D.

Natural History of In Situ Breast Cancer in a Defined Population

Temple WJ, Jenkins M, Alexander F, Hwang W-S, Marx LH, Lees AW, Williams HTG, Pambrun MG (Tom Baker Cancer Ctr, Calgary, Alta; Calgary Gen Hosp; Foothills Gen Hosp, Galgary; Cross Cancer Inst, Edmonton, Alta; Univ of Alberta Hosp)
Ann Surg 210:653–657, 1989   11–4

The increase in the diagnosis of in situ breast cancer by using screening mammography has created a therapeutic dilemma. Surgical treatment ranging from biopsy to modified mastectomy or even bilateral mastectomy with reconstruction has been suggested. The database concerning the natural history of in situ breast cancer is inadequate.

All cases of in situ breast cancer reported in Alberta, Canada, from 1953 to 1984 were reviewed. Of the 243 patients identified, 226 were available for review by 3 pathologists. The diagnosis of in situ disease was confirmed in 149 cases. Of these, 108 had 109 ductal carcinomas in situ and 38 patients had lobular carcinomas in situ. Three patients had both.

Treatments ranged from local excision to radical mastectomy. At a mean follow-up of 6 years survival was comparable in all treatment groups. Only 2 patients with a confirmed diagnosis of ductal carcinoma in situ died of clinically suspected systemic disease. In the group treated by local excision, ipsilateral cancers were noted in 12% of patients with ductal carcinoma in situ and 13% of those with lobular carcinoma in situ. Contralateral metachronous invasive cancers occurred in 6% of patients with ductal carcinoma in situ and in 3% of those with lobular carcinoma in situ. There was no lymph node involvement in any of these patients, either with prophylactic dissection or during follow-up.

Ductal carcinomas in situ and lobular carcinomas in situ have similar clinical courses. Lymph node dissection is unnecessary. Pathologic review is critical for accurate study of these types of cancer; 36% of the diagnoses in this series were changed. Different kinds of treatment do not appear to affect outcomes. Prospective, randomized trials are needed to determine the most appropriate treatment.

▶ The management of lobular carcinoma in situ remains a problem in view of the bilaterality and multicentricity of lobular carcinoma. Of breast specimens removed for in situ lobular carcinoma, 88% revealed other in situ lesions scattered throughout the specimen. Examination of the contralateral breast has demonstrated in situ lesions in 35% to 59% of specimens.—S.I. Schwartz, M.D.

Breast Biopsy for Calcifications in Nonpalpable Breast Lesions: A Prospective Study
Franceschi D, Crowe J, Zollinger R, Duchesneau R, Shenk R, Stefanek G, Shuck JM (Univ Hosps of Cleveland; Case Western Reserve Univ)
Arch Surg 125:170–173, 1990   11–5

The yield of carcinomas in biopsies for calcifications in nonpalpable breast lesions ranges from 12% to 30%. To identify patients at risk of early breast cancer, clinical and mammographic characteristics were correlated with histologic findings of biopsy specimens in 239 consecutive women (277 lesions) whose mean age was 58 years.

Most (76%) of the women had no history of clinical fibrocystic breast problems. The lesions were about equally distributed between the right (140) and left (137) breast, but nearly half (49%) were located in the upper outer quadrants. No significant patterns were observed between malignancy and lesion location, or between Wolfe's parenchymal pattern and malignancy.

Breast cancer was found in 65 biopsy specimens (24%) and lobular carcinoma in situ in 11. Small and numerous (more than 15) calcifications were frequently associated with cancer; only 1 patient with large calcifications had a malignant outcome. Calcifications in a linear or branching pattern were also significantly associated with malignancy. Of the cancers, 36% were found in lesions judged initially to have a minimal or low suspicion for malignancy. Based on clinical risk factor criteria such as family history and late age at first live birth, patients with malignant lesions were not different from those with benign lesions.

These findings emphasize the necessity for aggressive management of suspicious calcifications discovered at mammography. Lesions with a lower degree of suspicion should at least be monitored closely. The incidence of noninvasive ductal and lobular carcinoma in situ in this series confirms the significance of calcifications as a marker for early cancers.

▶ This procedure is an ever-increasing one, and it is well accepted, as the authors point out. But the yield of carcinoma from biopsies ranges between 12%

and 30%. The corollary is that a large percentage of patients undergo an operative procedure under general anesthesia for benign lesions. There is little question that mammography is a major addition to the management of patients with breast cancer. Although the possibility of identifying patients whose mammograms are highly associated with malignancy is an attractive one, this has not been substantiated by other investigators. There are no data to determine how frequently mammography should be performed. The English, who had been carrying out mammography on a routine basis every 3 years after age 50, have questioned the appropriateness of that frequency. An extended study of the interval, i.e., lesions detected between mammograms, must be carried out to assess the true value of mammography and determine the criteria for screening intervals.— S.I. Schwartz, M.D.

Outcome of Surgery for Non-Palpable Mammographic Abnormalities

Aitken RJ, MacDonald HL, Kirkpatrick AE, Anderson TJ, Chetty U, Forrest APM (Univ of Edinburgh; Royal Infirmary, Edinburgh)
Br J Surg 77:673–676, 1990   11–6

In 1980 two screening centers were established to offer mammography as part of the UK Trial of Early Detection of Breast Cancer. The Edinburgh screening center, 1 of the 2, also performed mammography on women aged 35 years or older attending the symptomatic breast clinic.

In all, 493 women had 515 localization biopsies for nonpalpable abnormalities found on mammography. In 509 cases the mammographic abnormality was found with a hooked wire. Specimen radiology was done on all tissue excised. The mammographic anomaly was visualized in the first piece of tissue excised in 78.1% of the cases. Complete excision was achieved in 92.4%. A palpable nodule was removed in 7.4% of the cases; in 44.7% of these, it was shown to contain a carcinoma. A mammographic abnormality was missed in 2.7% of the cases or only partly excised in 2.5%. Overall, 28% of the localization biopsies were malignant. Mammographic abnormality was not visualized on the specimen radiograph more often in women younger than 55 years, with dense breasts, whose mammographic anomaly contained only microcalcifications. Women found to have carcinoma underwent mastectomy or wide local excision. Residual carcinoma at the localization biopsy site was found in 44.4%. Ligand binding assay estrogen receptor analysis was possible in only 49.3% of the carcinomas.

Nonpalpable mammographic abnormalities are usually excised without difficulty. However, if not identified after 2 pieces of tissue are obtained, and if any palpable nodules have been excised and radiographed, it may be best to discontinue the localization biopsy. A repeat mammogram should be done 3 months later. A second localization biopsy is needed only rarely.

▶ Operations for mammographic abnormalities are increasing significantly. Efforts are being made to reduce the incidence of negative biopsies. The finding of residual carcinoma in 44% after localization biopsy indicates the need to routinely reexcise the biopsy site or perform a mastectomy. Future efforts should be directed to ensuring that mammograms are of excellent quality, and that a correlation is established between the types of mammographically defined lesions and the presence of malignancy.—S.I. Schwartz, M.D.

Level I and II Axillary Dissection in the Treatment of Early-Stage Breast Cancer: An Analysis of 259 Consecutive Patients

Siegel BM, Mayzel KA, Love SM (Faulkner Hosp, Jamaica Plain, Mass)
Arch Surg 125:1144–1147, 1990   11–7

Breast cancer is increasingly being treated by breast-conserving therapy. Although the extent of axillary surgery that should be a part of this therapy is controversial, the goals of axillary surgery include an accurate assessment of prognosis and local tumor control in the axilla. The accuracy, effectiveness, and toxic effects of limited (level I or I and II) axillary dissection with breast conservation were determined in a consecutive series of 259 patients treated from 1981 through 1988. The follow-up ranged from 1 month to 85 months (mean, 22.5 months). Patients underwent levels I and II axillary dissection on an outpatient basis without postoperative drainage of the axilla (Fig 11–2). Most patients also received a total dose of 6,100 cGy of radiation restricted to the breast.

Two to 24 nodes were removed from individual patients (mean, 9).

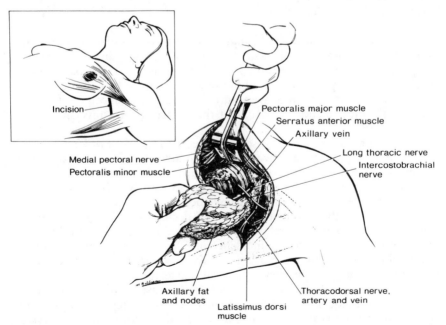

Fig 11–2.—Surgical approach to the axilla. (Courtesy of Siegel BM, Mayzel KA, Love SM: *Arch Surg* 125:1144–1147, 1990.)

The incidence of seroma was 4.2%, and that of lymphedema, 2.7%. Axillary recurrences developed in 2 patients, including 1 who had had 2 of 11 nodes positive and 1 who had had none of 11 nodes positive.

The results provide evidence that levels I and II axillary dissection can permit prognostic evaluation with limited morbidity and recurrence. The procedure does not require routine postoperative drainage of the axilla and avoids the need for axillary radiation therapy.

▶ The advantage of this approach is the ability to carry out the procedure on an outpatient basis without drains and a low incidence of seroma lymphedema. The question of whether there is a need for dissection or sampling with small T₁ lesions still requires answering. Winchester et al. (1) reported that flow cytometric determination of ploidy and S-phase fraction can provide valuable predictive information in node-negative breast cancer.—S.I. Schwartz, M.D.

Reference

1. Winchester DJ, et al: *Arch Surg* 125:886, 1990.

Segmental Mastectomy Without Radiotherapy for T1 and Small T2 Breast Carcinomas
Moffat FL, Ketcham AS, Robinson DS, Legaspi A, Ghandur-Mnaymneh L, Hilsenbeck S (Univ of Miami)
Arch Surg 125:364–369, 1990   11–8

Although there is little doubt that postoperative adjuvant radiotherapy abrogates the risk of local recurrence in patients with breast cancer undergoing segmental mastectomy, it is less certain that all such patients need radiotherapy. The potential for side effects must be considered. Segmental mastectomy, with or without radiotherapy, has been used to treat early infiltrating adenocarcinomas of the breast at the University of Miami since 1975.

Treatment results were assessed at a median follow-up of 72 months in 111 patients; radiotherapy was recommended as optional but not mandatory to 64 women based on 4 pathologic criteria: a primary tumor size of 2.5 cm or less, adequate resection margins, no lymphatic or vascular invasion in the segmental mastectomy specimen, and minimal associated in situ cancer. Fifty-one of these women decided to forgo radiotherapy; by the time of follow-up, relapse had occurred in the ipsilateral breast of 3 of these 51 patients, for an incidence of 6%. A retrospective pathologic study showed that tumor grade may also be important in determining who needs radiotherapy after segmental mastectomy.

Postoperative radiotherapy to the affected breast greatly reduces the incidence of subsequent local tumor recurrence in the breast. Relapse in the breast after conservative excision, however, does not prejudice survival, provided it is treated promptly, usually by completion mastectomy. Further research is needed to define which patients can be spared the potential morbidity, expense, and inconvenience of radiotherapy.

▶ The standard for patients undergoing conservative surgery is the addition of radiation. Haffty et al (1) quoted a 10-year actuarial survival of 67% and a breast recurrence-free rate of 91% at 5 years and 80% at 10 years. The question to be answered is whether recurrence of tumor in the ipsilateral breast has an impact on survival. Radiation therapy cannot be considered inocuous. Keidan et al. (2) reported on the incidence of delayed breast abscess as a complication; after treatment of breast carcinoma by lumpectomy and radiation therapy, a 6% instance of delayed breast abscess was noted.—S.I. Schwartz, M.D.

References

1. Haffty RG, et al: *Arch Surg* 124:1266, 1989.
2. Keidan, et al: *Am Surg* 56:440, 1990.

Systemic Therapy in Patients With Node-Negative Breast Cancer: A Commentary Based on Two National Surgical Adjuvant Breast and Bowel Project (NSABP) Clinical Trials
Fisher B, Redmond C, Wickerham DL, Wolmark N, Bowman D, Couture J, Dimitrov NV, Margolese R, Legault-Poisson S, Robidoux A (Natl Surgical Breast and Bowel Project Headquarters, Pittsburgh)
Ann Intern Med 111:703–712, 1989   11–9

Data from 2 trials were reviewed to determine whether there are groups of patients who do not require systemic therapy, or groups of patients who fail to benefit from such treatment. A total of 731 patients with estrogen-receptor-negative tumors either were untreated after surgery or received sequential methotrexate and fluorouracil followed by leucovorin. Another 2,834 patients with estrogen-receptor-positive tumors received placebo or tamoxifen. Disease-free survival over 4 years was analyzed.

When untreated patients in either trial were analyzed, women proved to have a disease-free survival rate of less than 80% through 4 years of follow-up. In both trials, all subgroups of women benefited from active treatment.

All node-negative women with breast cancer, whether estrogen-receptor-positive or estrogen-receptor-negative, should receive systemic treatment. Patients who are candidates for systemic treatment should have the opportunity to receive it, even if the potential benefit is limited.

▶ This is a provocative article. Although there is no significant survival advantage, the fact that there is a significant prolongation of disease-free survival is a marked psychological advantage to any patient population. We could ask for all patients about to receive chemotherapy or tamoxifen, regardless of their node positivity, whether there is any place for axillary dissection over and above intellectual curiosity.—S.I. Schwartz, M.D.

Combined Therapy for Inflammatory Breast Cancer

Donegan WL, Padrta B (Med College of Wisconsin, Milwaukee)
Arch Surg 125:578–582, 1990   11–10

Inflammatory breast cancer is a distinct clinical entity with an ominous progression. Mastectomy alone has proved useless against this virulent tumor, but the availability of modern chemotherapy regimens has improved the prognosis. To evaluate the current management of inflammatory breast cancer and identify prognostic determinants, data were reviewed on 25 women aged 27–80 years, in whom inflammatory breast carcinoma was diagnosed in 1967–1987. Five of the women had distant metastases at the time of diagnosis.

Of the 20 patients without dissemination, 16 underwent combination chemotherapy, which was administered before local treatment with radiotherapy or surgery in 10 patients and given after local treatment in 4. One patient was treated with chemotherapy alone. Another patient had chemotherapy only after relapse. Mastectomy was performed on 10 patients, 9 of whom had axillary nodes removed.

The 5-year survival rate for all patients was 20%, the 5-year survival rate for the 20 patients without initial dissemination was 24%, the 3-year survival rate was 40%, and the median survival, 30 months; the 5-year survival rate in the presence of clinically involved axillary nodes was 22%. Patients with dermal lymphatic invasion had a 5-year survival rate of 29% compared with 21% for those without. The 5-year survival rate for patients without a distinct breast mass was 37%, whereas none of the patients with a distinct breast mass survived for 4 years. The 5-year survival rate for patients with stage III disease who underwent chemotherapy at any time was 20%, compared with 34% for patients who received hormonal therapy instead of chemotherapy. If mastectomy was included in the treatment, the 5-year survival rate was 28%, compared with 23% if it was not used. The 5-year survival rate for the 11 patients in whom chemotherapy was initiated before local therapy was 40%, compared with 0% for the 5 patients who received local therapy first.

These survival rates are comparable with those reported from other centers and are considerably higher than survival rates reported before 1981. The data from this analysis support initiating chemotherapy before local treatment. The role of mastectomy in achieving local control or improving survival warrants further investigation.

▶ This excellent review of a difficult problem offers a glimmer of hope. In the combination of chemotherapy and mastectomy radiation therapy has resulted in cure. Israel et al. (1) reported a median survival of >72 months when patients were treated with initial chemotherapy followed by total mastectomy and 2 years of maintenance chemotherapy. Zylberberg et al. (2) recorded a median survival >56 months for patients who had initial chemoimmunotherapy followed by radical surgery and a year of postoperative chemotherapy.—S.I. Schwartz, M.D.

References

1. Israel L, et al: *Cancer* 57:24, 1986.
2. Zylberberg B, et al: *Cancer* 49:1537, 1982.

12 The Head and the Neck

Malignant Tumors of Major Salivary Gland Origin: A Matched-Pair Analysis of the Role of Combined Surgery and Postoperative Radiotherapy
Armstrong JG, Harrison LB, Spiro RH, Fass DE, Strong EW, Fuks ZY (Mem Sloan-Kettering Cancer Ctr, New York)
Arch Otolaryngol Head Neck Surg 116:290–293, 1990   12–1

Malignant tumors of the major salivary glands are rare, making up 6% of all head and neck cancers. A review of 35 years' surgical experience at the Memorial Sloan-Kettering Cancer Center indicated that local-regional recurrence followed surgical treatment alone in 39% of 623 patients with malignant parotid tumors and in 60% of 129 with submandibular primaries. These results reveal the high incidence of recurrence, particularly in patients with more advanced disease, and indicate the need for an adjuvant treatment that can improve on the results of surgery alone.

In a group of 155 patients with previously untreated, nonmetastatic malignant tumors of major salivary gland origin who had definitive treatment between 1966 and 1982 at Memorial Sloan-Kettering Cancer Center, 46 patients were treated with combined surgery and postoperative radiotherapy. Radiation dosage ranged from 4,000 to 7,740 cGy (median, 5,664 cGy). A comparison was made with 46 patients from a total of 319 patients treated surgically without postoperative radiotherapy between 1939 and 1965.

The 5-year determinate survival rate for the patients with stages I and II disease receiving combined therapy vs. patients undergoing surgery alone was 81.9% vs. 95.8%, whereas for those with stage III or IV disease it was 51.2% vs. 9.5%, respectively. The local control for stages III and IV in those given combined therapy compared with those receiving only surgery at 5 years was 51.3% vs. 16.8%. In patients with nodal metastases, the 5-year determinate survival rate in the combined-therapy group vs. the surgery-only group was 48.9% vs. 18.7%, and the corresponding local-regional control was 69.1% vs. 40.2%. Postoperative radiotherapy significantly improves the outcome for patients with stage III or IV disease and for those patients with lymph node metastases.

▶ This typically large series from Memorial Sloan-Kettering Cancer Center provides interesting data for the surgeon dealing with salivary gland tumors. Although it suffers from the use of 2 comparative time periods instead of simultaneously randomized groups, the evidence appears overwhelming that postoperative radiotherapy is useful in stage III and stage IV tumors.—M.C. Robson, M.D.

Multiple Synchronous and Metachronous Cancers of the Upper Aerodigestive Tract: A Nine-Year Study

Panosetti E, Luboinski B, Mamelle G, Richard J-M (Kantonsspital, Luzern, Switzerland; Inst Gustave Roussy, Villejuif, France)
Laryngoscope 99:1267–1273, 1989   12–2

There has been renewed interest in multiple primary cancers associated with the recent development of screening endoscopy. A retrospective review of 9,089 patients treated for cancer of the head and neck included 855 patients with multiple primary cancers treated between 1975 and 1983, for an incidence of 9.4%. Men comprised almost 94% of the patients. The mean age was 55.5 years. Of the multiple cancers, 350 (42%) were judged to be synchronous, whereas 480 (58%) were classified as metachronous.

Of the metachronous cancers, 50% developed within 31 months after the first primary; the mean time between development of the first and second primary tumors was 45 months. About 22% of second primary tumors were diagnosed more than 5 years after the initial tumor.

The 5-year survival rates were higher for metachronous cancer patients (55%) than for those with synchronous cancers (18%). The patient's age was not a statistically significant factor in survival. Survival rates varied according to the treatment. In 49% of synchronous tumors, treatment had to be modified because of the presence of 2 cancers. In these patients the 5-year survival rates were as low as 8%. For patients with synchronous cancers that needed no modification of therapy, the prognosis was better and the survival rate was 28%.

In multiple synchronous cancers (350 cases), endoscopy was significantly useful in diagnosis of cancers of the hypopharynx, larynx, esophagus, and lung. For cancers in the oropharynx and oral cavity, clinical evidence indicated the diagnosis in about 50%. The initial tumor in synchronous cancers was located in the oropharynx in 100 cases (29%), in the oral cavity in 95 (27%), in the hypopharynx in 80 (23%), and in the larynx in 32 (9%). In 36 cases, the initial tumor was outside the ear, nose, or throat; 9 were in the lung, 11 in the esophagus, and 16 in other areas. These findings led to the conclusion that synchronous cancer will usually be located in adjacent, rather than in more distant, areas. Treatment consisted of radiotherapy in 234 patients, primary surgery alone in 31, and surgery with radiotherapy in 57. Chemotherapy was administered to 10 patients. In 18 patients no therapy was considered.

In metachronous cancers, the site of the first primary was the oropharynx in 120 patients, the oral cavity in 103, the larynx in 87, and the hypopharynx in 92. In 61 patients the primary tumor was not in the otorhinolaryngologic area. When the first cancer was in the oral cavity, the second primary occurred most often in the oropharynx, hypopharynx, or oral cavity itself. If the first cancer was noted in the oropharynx, the second was generally in the oral cavity and the lung. In treatment of metachronous cancers, the protocol for the second tumor could be used in 82% of the patients. The 5-year survival rate for simultaneous cancers (273 patients) treated as if they were the only known cancer was 22%. The 5-year survival rate fell to 15% for the 77 patients whose second tumor was noted after treatment of the first cancer was started or after therapy was concluded.

There is a fundamental difference between the prognosis for synchronous cancers and that for metachronous cancers. Treatment of multiple cancers should include, in addition to the classic therapy of surgery and radiotherapy, new methods such as chemotherapy and immunomodulation.

▶ This large series shows how poorly the patient with synchronous tumors fares and how relatively well the one with metachronous tumors might do. As might be expected, the longer the period between metachronous lesions, the better the prognosis. When possible, synchronous tumors should each receive full therapeutic treatment. Because this is often not possible, new modalities appear to be required if synchronous tumors are to be controlled. What is not discussed in this article are novel approaches at immunostimulation in patients with synchronous tumors.—M.C. Robson, M.D.

Patterns of Cervical Node Metastases From Squamous Carcinoma of the Oropharynx and Hypopharynx

Candela FC, Kothari K, Shah JP (Mem Sloan-Kettering Cancer Ctr, New York)
Head Neck 12:197–203, 1990   12–3

Radical neck dissection with comprehensive clearance of neck levels I through V has been the traditional approach to excision of neck node metastases in patients with squamous cell carcinoma of the oropharynx and hypopharynx. Modifications in the extent of lymphadenectomy have been suggested, especially for N_0 and N_1 patients.

A retrospective review was undertaken to determine the prevalence and patterns of regional lymph node metastases in a series of 333 patients selected from among 646 patients with oropharyngeal and hypopharyngeal carcinoma treated at a single institution during a 22-year period. The selected patients were previously untreated and had undergone classic radical neck dissection. They ranged in age from 12 to 84 years; 234 were males (70%) and 99 were females (30%). At the time of surgery, 71 had elective dissection in the N_0 neck and 259 underwent immediate therapeutic dissection in the N+ neck.

Neck levels II, III, and IV were at greatest risk of nodal metastases from primary squamous cell carcinoma of the oropharynx or hypopharynx (Fig 12–1). Clinical N_0 patients rarely had involvement of neck level I (1.4%) or V (1.4%). Such involvement was significantly higher in the N+ group—12.6% for neck level I and 9.7% for neck level V. Level V involvement, always associated with nodal metastases at other neck levels, occurred only in N_2 or more involved necks.

The findings appear to support the current trend toward modified neck dissection in N_0 patients. In these cases, an anterior neck dissection com-

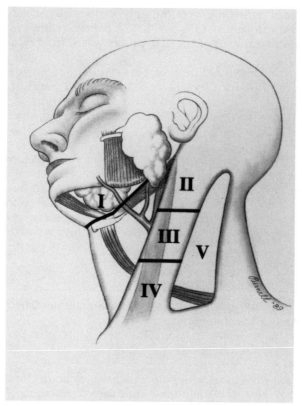

Fig 12-1.—Cervical lymph node levels used for description of clinical and pathologic findings. (Courtesy of Candela FC, Kothari K, Shah JP: *Head Neck* 12:197-203, 1990.)

prising levels II–IV should remove most nodal metastases. Any patients with N+ disease or histologic evidence of nodal metastases should undergo a comprehensive neck dissection.

▶ Further evidence is provided by the authors that the standard radical neck dissection is not always necessary. As all of these patients had a complete dissection, it allowed an exact comparison of the primary and the resultant histologic metastases. The data clearly support modified neck dissections for clinical N_0 patients.—M.C. Robson, M.D.

Squamous Cell Carcinoma of the Supraglottic Larynx Without Clinically Detectable Lymph Node Metastases: Problem of Local Relapse and Influence of Overall Treatment Time
Hoekstra CJM, Levendag PC, van Putten WLJ (Dr Daniel den Hoed Cancer Ctr/ Univ Hosp Dijkzigt, Rotterdam)
Int J Radiat Oncol Biol Phys 18:13–21, 1990

12–4

The management of patients with supraglottic carcinoma of the larynx without clinically detectable lymph nodes is controversial. Patients were followed for a mean of 10 years to assess results of treatment on the control rate of the primary tumor and the influence of overall treatment time.

During a 15-year period, 212 patients were treated for primary supraglottic carcinoma T_{1-4} N_0 M_0. The 203 patients with squamous cell carcinoma were studied. The mean age was 61 years, and most (184) were men. Seven tumors were T_1, 101 were T_2, 36 were T_3, and 59 were T_4.

Curative treatment was undertaken with radiation therapy only, reserving surgery for those in whom radiation failed. A total dose of 40 Gy was delivered. The 132 patients who had a good response to radiation therapy continued to a full dose of 60–70 Gy. Of the patients having a poor response who were eligible for surgical treatment, 23 eventually underwent surgery. Thirty-three patients, however, refused surgery or were unable to undergo an operation and received a second course of radiation.

Advancing T stage was associated with a lower rate of survival and a higher rate of local relapse. The 5-year relapse-free survival rate was 53% for T_2 tumors and 39% for T_4 tumors. Age was also a factor: patients older than age 60 years had a 2.2 times higher risk of dying of laryngeal cancer. Although relapse-free survival was similar for those who responded initially to radiation or had a second course, corrected survival for the latter group was worse (44% vs. 69%). Corrected survival was comparable for the patients who responded to radiation or radiation plus surgery (64% vs. 69%).

Seventy-one patients died of intercurrent disease—a mortality rate 1.8 times as high as might be expected in the normal population. More than half of these patients had a second primary tumor. Although no influence of radiation dose was found on local relapse rate, there was a positive association between this rate and overall treatment time.

▶ This sizable series of supraglottic laryngeal cancers clinically localized allows some therapeutic conclusions. The main one is that T_1–T_3, N_0 M_0 lesions respond well to radiotherapy alone, allowing voice preservation. The data must not be overinterpreted, however, because there was no randomization and surgery was used only after radiation failed.—M.C. Robson, M.D.

Morphometric Evaluation of Intracytoplasmic Lipid in Normal and Pathological Parathyroid Glands
Cinti S, Sbarbati A, Zancanaro C, Morroni M, Franceschini F, Carboni V, Lo Cascio V (Univ of Ancona, Italy; Univ of Verona, Italy)
J Pathol 160:31–34, 1990   12–5

The cytoplasmic content of lipid has been the chief morphological criterion for classifying parathyroid glands as "normal," "suppressed," or "activated." To assess the validity of this criterion, 10 normal parathyroid glands from patients undergoing thyroidectomy, 20 enlarged "adenomatous" glands from patients with primary hyperparathyroidism, and 20 glands of normal size from the same hyperparathyroid patients were studied.

In normal parathyroid glands, cytoplasmic lipid comprised almost 2.5% of the total parenchymal area. A similar result was found in the "normal" parathyroid glands of hyperparathyroid subjects (2.2%) but with a wider range of values. The mean value of lipid in the "adenomatous" glands was significantly lower (1.3%) than that in the other 2 groups.

The "normal" glands removed from hyperparathyroid patients contained chief cells that appeared active despite abundant cytoplasmic lipid. Signs of cell activation included well-developed rough endoplasmic reticulum, hypertrophy of the Golgi apparatus, and interdigitation of plasma membranes.

When individual data were considered, there was considerable overlap in lipid content values between normal and pathologic parathyroid glands. Thus one must be cautious in using the lipid content criterion to assess the functional status of the parathyroid gland, mainly when differentiating between adenoma and hyperplasia.

▶ What has been regarded as a diagnostic aid in determining normal as opposed to suppressed or activated parathyroid glands is challenged by this article (1). Cytoplasmic lipid or fat was shown not to be diagnostic. The surgeon must question his pathologist as to his diagnostic criteria for determining a normal or abnormal gland.—M.C. Robson, M.D.

Reference

1. Roth SI, et al: *Am J Pathol* 84:521, 1976.

Blood Use in Head and Neck Tumor Surgery: Potential for Autologous Blood

McCulloch TM, Glenn MG, Riley D, Weymuller EA Jr (Univ of Washington)
Arch Otolaryngol Head Neck Surg 115:1314–1317, 1989   12–6

Patients who undergo scheduled surgery may be able to use their own previously donated blood should a transfusion be necessary. This method avoids potential exposure to blood that is contaminated, as well as transfusion reaction and immunosuppression. The blood product requirements of patients with head and neck tumors were examined to determine whether this patient group could make use of autologous blood.

During 1987 a total of 77 patients at 3 hospitals underwent major surgical resections for head and neck carcinoma. The parameters examined included tumor site and stage, surgical procedure, preoperative and postoperative hematocrit values, estimated blood loss, operative and postoperative blood product use, and operative time.

Maxillectomy-midface procedures led to the highest average estimated blood loss (1,037 mL) and the highest average blood use (1.5 units), followed by composite resections and laryngectomies. In the assessable groups, previous radiation therapy did not make a significant difference in blood loss or procedure time. Estimated blood loss, however, had a positive correlation with procedure time in all groups.

A review of the patients' medical history and preoperative hematocrit values indicated that 84% met all donor requirements and 65% satisfied all criteria for autologous blood product use with a well-planned preoperative donation of 2 units of blood. Thus with proper planning and timing the use of autologous blood appears to be reasonable and safe in head and neck surgery.

▶ In this era of fear of blood-transmitted diseases, this article is of practical use. The authors reviewed their blood loss and transfusion requirements to predict future usage. However, the usefulness is mainly to suggest that each surgeon must determine his or her own practice, because the values of other surgeons may not apply universally.— M.C. Robson, M.D.

Intraoperative Radiotherapy of Head and Neck Cancer
Freeman SB, Hamaker RC, Singer MI, Pugh N, Garrett P, Ross D (Naval Hosp, Portsmouth, Va; Head and Neck Surgery Associates, Indianapolis; Methodist Hosp of Indiana, Indianapolis)
Arch Otolaryngol Head Neck Surg 116:165–168, 1990   12–7

Advances in endotracheal anesthesia and electronic monitoring have made intraoperative radiation therapy (IORT) feasible. The delivery of radiation during surgery allows direct exposure of all margins to maximum radiation without significant exposure of surrounding tissue. The value of IORT in treating aggressive, extensive, or recurrent cancers of the head and neck was assessed in 104 patients (mean age, 59 years) who were treated from 1982 to 1988.

Seventy-four patients had epidermoid carcinomas originating in the mucosa of the upper aerodigestive tract and 24 had salivary gland tumors. In 40 patients surgery plus IORT was the initial treatment; 64 patients received IORT during attempts at surgical salvage.

Technique.—After resection is complete the patient is transported to the radiation department while anesthesia is maintained intravenously. Areas of skin, mucosa, and bone that do not require radiation are protected with lead shielding. The surgical and radiation therapy teams leave the room and radiation is started. Areas in the oral cavity, salivary gland, and skull base are then treated (in this series, 15–20 Gy of radiation). The wound is then covered and the patient is returned to the operating room.

In 35 patients with squamous cell carcinoma who were followed for 2 or more years, 14 remained free of local recurrence (40%). Autopsies showed that local recurrence was outside the margin of the port in 22 of 25 patients who died with local disease. At a mean follow-up of 21 months, there had been no local recurrence of 4 adenocarcinomas and 8 adenoid cystic carcinomas treated with IORT.

These cancers that have a history of poor prognosis have in the past been treated with radioactive implants, but IORT has several advantages over this modality. Noninvolved tissue can be avoided, and delivery techniques are familiar to all radiation oncologists. The number of complications was acceptable, given the advanced nature of the disease. Overall, IORT is a safe and beneficial adjunctive therapy for aggressive or advanced cancer of the head and neck.

▶ This paper describes the logistics required for intraoperative radiotherapy. The figures are not convincing that the complexity of transfer is justified. Most disturbing is the number of local recurrences, which the authors state occurred "outside the margin of the port." Possibly in an attempt to cone down on the operative site, microscopic foci were not included. Another possibility is that the effect of postoperative angiogenesis and tumor growth is wider in the healing wound than would be supposed at the time of operation.—M.C. Robson, M.D.

Functional Effects of Intraoral Reconstruction With a Free Radial Forearm Flap

Michiwaki Y, Ohno K, Imai S, Yamashita Y, Suzuki N, Yoshida H, Michi K (Showa Univ, Tokyo)
J Craniomaxillofac Surg 18:164–168, 1990   12–8

Few studies have attempted to illuminate the characteristics of speech dysfunction after ablative surgery of the tongue and floor of the mouth; nor has surgical rehabilitation of this dysfunction been widely addressed. Patients undergoing glossectomy were studied to investigate speech impairment and evaluate the function of reconstruction with free radial forearm flaps.

Five men with oral cancer had hemiglossectomy or partial glossectomy, extirpation of the ipsilateral floor of the mouth, and upper neck dissection. These procedures were followed immediately by intraoral reconstruction with a free radial forearm flap. To evaluate the effects of reconstruction on the intelligibility of speech, 100 Japanese syllables and 3 groups of glossal sounds were used. The glossal sounds were chosen to evaluate anterior, middle, and posterior portions of the tongue.

Overall intelligibility scores ranged from 46% to 82% after hemiglossectomy, excluding the root of the tongue. Two patients scored particularly low for sounds produced by the rear part of the tongue, which suggests that suspension slings might prevent depression of the reconstructed tongue and floor of the mouth. A patient who had partial glossectomy achieved a score of 80.5% and excellent glossal sounds 1 year postoperatively. A patient who also had partial mandibulectomy had a score of 69%.

Many factors affect articulation after intraoral reconstruction. Intelligibility scores appear to plateau within 6 months to 1 year after surgery, probably because of compensatory efforts on the patient's part. Rear glossal sounds are difficult to compensate for, although some compensation has been noted. Articulation is affected by the condition of the teeth and oral tissues.

▶ Function has been used to assess reconstruction of the head and neck cancer patient much too infrequently. This paper attempts to evaluate speech postoperatively in the same detail used for cleft palate patients. Although not too many conclusions can be reached because of the small series reported here, I believe that this should be a landmark publication in that it suggests more rigid standards by which to assess functional operative results.—M.C. Robson, M.D.

Prevention of Second Primary Tumors With Isotretinoin in Squamous-Cell Carcinoma of the Head and Neck

Hong WK, Lippman SM, Itri LM, Karp DD, Lee JS, Byers RM, Schantz SP, Kramer AM, Lotan R, Peters LJ, Dimery IW, Brown BW, Goepfert H (Univ of Texas, Houston; Boston Veterans Affairs Hosp; Hoffman-LaRoche, Nutley, NJ)
N Engl J Med 323:795–801, 1990   12–9

Patients with head and neck cancer are at high risk for recurrent and second primary tumors even when they are disease free after local therapy. Retinoids are valuable in the treatment of premalignant oral lesions and hold promise for the prevention of epithelial carcinogenesis. A randomized, placebo-controlled study was made of the synthetic retinoid isotretinoin to test its efficacy in oral premalignant lesions.

The series comprised 103 patients who were disease free after primary treatment for squamous cell cancers of the larynx, pharynx, or oral cavity. After they completed surgery and/or radiotherapy, they were randomly assigned to either isotretinoin, $50–100$ mg/m^2/day, or placebo, both taken daily for 12 months.

No significant differences between groups were found with regard to number of local, regional, or distant recurrences of the primary disease. However, patients given isotretinoin had significantly fewer second primary tumors. After a median 32 months' follow-up, only 4% of those given isotretinoin had second primary tumors, compared with 24% given placebo. Four patients, all of whom were given placebo, had multiple second primary tumors. Of the 14 second cancers that occurred, 13 were in the head and neck, esophagus, or lung.

Daily therapy with high doses of isotretinoin effectively prevents second primary tumors in patients who have had treatment for squamous cell carcinoma of the head and neck. However, isotretinoin treatment does not prevent recurrences of the original tumor.

▶ As noted in a previous review, metachronous cancers of the upper aerodigestive tract are a problem. Because treatment of the second primary is not always successful, prevention is an obvious goal. This paper, suggesting that isotretinoin can prevent a second primary tumor, bears close scrutiny; if the data hold up in a larger population, this therapeutic approach will represent a significant advance.— M.C. Robson, M.D.

Treatment of Craniomaxillofacial Fibrous Dysplasia: How Early and How Extensive?
Chen Y-R, Noordhoff MS (Chang Gung Memorial Hosp, Taipei, Taiwan)
Plast Reconstr Surg 86:835–844, 1990   12–10

The progression of fibrous dysplasia generally stops after adolescence, but in some patients the lesions may keep on growing, causing both deformity and functional problems. Also, there have been more than 30 reports of malignant degeneration of this normally benign pathologic condition. A treatment policy was developed for patients with craniomaxillofacial fibrous dysplasia.

The craniomaxillofacial bone was classified into 4 major zones and treatment principals were developed for each of the zones (table). In zone 1—the facial area above the maxillary alveolar bone—dysplastic bone is excised and the defect reconstructed with autogenous bone graft. In zone 2—the hair-bearing cranium—only conservative shaving is performed, except in small areas connected to zone 1, where radical excision is continued. If there are no symptoms, no surgery is performed in zone 3, the central cranial base. If there is optic nerve compression, surgeons perform optic canal unroofing. Zone 4 includes the tooth-bearing bones. Only conservative shaving is done in this area.

Twenty-eight patients with craniomaxillofacial fibrous dysplasia were treated according to the plan as soon as symptoms occurred. Patients were followed from 1 to 11 years. There was no recurrence or invasion of fibrous dysplasia into grafted bone. One patient required orthognathic maxillary osteotomy on the reconstructed maxilla 6 years after initial treatment. Of 19 patients with alveolar dysplasia, 5 had recurrences that required reshaping. One patient needed mandibular sagittal osteotomies to set back a prognathic fibrous dysplastic mandible when conservative shaving failed after 3 attempts. Another patient with mandibular fibrous dysplasia had recurrence with pain. A hemimandibulectomy and immediate free vascularized iliac bone-graft reconstruction was successful.

In this plan, the principles of surgical treatment are based on the zones of involvement. There was no invasion of dysplasia into reconstructed bones in this series, and the reconstructed bones retained their contour satisfactorily at long-term follow-up.

Treatment Principles Related to Dysplastic Zones

	Reconstruction Importance	Anatomic Location	Treatment Procedure
Zone 1	Most evident facial part; can be completely excised; can be adequately reconstructed	Frontal, orbital, nasal, ethmoid, zygoma, upper maxilla	Radical excision and reconstruction
Zone 2	Hair-covered cranium	Parietal, part of occipital, temporal (lateral cranial base)	Optional: Conservative or radical
Zone 3	Difficult or dangerous	Central cranial base, petrous, mastoid, pterygoid, sphenoid	Observing; No surgery when no symptoms*
Zone 4a	Teeth-bearing	Maxillar alveolar bone	Conservative
4b	Teeth-bearing	Mandible	Conservative

*When there is optic nerve compression, optic canal unroofing is done.
(Courtesy of Chen Y-R, Noordhoff MS: *Plast Reconstr Surg* 86:835–844, 1990.)

▶ This large experience of craniomaxillofacial fibrous dysplasia attempts to set forth principles for operation based on regions of occurrence. It also explains that the disease process is not limited to children, as once thought. The discussion of this paper by Dr. Munro is worth reading to give a more complete treatise of the subject.—M.C. Robson, M.D.

13 The Thorax

Survival After Conservative Resection for T1 N0 M0 Non-Small Cell Lung Cancer
Read RC, Yoder G, Schaeffer RC (John L McClellan Mem Veterans Hosp, Little Rock, Ark; Univ of Arkansas)
Ann Thorac Surg 49:391–400, 1990   13–1

Lobectomy has long been standard procedure in the treatment for cure of primary lung cancer, whereas the role of conservative resection for cure is controversial. Between 1966 and 1988, conservative resection for $T_1N_0M_0$ non–small-cell lung cancer was attempted in 244 veterans aged 40–83 years (mean, 62 years). Lung cancer had been diagnosed on routine radiography during hospitalization or in medical, preoperative, or pension evaluations. All except 1 were smokers, and all except 2 were men. Most (68%) were asymptomatic for pulmonary disease. The patients underwent 131 lobectomies, 107 segmentectomies, and 6 wedge resections.

The 30-day mortality was 2.9%. The overall survival rates were 95% at 1 year, 83% at 3 years, and 78% at 5 years. The absolute 5-year survival rate, when only deaths from the initial lesion were considered, was 51%. There were 15 local recurrences in the lobectomy group and 5 in the segmentectomy group. New lung cancer developed in 21 patients, 6 of whom underwent reoperation; 14 of these died. The average lesion diameter was 2 cm. Patients with small tumors had a better chance of survival than those with lesions greater than 2 cm. Routine preoperative CT staging and intraoperative sampling of even normal-sized hilar and mediastinal nodes, conducted after 1982, improved survival. Squamous histology was more favorable than nonsquamous. All nonsquamous deep-seated bronchial tumors were highly malignant.

The $T_1N_0M_0$ category of lung cancer is not uniform. Survival after curative resection is significantly influenced by comorbidity, metachronous lung cancer, and staging. Whereas deep-seated lesions require lobectomy, conservative resection can be used to treat the other lesions, with minimal risk of local recurrence. In this patient population, the results of conservative resection were similar or actually better than those of lobectomy.

▶ The value of conservative resection in this favorable group of lung neoplasms, less than 2 cm in size, is documented in this report, describing experiences with 244 patients treated over a period of 19 years. The 5-year survival rate from a cancer-related death was 78%.—F.C. Spencer, M.D.

Selection Factors Resulting in Improved Survival After Surgical Resection of Tumors Metastatic to the Lungs

Marincola FM, Mark JBD (Stanford Med Ctr, Calif)
Arch Surg 125:1387–1393, 1990   13–2

A number of studies have reported 5-year cure rates of 25% to 40% after resection of metastatic tumor from the lung. A review was made of experience with 140 patients who had 184 operations for this purpose between 1973 and 1987. Five-year follow-up was achieved in 102 cases. Many of the patients had sarcomas, and 44% had solitary metastatic lesions. Only 18% were symptomatic.

Overall survival rates were 63% at 3 years and 48% at 5 years. All groups of patients, except for those with melanoma and breast cancer, had 3-year rates exceeding 50% and 5-year survival rates of more than 40%. Conservative resection was the rule; there were only 3 pneumonectomies. No patients died postoperatively while hospitalized. Patients with smaller lesions and those free of disease for more than a year tended to do well, but survival was unrelated to age or number of metastatic lesions present.

At present, patients are selected for pulmonary metastectomy if it appears that all tumor can be removed, that the patient can tolerate the planned operation, and that the primary tumor is controlled. In addition, there should be no tumor elsewhere in the body, and no other reasonable treatment should be available. Possibly more stringent criteria should apply to melanoma patients.

▶ This report details experiences at Stanford with 140 patients undergoing surgical removal of pulmonary metastases over a period of 14 years. Slightly more than half of the patients had multiple metastases. A conservative resection was usually done, with single or multiple wedge resections performed in the majority of patients. A median sternotomy incision was preferred for bilateral metastases. The authors make the important observation that many patients thought to have unilateral lesions are found to have bilateral lesions at the time of sternotomy. The 5-year survival was near 50%, with the exception of those with melanoma and breast cancer, who seemed to derive little benefit from resection. Hence, these data reaffirm that surgical removal of multiple pulmonary metastases gives excellent results in carefully selected patients, especially those who have no sign of tumor elsewhere.—F.C. Spencer, M.D.

Systemic Arterial Air Embolism in Penetrating Lung Injury

Estrera AS, Pass LJ, Platt MR (Univ of Texas, Dallas)
Ann Thorac Surg 50:257–261, 1990   13–3

Systemic arterial air embolism may be an unrecognized cause of death in patients having isolated penetrating lung injury. Nine patients with such injuries were seen from 1975 to 1983. Six had gunshot and 3 had stab wound injuries. Arterial air embolism developed after lung injury in these patients.

All but 1 of the patients were in profound shock or had cardiac arrest. All received positive-pressure ventilation. Air was directly visualized in the coronary vessels and, in 3 patients, it was aspirated from the left ventricular apex and aortic root. Five patients had significant hemoptysis. Each patient was found to have a deep puncture or a through-and-through wound of the lung close to the hilum. In 5 cases a massive amount of blood was suctioned from the endotracheal tube, compromising ventilation. Four patients survived surgery and 3 recovered completely.

Sudden hemodynamic collapse of a previously stable patient should suggest the possibility of systemic arterial air embolism, as should hemoptysis or recovery of blood from the endotracheal tube. An air leak with foamy air-blood admixed together also suggests arterial air embolism. Once suspected, the hilus or pedicle of the involved lobe or lung should be clamped immediately. This is the one traumatic setting in which evaluation and resuscitation must proceed simultaneously.

▶ This unusual report seems very significant for patients with penetrating thoracic injuries. The 9 case reports tabulated in Table 1 of the full-length article should be studied in detail. In brief, systemic arterial air embolism was documented in 9 patients with penetrating injuries of the lung, only 3 of whom survived. The diagnosis was established by direct observation of air in the coronary arteries; the true frequency is unknown. The significant factors that can produce this serious complication include a penetrating injury near the hilum that simultaneously injures a bronchus and a large pulmonary vein. Hence, hemoptysis is frequent. Positive-pressure ventilation with pressures of more than 40–50 mm may force air into the pulmonary veins, with resultant entry into the arterial circulation. In these circumstances the syndrome can be suspected by the sudden onset of ventricular fibrillation, resulting from coronary emboli.

Once diagnosed, the hilum to the injured lung segment should be clamped immediately, after which measures can be undertaken for removal of air from the heart and defibrillation. To repeat, the sudden onset of ventricular fibrillation in such patients should alert the operating surgeon to the possibility of coronary embolism. The authors are to be complimented for documenting this unusual syndrome. It may occur far more frequently than is currently recognized.— F.C. Spencer, M.D.

Empyema Thoracis: A Review of a 4½ Year Experience of Cases Requiring Surgical Treatment

Forty J, Yeatman M, Wells FC (Papworth Hosp, Cambridge, England)
Respir Med 84:147–153, 1990
13–4

Empyema thoracis is a relatively common and severely debilitating illness caused by drainage of pus from an intrathoracic abscess. Although the literature of the past 7 years is controversial about the role of surgery in the treatment of an established empyema, early surgical treatment may significantly shorten the length of postoperative recovery.

Between 1985 and 1989, 37 males and 16 females aged 16–77 years were referred from elsewhere for the surgical treatment of empyema thoracis. Twenty-seven patients had empyema after bronchopneumonia, and 6 patients had primary lung disorders. Thirty-five patients had associated illnesses. The duration of symptoms on admission ranged from 4 days to 3 years (mean, 40 weeks). Forty-seven patients underwent thoracotomy, decortication, and excision of empyema as their primary treatment; 6 patients were treated by rib resection. Twenty patients had undergone previous tube drainage for 7–42 days. All patients were treated with intravenously administered antibiotics to control systemic sepsis before and during operation, but antibiotic therapy contributed little to the treatment of the intrapleural abscess.

Five patients with significant accompanying debilitating disease who underwent decortication died within 7 days of operation. None of the patients having rib resection died. Major wound infections developed in 3 patients. Chest drains placed at the time of operation were removed after a median of 7 days (mean, 12 days). The median postoperative in-hospital stay was 13 days (mean, 20 days). This is in stark contrast to the mean hospital stay of 103.6 days before referral for surgical treatment. None of the patients had a recurrence of empyema or any other major complications during a postoperative follow-up of 1 year.

Although thoracotomy, decortication, and excision of the empyema remains a major surgical procedure, this approach achieves excellent results with minimal morbidity and mortality in patients with empyema thoracis without other chronic underlying illnesses. Tube drainage or rib resection should be first considered in those with accompanying chronic or debilitating illness.

▶ The data in this short report from a regional thoracic surgical center in England are impressive. In a period of about 4 years, 53 cases of empyema were treated, 47 by decortication. Twenty patients had previous tube drainage for nearly 3 weeks before referral.

Recovery after decortication was prompt, with cessation of chest drainage within about a week and discharge from the hospital in 2–3 weeks. Five deaths occurred, all in severely debilitated patients with chronic illness.

These results reaffirm the safety and efficacy of decortication when empyema is refractory to simpler forms of treatment. The prolonged morbidity from continued ineffective tube drainage should be avoided; decortication can be undertaken as soon as it becomes clear that tube drainage will not be successful.—F.C. Spencer, M.D.

Postpneumonectomy Emphysema: The Role of Intrathoracic Muscle Transposition
Pairolero PC, Arnold PG, Trastek VF, Meland NB, Kay PP (Mayo Clinic and Found, Rochester, Minn)
J Thorac Cardiovasc Surg 99:958–968, 1990   13–5

Empyema developing after pneumonectomy is infrequent but serious; it often is associated with bronchopleural fistula. The results of surgical management were reviewed in 45 consecutive patients seen from 1980 to 1989 with postpneumonectomy empyema. About 75% of the patients had undergone pneumonectomy for cancer. The median time between pneumonectomy and the diagnosis of empyema was 4 weeks.

All patients were managed initially by open pleural drainage. A bronchopleural fistula was closed in 28 patients and the closure reinforced by muscle transposition. Seven patients received multiple flaps. The serratus anterior muscle was transposed most often, followed by the latissimus dorsi and the pectoralis major. The pleural cavity was then obliterated with antibiotic solution and the pleural window closed. The median number of procedures was 5.

Operative mortality was 13%. All perioperative deaths occurred in patients whose chest wall was never closed. During a median follow-up of 22 months, 26 of 31 patients having the complete Clagett procedure gained a healed chest wall without evidence of recurrent infection. The bronchopleural fistula remained closed in 24 of 28 cases. No late deaths were related to postpneumonectomy empyema. Transposition of extrathoracic skeletal muscle, in conjunction with the Clagett procedure, is an effective approach to postpneumonectomy empyema.

▶ This report provides a lot of valuable data for the serious complication of postpneumonectomy empyema. This is especially a problem when an associated bronchopleural fistula is present. In this series of 45 patients with empyema, 28 had an associated bronchopleural fistula closed with a muscle transposition at the time of open drainage. After the fistula was closed and the pleural cavity cleaned, the second stage of the Clagett procedure was performed. The length of hospitalization ranged widely (average, 34 days), and the operative mortality rate was about 13%. Among the 39 survivors, 84% had a healed chest wall, with the bronchopleural fistula remaining closed in about 86%. These data well support the approach of pleural drainage, closure of the fistula with a muscle flap, and subsequent closure of the clean pleural cavity.—F.C. Spencer, M.D.

Primary Tracheal Tumors: Treatment and Results
Grillo HC, Mathisen DJ (Massachusetts Gen Hosp, Boston; Harvard Med School)
Ann Thorac Surg 49:69–77, 1990   13–6

Primary tumors of the trachea are rare. In a 26-year period 196 patients with primary tracheal tumors were evaluated. A total of 147 tumors were excised, including 132 by resection and primary reconstruction, 7 by laryngotracheal resection or cervicomediastinal exenteration, and 8 by staged procedures. Eleven tumors were explored. Forty-four squamous cell carcinomas, 60 adenoid cystic tumors, and 43 other benign or malignant tumors were resected.

Among the 132 patients who underwent primary resection and reconstruction there were 7 operative deaths (5%). One death occurred among the 82 tracheal reconstructions and 6 among the 50 carinal reconstructions. There were 6 stenoses after tracheal or carinal resections, and all patients successfully underwent reresection. There were 5 deaths in the 8 patients who underwent staged reconstruction, and the procedure was abandoned.

Twenty of 41 survivors of resection of squamous cell carcinomas are alive and free of disease (some for more than 25 years). Thirty-nine of 52 patients with adenoid cystic carcinoma and 35 of 42 with other tumors (5 were lost to follow-up) are also alive and free of disease. Analysis of survival showed a sharp decrease in the number of patients free of squamous cell carcinoma 3 years after resection, with little disease thereafter; patients with adenoid cystic carcinoma remained disease free for many years but appeared to be threatened by late recurrence.

Positive lymph nodes or invasive diseases at resection margins were associated with poor prognosis in patients with squamous cell carcinoma but had little effect on patients with adenoid cystic carcinoma. Resection combined with irradiation provided tripled survival time for those with squamous cell carcinoma and at least tripled survival time for those with adenoid cystic carcinoma.

Based on this 26-year experience, the following therapeutic recommendations for the treatment of primary tracheal tumors appear to be justified. Benign primary tumors of the trachea and tumors of intermediate aggressiveness should be treated by surgical resection with reconstruction of the airway. Primary squamous cell carcinoma, adenoid cystic carcinoma, and malignant primary tracheal tumors of other types should be treated by resection when primary reconstruction can be accomplished safely. Resection should probably be followed by full-dose mediastinal irradiation in most patients.

▶ This extensive report by Grillo, certainly one of the world's authorities on tracheal surgery, represents a vast experience with primary tracheal tumors—198 treated in a 26-year period. About two thirds, 132, were treated by resection, and 50 of these required carinal resection. Mortality was very low with tracheal resection, with only 1 death, rising to an overall mortality rate of near 5% with carinal repair.

Quite encouraging is the fact that long-term survival was very good—more than 50% with squamous carcinoma and nearly 80% with adnoid cystic carcinoma.—F.C. Spencer, M.D.

Clinical Experience With the Silicone Tracheal Prosthesis
Neville WE, Bolanowski PJP, Kotia GG (UMDNJ–New Jersey Med School, Newark)
J Thorac Cardiovasc Surg 99:604–613, 1990   13–7

It is best to use autologous tissue for tracheal reconstruction, but an alternative method is required when this is not feasible. In 62 patients seen from 1970 to 1988 with benign or malignant tracheal stenosis, airway continuity was reestablished with a silicone tube.

The molded silicone prosthesis used was a straight graft in 48 cases; 14 patients received a bifurcated unit. The involved tracheal segments were removed from 27 of the former patients, 7 of whom had a primary malignancy. Six of 21 patients in whom the stent was placed intraluminally, rather than being sutured to the luminal margins, had primary malignancy. All patients given a bifurcated graft had tracheocarinal cancer.

Suture-line granulations were managed by intermittent fulguration or laser vaporization. Subglottic granulomas developed in 2 patients. There was 1 instance of graft dehiscence, which was managed by replacement with a silicone T tube. No patient acquired mediastinal infection or had impeded pulmonary secretions across long tubular segments.

Silicone tubes function satisfactorily as an airway in patients with benign or malignant tracheal stenosis. Ciliated epithelium appears not necessary to prevent mucus encrustations within the prosthesis.

▶ This report summarizes 18 years of experience by Dr. Neville with 62 patients who had airway continuity established with a silicone tube. Dr. Neville has studied the possibilities of silicone tracheal prostheses for more than 2 decades, and his cumulative experiences are thus uniquely valuable.

Although may problems developed in patients with critical illnesses, the silicone tubes continued to function for many years without disastrous complications developing. Clearly, sputum can be expectorated across the silicone tube, even though these are not covered by epithelium. In serious illnesses, when direct resection and anastomosis are not feasible, silicone tubes seem to be a reasonable alternative.—F.C. Spencer, M.D.

Primary Mediastinal Nonseminomatous Germ Cell Tumors: Results of a Multimodality Approach
Wright CD, Kesler KA, Nichols CR, Mahomed Y, Einhorn LH, Miller ME, Brown JW (Indiana Univ, Indianapolis)
J Thorac Cardiovasc Surg 99:210–217, 1990   13–8

Primary mediastinal nonseminomatous germ cell tumors account for 1% to 3.5% of all tumors of the mediastinum and 1% to 2% of all germ cell tumors in men. Before cisplatin-based chemotherapy was developed, long-term survival was rare. Presently, the main treatment is chemotherapy with surgery as an adjuvant to achieve a complete response.

Between 1976 and 1988, 48 males aged 14–46 years underwent multimodality treatment for primary mediastinal nonseminomatous germ cell tumor. Twenty-eight patients received initial therapy and 20 were referred for salvage chemotherapy after initial chemotherapy received elsewhere had failed. All patients had a large symptomatic mass in the anterior part of the mediastinum ranging in size from 6 × 6 cm to 20 × 25 cm on chest radiographs. Forty-four patients had elevated serum tumor marker levels at the time of diagnosis. Seven patients had pulmonary metastases on initial examination. The diagnosis was established by biopsy alone in 32 patients. Chemotherapy was individualized, but it commonly consisted of cisplatin and etoposide-based regimens before 1983, and cisplatin plus ifosfamide plus either vinblastine or etoposide after 1983.

There was no surgical mortality and no initial mortality from induction chemotherapy. Twenty-two of the 28 patients treated initially had a complete response, as defined by normal serum tumor marker levels and absence of residual tumor; 16 of these underwent resection of residual disease after chemotherapy, 4 had total or near total resection before chemotherapy, and only 2 had chemotherapy alone. Seventeen patients were alive after this treatment, with a median survival of 64 months and a Kaplan-Meier 5-year survival rate of 57%. Ten patients had a relapse after complete remission and required salvage chemotherapy; 2 subsequently had a complete response, but only 1 survived. Only 1 of the 20 patients referred from elsewhere for salvage treatment was a long-term, disease-free survivor. The keys to a successful outcome in patients with primary mediastinal nonseminomatous germ cell tumor include intensive cisplatin-based chemotherapy, salvage chemotherapy if necessary, and aggressive surgical resection to remove residual tumor.

▶ The development of cisplatin-based chemotherapy dramatically changed the outlook in unusual patients with a primary mediastinal nonseminomatous germ cell tumor. Such tumors account for only 25% of all tumors of the mediastinum. Survival after either radiation or surgical resection was unusual before effective chemotherapy. In this series of 28 patients who received their initial therapy at Indiana University, 22 of 28 had a complete response to treatment, measured by normal serum tumor markers. Of this group, 16 had resection of residual disease after chemotherapy, 4 beforehand. The preferred practice is to administer chemotherapy beforehand, then proceed with operation. The 5-year survival was 57%. By contrast, of 20 patients referred after initial unsuccessful therapy elsewhere, only 1 survived.—F.C. Spencer, M.D.

A Comparison of Transhiatal and Transthoracic Resection for Carcinoma of the Thoracic Esophagus
Fok M, Siu KF, Wong J (Univ of Hong Kong)
Am J Surg 158:414–419, 1989   13–9

Most patients with carcinoma of the esophagus are incurable. Although it is generally agreed that surgical resection offers the best palliation, the relative merits of using the transhiatal nonthoracotomy approach or the transthoracic route have not been well studied.

During a 4½-year period, 294 patients underwent resection for carcinoma of the esophagus; 210 of these had tumors located in the middle and lower thirds of the thoracic esophagus. Of these 210 patients, 172 (82%) (mean age, 60 years) had transthoracic resection and 38 (18%) (mean age, 67 years) had transhiatal resection. The latter took an average of 190 minutes to complete, whereas the average duration of a transthoracic resection was 240 minutes. The average blood loss with both operations was similar.

A significant number of intraoperative complications occurred when the transhiatal route was used, including excessive bleeding and tumor perforation as a result of blunt dissection (7 patients, 18%) and recurrent nerve injury (5 patients, 13%). Tracheal damage or chylothorax did not occur. The incidence of postoperative complications was similar with either approach.

The hospital mortality was 18% with transhiatal resection and 16% with transthoracic resection. The 30-day mortality was 8% with transhiatal resection and 5% with transthoracic resection. Malignant cachexia, respiratory failure, and sepsis, the 3 most common causes of in-hospital death, also accounted for all deaths after 30 days. The late mortality was 11% after transhiatal resection and 12% after transthoracic resection. Actuarial survival analysis showed a survival advantage for the transthoracic approach: The median survival was 6.3 months after the transhiatal approach and 11.3 months after the transthoracic approach. The latter approach would appear to be preferred unless there are serious adverse factors that contraindicate its use.

▶ With the current interest in transhiatal esophagectomy, this report from Hong Kong of experiences with 210 patients is of particular interest. Results with 172 transthoracic resections were compared with 38 performed by the transhiatal method. Although operative mortality and morbidity were similar in both groups, late survival by life-table analysis showed the transhiatal approach to be significantly inferior. Such results are certainly consistent with the thesis that a more effective tumor operation can be performed by the transthoracic approach even though the 5-year survival is small, no matter what technique is used.—F.C. Spencer, M.D.

Tracheobronchial Obstructions in Infants and Children: Experience With 45 Cases
deLorimier AA, Harrison MR, Hardy K, Howell LJ, Adzick NS (Univ of California, San Francisco)
Ann Surg 212:277–289, 1990   13–10

The management of high-grade intrathoracic tracheo-bronchial obstructions was evaluated in 45 infants and children. Six infants had segmental stenosis of the trachea, defined as involvement of less than half the length of the airway. Twelve infants had elongated stenosis involving more than half the length of the trachea, and 11 had complete annular cartilage rings along the entire length of the trachea. Sixteen patients had severe tracheomalacia, including 6 with associated aortic arch and branch vessel anomalies and 9 with associated esophageal atresia.

Segmental tracheal resection was performed in 17 patients, including 7 with complete ring stenosis, 1 with an intact membranous trachea, 4 with localized severe tracheomalacia, 1 with a polypoid hamartoma, and 2 with recurrent granulomation tissue in a rib cartilage graft. Resection of bronchial stenosis in 2 patients resulted in a widely patent bronchus. Three anastomotic strictures occurred in 3 infants less than 23 weeks old. The stricture was related to excessive tension on the anastomosis when 50% of the trachea was resected, and another was related to an elongated and narrow lumen. The other patient with a stricture had tracheomalacia associated with a double aortic arch. Resection of the stricture resulted in an excellent airway in 2 infants and recurrence of the stricture in 1. Rib cartilage grafts were used in 5 patients. Three had elongated stenosis with complete tracheal rings, 2 of whom subsequently required resection. The other 2 patients had tracheomalacia, and 1 had excellent outcome.

Primary segmental tracheobronchial resection and re-resection of recurrent stenosis are highly successful. It appears that approximately 50% of an infant's trachea can be resected, but rib cartilage can be used for elongated stenosis. When using the latter, normal epithelialization can be expected when the rib cartilage graft amounts to approximately 25% or less of the circumference of the airway, but not when 30% or more of the circumference is rib graft.

▶ Intrathoracic tracheobronchial obstructions represent a serious problem in infants and children. These data provide a valuable reference source for such problems. Particularly noteworthy was the fact that about 50% of the infant's trachea could be resected. With more extensive stenosis, cartilage grafts were used. If the cartilage grafts involved less than 25% of the circumference of the airway, they were readily resurfaced with epithelium; more extensive replacement was not always satisfactory.—F.C. Spencer, M.D.

Fetal Diaphragmatic Hernia: Ultrasound Diagnosis and Clinical Outcome in 38 Cases

Adzick NS, Vacanti JP, Lillehei CW, O'Rourke PP, Crone RK, Wilson JM (The Children's Hosp, Boston; Harvard Med School)

J Pediatr Surg 24:654–658, 1989   13–11

The natural history and clinical outcome of congenital diaphragmatic hernia (CDH) were reviewed in 94 patients. Prenatal diagnosis appears to be accurate and the mortality high; polyhydramnios is a prenatal indicator of a poor clinical outcome. A follow-up study of 38 consecutive patients was undertaken to assess prognostic factors and the role of extracorporeal membrane oxygenation (ECMO) on outcome.

Fetal CDH was diagnosed by ultrasound at 15–41 weeks' gestation. None of the 14 fetuses in whom the diagnosis was made before 25 weeks' gestation survived. Polyhydramnios was present in 69% of fetuses but usually did not appear until the third trimester. Only 18% of fetuses with polyhydramnios survived. Chromosomal abnormalities, present in 16% of the fetuses, included trisomy 18 in 3, and in 1 each, trisomy 21, tetrasomy 21, and tetrasomy 12p. Twelve infants were managed with

ECMO either before or after CDH repair. Nine of these infants died, and ECMO complications were significant. The overall survival rate was 24% (9 of 38 infants), and this increased to 33% (9 of 27) among fetuses surviving beyond delivery. The diagnosis was made later in gestation in the 9 survivors. Of these, 7 had diaphragmatic defects that could be closed primarily, all were responders, and only 3 required ECMO. The remaining 2 were responders who required ECMO before delayed surgical repair.

Improved postnatal therapy or surgical intervention before birth is necessary to salvage the CDH fetus with an early gestational diagnosis of associated polyhydramnios. Despite optimal postnatal therapy including ECMO, survival is poor in CDH. Polyhydramnios correlates highly with poor outcome, and associated anomalies are also a significant mortality factor. Amniocentesis is indicated when CDH is diagnosed antenatally to rule out chromosomal abnormalities.

▶ How much ideal surgical therapy can decrease the high operative mortality associated with CDH has been debated for decades. Hence, this report of 38 cases diagnosed in utero and treated by the same surgical team is of particular significance. Despite prompt operation and the use of ECMO, survival in general was poor. Polyhydramnios was present in 69%, and only 18% survived. All 14 fetuses in whom the diagnosis was made before 25 weeks' gestation died. These data indicate the severity of the embryologic defect, which may preclude effective surgical therapy in many of these infants.—F.C. Spencer, M.D.

Chest Injuries in Childhood
Nakayama DK, Ramenofsky ML, Rowe MI (Children's Hosp of Pittsburgh; Univ of Pittsburgh)
Ann Surg 210:770–775, 1989   13–12

Because thoracic injuries are uncommon in children, physicians may have difficulty in recognizing and treating such injuries. In addition, children differ from adults with similar injuries because of variations in anatomy and in mechanisms of injury. In a review of admissions to a children's hospital from January 1981 through June 1988, 105 significant chest injuries were identified.

The mean age of the 78 boys and 27 girls was 7.5 years. Blunt trauma caused 102 injuries (97%). More than half of the injuries were traffic related. Contusions (53%) and rib fractures (49.5%) were the most common types of blunt thoracic trauma. Pneumothorax (37%) and hemothorax (13%) occurred less frequently. Fifty-six children had more than 1 type of chest injury, and about 69% had associated head, abdominal, and orthopedic injuries. Endotracheal intubation and ventilatory support were required in 22 children (21%), generally for a brief period.

Only 6 children underwent surgery; 2 had penetrating and 4 had blunt injuries. The overall mortality was 6.7%. One child died of a penetrating injury and 5 of blunt trauma. Until age 4 years, abuse and motor vehicles were the most common causes of injury. Pedestrian injuries predominated in those aged 5−9 years, and bike injuries predominated in those aged 10−17 years.

Because children's ribs are pliable, chest trauma often causes them to bend but not break. Pulmonary contusion and pneumothorax are relatively common, however, because children have a soft chest wall. Children generally sustain a less severe high-speed chest impact than adults in motor vehicle crashes and are less likely than adults to be exposed to gunshot and stab wounds. Nevertheless, the potential for morbidity and death is high in children who sustain thoracic trauma.

▶ This experience with 105 children hospitalized for thoracic trauma in Pittsburgh over a period of 7 years is of particular interest. Blunt trauma was cause of injury in 97% of these children, and 5 deaths occurred.

There are noteworthy differences between the type of injury seen in children and that in adults. About half of the chest injuries occurred without rib fractures. Traumatic aortic injury, cardiac contusion, or rupture of the diaphragm were uncommon. Thoracotomy was needed in only 5 patients.— F.C. Spencer, M.D.

Congenital Bronchopulmonary Malformations: Diagnostic and Therapeutic Considerations
Bailey PV, Tracy T Jr, Connors RH, deMello D, Lewis JE, Weber TR (Cardinal Glennon Children's Hosp, St Louis; St Louis Univ)
J Thorac Cardiovasc Surg 99:597−603, 1990   13−13

Forty-five children aged 13 years or younger, who were evaluated and treated for bronchopulmonary malformations in 1970−1988, were studied. No sex predominance was evident. Thirty-seven children had solitary lesions, the most frequent being bronchogenic cyst and cystic adenomatoid malformation. Eight patients had 2 abnormalities simultaneously, most often sequestration plus cystic adenomatoid malformation.

Twenty-one patients had respiratory symptoms, which were pronounced in 7 cases. Twelve patients had pulmonary infection. Ultrasonography was helpful in diagnosing cystic adenomatoid malformation and pulmonary sequestration. Forty-two patients survived excision of the lesion by lobectomy or pneumonectomy. Three neonates died of pulmonary hypoplasia and hypertension; 2 had a concomitant diaphragmatic hernia.

Combinations of different types of bronchopulmonary malformation are not infrequent. All of these lesions can be managed operatively shortly after diagnosis. Surgery is well tolerated if significant pulmonary hypoplasia and hypertension are absent.

▶ This report from St. Louis University describes experiences with 45 congenital bronchopulmonary malformations treated in a period of 19 years. Diagnosis was possible in the majority with plain chest x-ray studies. Six different types of lesions were found, among which bronchogenic cysts and cystic adenomatoid malformation were the most common.—F.C. Spencer, M.D.

Recurrent Tracheo-Oesophageal Fistula: Experience With 24 Patients
Ghandour KE, Spitz L, Brereton RJ, Kiely EM (Hosp for Sick Children, London)
J Paediatr Child Health 26:89–91, 1990   13–14

The reported incidence of recurrent tracheoesophageal fistula after primary repair of esophageal atresia ranges from 5% to 14%. Surgical correction of a recurrent fistula is associated with significant morbidity and mortality.

During an 11-year period, 275 infants underwent primary repair for esophageal atresia and tracheoesophageal fistula; 22 of these (8%) had a recurrent fistula. Another 2 infants with an established recurrent fistula were referred for secondary operation. Twenty of the 22 initially treated infants who had a recurrence had respiratory problems, and 2 had evidence of swallowing difficulties. The mean age at symptom onset was 20 weeks. The average period before the diagnosis of recurrence was confirmed was 6 weeks. Diagnostic investigation included cine-tube esophagography and bronchoscopic cannulation of the fistula with methylene blue dye injection, followed by esophagoscopy.

Of 24 infants operated on for a recurrent tracheoesophageal fistula, 1 died during operation and 1 died of an unrecognized esophageal perforation; a third infant died at age 10 months of "crib death." Eighteen patients underwent division and repair of the recurrent fistula, of whom 4 had a second recurrence. Four patients underwent esophageal replacement by cervical esophagostomy and gastrostomy. The esophageal closure leaked in 5 patients, who then underwent secondary esophageal replacement. None of the patients had a third recurrence, but 7 required additional Nissen fundoplication or aortopexy, or both.

▶ This report from the Great Ormond Street Hospital in London, a world-famous institution for pediatric surgery, describes experiences with the unusual problem of recurrence of tracheoesophageal fistula. Twenty-two such patients were treated in a period of 11 years, during which time about 275 infants were operated on.

The complexity of the problem is clearly evident from the results, with repeat operation required in 24 patients. There were 3 deaths, a second recurrence developed in 4 patients, and a secondary esophageal replacement was required in 5. Clearly, these are unusually complex problems. The experiences described in this report should be studied carefully by anyone working with this severe congenital malformation.—F.C. Spencer, M.D.

14 Congenital Heart Disease

Outcome After a "Perfect" Fontan Operation

Fontan F, Kirklin JW, Fernandez G, Costa F, Naftel DC, Tritto F, Blackstone EH (Hôp Cardiologique du Haut-Leveque, Bordeaux, France; Univ of Alabama, Birmingham; Servico de Cirurgia Cardiaca, Curitiba, Brazil)

Circulation 81:1520–1536, 1990   14–1

The Fontan operation creates a state in which the force driving the pulmonary blood flow is solely or largely a residue, in the systemic venous pressure, of the main ventricular chamber's contractile force. Despite the excellent early clinical results, some studies suggest that the Fontan state may ultimately have deleterious effects. The early and long-term outcomes dictated by the Fontan state per se and the transition to it, by surgery, from the state of congenital heart disease under optimal conditions (after a "perfect" Fontan operation) were evaluated in 334 patients. The median follow-up time was 5 years (range, 1 month to 20 years).

In the primary study design, the multivariate risk factor equation for death was used to determine the time-related survival and hazards functions after a perfect Fontan operation. The survival rates were predicted to be 92%, 89%, 88%, 86%, 81%, and 73% at 1 month, 6 months, and 1, 5, 10, and 15 years, respectively. The hazard function (instantaneous risk of death at each moment in time after the operation) had an early rapidly declining phase, which at about 6 months led to a late hazard phase, which gradually increased about 6 years after surgery. Functional capacity, as defined by the New York Heart Association functional classification, was less the longer the period of follow-up. Other than older age at the time of surgery, no risk factors were found for the late decline in survival or functional status. A secondary design, using the theory of competing risks, yielded similar survival and hazard function information. The highest instantaneous risk of death was of heart failure, followed by sudden or arrhythmic death.

These data suggest that the Fontan state per se imposes a gradually declining functional capacity and premature decline in survival after initial, often excellent, palliation. The inference is that the Fontan operation is palliative and not curative.

▶ This important paper by Fontan and colleagues analyzes the significant question of long-term prognosis for morbidity and mortality after the influence of different risk factors is evaluated. The data included 334 patients from 3 different institutions in different parts of the world. Statistical mathematical analyses were performed. These defined a "late hazard phase," developing about 6 years after surgery. After 6 years there was a gradual decline in functional capacity and an increase in mortality. The predicted survival was 86% 5 years after operation, declining to 81% at 10 years and to 73% at 15 years. This late deterioration is apparently attributable to the abnormal physiologic state in which the force driving the pulmonary blood flow is determined by systemic venous pressure rather than by the contractile force of the right ventricle.— F.C. Spencer, M.D.

A Reconsideration of Risk Factors for the Fontan Operation
Myers JL, Waldhausen JA, Weber HS, Arenas JD, Cyran SE, Gleason MM, Baylen BG (Pennsylvania State Univ, Hershey)
Ann Surg 211:738–744, 1990   14–2

The Fontan operation is used in the treatment of complex congenital univentricular cardiac malformations. During a 12-year period, 38 patients underwent the Fontan operation. All operations were performed with cardiopulmonary bypass, direct caval cannulation, and deep or moderate hypothermia. Follow-up ranged from 1 month to 8.4 years, and complete follow-up data were available for all 38 patients.

In the first 5 patients (aged 7.5–23 years) a conduit was placed from the right atrium to the small right ventricle or pulmonary artery (PA). The other 33 patients (aged 7 months to 14 years) had a modified Fontan operation with a direct systemic venous or right atrial to pulmonary artery anastomosis. Indications included tricuspid atresia in 14 patients, single ventricle in 10, hypoplastic right or left ventricle in 9, double-outlet right ventricle with inlet ventricular septal defect and pulmonary atresia or stenosis in 3, crisis-cross ventricles and transposition of the great arteries in 1, and atrioventricular canal and anomalous pulmonary venous connection in 1. Thirty-two patients had undergone operations previously.

There were 4 operative deaths (10.5%), 3 as a result of low cardiac output and 1 caused by subaortic obstruction. There was no significant association between mortality and anatomical diagnosis or between previous surgery and subsequent mortality. There was no association between operative death and aortic arterial saturation, mean pulmonary artery pressure, left ventricular end-diastolic pressure, or preoperative hematocrit. Subaortic obstruction developed in 6 of the 7 patients who had pulmonary artery banding. Three of these 6 patients died more than 30 days after operation.

Because subaortic obstruction is a major risk factor for late death, a Damus-Kaye-Stansel anastomosis combined with a systemic to pulmonary artery shunt is now performed in all children with excessive pulmonary blood flow who are likely on anatomical grounds to have subaortic obstruction. The Fontan operation should be performed any time after 1 year of age, ideally during the second year of life.

▶ A retrospective review was made of findings in 38 patients undergoing a Fontan operation. In the majority of patients the conduit was placed directly to the pulmonary artery. There were 4 postoperative deaths. The subsequent development of subaortic obstruction was a major risk factor for late death; this occurred in 6 of 7 patients with pulmonary artery banding and led to 3 deaths. Analysis of the data concluded that a modified Fontan operation can be performed any time after 1 year of age, providing the patient's anatomy and physiology are acceptable.—F.C. Spencer, M.D.

Effect of Transannular Patching on Outcome After Repair of Tetralogy of Fallot

Kirklin JK, Kirklin JW, Blackstone EH, Milano A, Pacifico AD (Univ of Alabama, Birmingham)
Ann Thorac Surg 48:783–791, 1989   14–3

To determine the effect of transannular patching on early and intermediate-term survival, functional status, and freedom from reoperation, data on 814 patients who underwent repair of tetralogy of Fallot with pulmonary stenosis were reviewed. At the time of operation, most patients (75%) were aged 11 years or younger. Surgical repair was performed through a right ventriculotomy in 707 patients and from the right atrium or by a combined right atrial and pulmonary arterial approach in 107. The mean follow-up after initial repair was 9 years. All but 68 patients were traced during follow-up or had died.

Although transannular patching was a risk factor for death early after repair of tetralogy of Fallot, it did not remain a risk factor thereafter. The risk of early death decreased in operations performed in recent years. At the last follow-up, 96% of survivors were in New York Heart Association functional class I. Transannular patching was not a risk factor for reoperation in general but was clearly a risk factor for reoperation for pulmonary regurgitation. However, when an obstructing lesion beyond the transannular patch was not present, patching rarely resulted in reoperation for pulmonary regurgitation within 20 years. The incidence of reoperation increased to about 20% with important distal stenoses.

Transannular patching may be indicated when the predicted postrepair ratio between peak pressure and that in the left ventricle late postoperatively is greater than about .65 long after operation. Because clinical evidence of the adverse effects of transannular patching is delayed for at least 20 years in most patients, widespread use of the technique in those with tetralogy of Fallot with pulmonary stenosis is not indicated.

▶ The series discussed in this short report must be one of the largest in the world: 814 patients operated on in a period of 20 years. The data clearly show a slight influence of transannular patching on operative mortality: 4% vs. 1.4%. Quite significant, however, is the fact that the need for reoperation because of pulmonary regurgitation in the following 20 years was small regardless of the use of a transannular patch, unless distal stenoses were present. These data are particularly relevant in deciding on the indications for insertion of a pulmonary homograft to correct pulmonic insufficiency.—F.C. Spencer, M.D.

Pulmonary Allograft Conduit Repair of Tetralogy of Fallot: An Alternative to Transannular Patch Repair

Clarke DR, Campbell DN, Pappas G (Univ of Colorado)
J Thorac Cardiovasc Surg 98:730–737, 1989   14–4

Cryopreserved allograft valves and valved conduits were used to repair congenital heart defects in 122 patients since 1985. In 55 patients the right ventricular outflow tract was reconstructed with a pulmonary allograft valved conduit. They included 12 patients with tetralogy and no pulmonary atresia or absent valve syndrome. Indications for the conduit repair included pulmonary artery problems and increased pulmonary vascular resistance. The mean internal diameter of the conduit was 22 mm. Distal pulmonary artery reconstruction beyond the bifurcation was necessary in 9 patients.

Early postoperative problems were fewer than in patients having transannular patch repairs. Several of these patients subsequently required pulmonary artery conduit reconstruction. Perioperative mortality in patients given a pulmonary artery conduit was 8%. The 11 survivors have mild pulmonary regurgitation, but right ventricular function was good and all patients were active without cardiac symptoms.

Pulmonary artery conduit repair of tetralogy of Fallot is no less safe than transannular patch repair. Pulmonary regurgitation is avoided. Conduit repair is especially useful when distal reconstruction is required or when the pulmonary vascular resistance is increased.

▶ Experiences with cryopreserved allograft valves and conduit in 122 patients in the past 3 years are described in this report. In 55 of the group the right ventricular outflow tract was reconstructed with a pulmonary allograft conduit. An unanswerable clinical question at present is when an allograft valve should be used rather than conventional transannular patch repair for complex tetralogy. The excellent results with transannular patch repairs for at least 10–15 years indicate that a long period of follow-up would be needed to prove that initial pulmonary allograft repair is preferable.—F.C. Spencer, M.D.

A Technique for Correction of Truncus Arteriosus Types I and II Without Extracardiac Conduits

Barbero-Marcial M, Riso A, Atik E, Jatene A (Univ of São Paulo, Brazil)
J Thorac Cardiovasc Surg 99:364–369, 1990   14–5

Seven patients with truncus arteriosus type I or type II underwent a new repair that does not require use of an extracardiac conduit. The patients, 6 with a type I defect, were aged 2–9 months. The common trunk is septated into aortic and pulmonary segments with a pericardial patch, and the ventricular septal defect is closed via a ventriculotomy. A direct anastomosis then is made between the pulmonary arteries and right ventricle. The anterior wall is constructed with a patch having a pericardial monocusp valve attached.

There was 1 postoperative death, but no patient had low output or other complications. The 6 survivors were free of symptoms after 1–14 months. Ventricular function was normal, and the monocusp valve performed normally. Only 1 patient had significant pulmonary regurgitation. On cardiac catheterization, only 1 of 5 patients had a moderately elevated right ventricular/left ventricular peak systolic ratio.

Two more recent operations for type I truncus arteriosus have been successful. This technique is best suited to neonates and infants having type I or II truncus arteriosus—comprising more than 80% of all cases—if congestive heart failure and low body weight are present. Pulmonary artery banding or repair with an extracardiac conduit are followed by immediate and late complications and deaths.

▶ This interesting report from the Cardiac Institute in São Paolo is from the cardiac group headed by Jatene, the pioneer who launched the current era of corrective operation for transposition. Preliminary results with a new procedure for correction of truncus arteriosus in 7 patients are described. The common truncus was septated with a patch and reconstruction performed without the use of an extracardiac conduit. If further experiences are favorable, this type of procedure would be far better than insertion of a conduit in infancy, as all such infants require reoperation within a few years.—F.C. Spencer, M.D.

Appraisal of Resection and End-to-End Anastomosis for Repair of Coarctation of the Aorta in Infancy: Preference for Resection
van Son JAM, Daniëls O, Vincent JG, van Lier HJJ, Lacquet LK (Academic Hosp Nijmegen, The Netherlands)
Ann Thorac Surg 48:496–502, 1989   14–6

The use of resection and end-to-end anastomosis (RETE) for coarctation of the aorta is being reappraised in the light of higher rates of early recurrence in patients treated with the newer subclavian flap angioplasty (SFA). A 14-year experience was reviewed retrospectively, including assessment of left upper limb function.

The sample consisted of 70 infants who consecutively underwent surgical repair of coarctation of the aorta. The mean age at surgery was 80 days and the mean weight, 3 kg. Subclavian flap angioplasty was done in 19 patients and RETE in 51. The overall operative and hospital mortality rate was 20%. The mortality rate for children who had SFA was 11% compared with 24% for children who had RETE; this difference was not significant. In the SFA group, 87% of patients needed no repeat intervention for recoarctation after 5 years, compared with 95% in the RETE group.

The 5-year survival rate was 100% for patients with isolated coarctation, 73% for those with coarctation plus ventricular septal defect, and 28% for those with coarctation plus intracardiac defects other than ventricular septal defect. Complications of SFA included detrimental effects of the sacrifice of the left subclavian artery. One patient had a 2.5-cm shortening of the left arm 6 years postoperatively. Five others complained of claudication in the arm after strenuous exercise.

Neither technique, RETE or SFA, appears to have a major advantage in terms of mortality and recoarctation, but SFA carries the risk of late contracture of isthmic ductal tissue and resultant detrimental effects on the left arm. Satisfactory performance of the RETE procedure, with preservation of the aorta's growth potential, is recommended as a hemodynamically adequate repair.

▶ The best operation for coarctation of the aorta in infants is unclear. Hence, this report from Holland of experiences with 70 infants operated on in a period of 14 years is of particular significance. Subclavian flap angioplasty was performed in 19 patients and resection and end-to-end anastomosis in 51. Five years after operation 13% of the subclavian flap patients required reoperation, as opposed to only 5% of those with resection and end-to-end anastomosis. Furthermore, 6 of the 19 subclavian flap patients had symptoms in the left arm, including a 2.5-cm shortening in 1. For these reasons, end-to-end anastomosis is preferred.— F.C. Spencer, M.D.

Coarctation of the Aorta: Long-Term Follow-Up and Prediction of Outcome After Surgical Correction
Cohen M, Fuster V, Steele PM, Driscoll D, McGoon DC (Mt Sinai School of Medicine of City Univ of New York; Mayo Clinic and Found, Rochester, Minn)
Circulation 80:840–845, 1989   14–7

To determine the long-term outlook after isolated repair of aortic coarctation, the records of 646 patients operated on in 1946–1981 were reviewed. In 87% of patients the coarcted segment was resected and end-to-end anastomosis was performed. The other patients either had prosthetic material implanted or underwent a subclavian artery flap procedure.

At last follow-up, 82% of the patients were alive at a mean age of 34 years, and most functioned normally. Only 3% of the patients were severely symptomatic. There were 17 perioperative deaths. Later cardiovascular surgery was necessary on long-term follow-up in 11% of patients, and hypertension developed in 25%. Survival to 20 years was best for patients operated on when younger than 14 years of age, especially those aged 9 years and younger. Late deaths were most frequent in patients with higher postoperative systolic pressures. Of the patients operated on after age 14 years, 33% became hypertensive, as defined by a blood pressure of 150/90 mm Hg or greater.

Age at initial repair is an important predictor of long-term survival in patients with coarctation of the aorta. The most frequent cause of late death is coronary artery disease. Coarctectomy at the time of diagnosis appears wise. In this series, 93% of patients treated before age 1 year survived; at this age the decision to operate should be made by weighing the blood pressure against the risk of reoperation.

▶ This series of 646 patients, the largest group ever reported, underwent repair of coarctation of the aorta with a subsequent mean follow-up of as long as 20 years. Patients operated on before 14 years of age had a 20-year survival rate of 91%, considerably better than that in older patients, whose survival rate at 20 years was only 79%. The best results were in those operated on before age 9 years. These data provide clear evidence that operation should be performed as soon as possible after 1 year of age, especially if severe hypertension is present.—F.C. Spencer, M.D.

15 Valvular Heart Disease

Allograft Aortic Valve Implantation: Techniques for All Types of Aortic Valve and Root Pathology
O'Brien MF, McGiffin DC, Stafford EG (Prince Charles Hosp, Brisbane, Australia)
Ann Thorac Surg 48:600–609, 1989   15–1

The allograft aortic valve can be used to manage the full spectrum of aortic valve and valve root pathology. Standard valve replacement methods apply to valve annuli 22–29 mm in diameter. Surgery is done under cardiopulmonary bypass and cardioplegia, supplemented by pericardial ice slush and intracavity cold Ringer's solution. The valve is turned inside out and inverted before being sutured into place. Equidistant placement of 3 double-armed 3-0 braided polyester sutures in both the host annulus and graft is a critically important step.

Technique.—A small annulus is enlarged with a pericardial or Dacron gusset. The allograft is not inverted when placing the proximal suture line. With a large asymmetric noncoronary sinus, the noncoronary sinus aortic wall of the graft is retained. The distal suture line is placed horizontally around the host sinotubular ridge. Usually, the aneurysmal sinus is incorporated into the aortotomy closure. If the valve annulus exceeds 30 mm, competence can be assured by using the allograft valve intact with its aortic sinuses as a small cylindrical tube or miniroot. If aortic root replacement is indicated for a large annulus, with or without primary aortic wall aneurysm, the aortic incision includes a medial extension toward the left side of the right coronary ostium to widely expose the aortic root. The proximal muscle cuff is left 3–4 mm thick and 4–5 mm long.

If active aortic valve endocarditis is present with annular or subannular abscesses, these can be closed, left open to the circulation, or excluded from the circulation and aortic root. No infected pocket should be left in place. Total allograft root replacement is used if the root is extensively destroyed and there is some left ventriculoaortic discontinuity. With a less damaged root, the subcoronary implantation technique may be used.

▶ There is growing interest in and usage of aortic valve allograft, especially in children. Hence, this report from Brisbane, Australia, by Mark O'Brien, a leading investigator of allograft aortic valves for more than 20 years, is of particular interest.—F.C. Spencer, M.D.

Homograft Valve Durability: Host or Donor Influence?

Gonzalez-Lavin L, Spotnitz AJ, Mackenzie JW, Gu J, Gadi IK, Gullo J, Boyd C, Graf D (Robert Wood Johnson Univ Hosp, New Brunswick, NJ; Deborah Research Inst, Browns Mills, NJ)

Heart Vessels 5:102–106, 1990

15–2

Antibiotic-sterilized homograft valves for use in aortic valve replacement are more durable than chemically sterilized valves, but the reason remains obscure. Some physicians have attributed long-term valve durability to the retention of viable donor fibroblasts capable of repairing the grafted valve, whereas others attribute it to ingrowth of host fibroblasts into and onto the leaflet ground substance. The presence, distribution, and origins of cells in a cryopreserved homograft aortic valve were studied after its explantation for technical malalignment.

A cryopreserved aortic homograft from a 21-year-old, brain-dead organ donor was sterilized in antibiotic solution and later inserted in a 20-year-old woman who had congenital aortic regurgitation. Ten months after operation the patient required reoperation for replacement of the aortic homograft because of moderate aortic regurgitation. The explanted valve was subjected to immunocytochemistry, tissue culture, and karyotyping.

The leaflet bases showed normal morphology with an intact endothelium. The distal one third of the leaflets contained no fibroblasts. Cytogenetic analysis of culture-derived fibroblasts from the leaflet bases revealed the fibroblasts to be of host origin. In this case, the homograft appeared to have been implanted with an intact ground substance that allowed for host cell repopulation of the inner third of the leaflets.

Perhaps donor cell viability in itself is not as important to long-term valve durability as is preservation of the leaflet ground substance to enhance host cell infiltration. Further investigation into preservation of donor endothelial tissue and the role of immunogenicity in homograft degeneration is indicated. The use of immunocytochemistry and karyotyping of culture-derived fibroblasts from excised leaflets is recommended so that more data on this issue can be collected and analyzed.

▶ This short case report describes the implications of a cryopreserved aortic homograft that was explanted after 10 months and studied with tissue culture and karyotyping. The leaflets exhibited normal morphology with intact endothelium. Cytogenetic analysis of cultured derived fibroblasts from the leaflet bases showed them to be of host origin.

The authors review the 2 prevailing theories of whether the better survival of allografts with antibiotic-sterilized valves is attributable to preservation of donor cells or better preservation of ground substance that facilitates ingrowth of host cells. Present evidence seems to favor the latter theory, but the issue is by no means settled.—F.C. Spencer, M.D.

The Carpentier-Edwards Standard Porcine Bioprosthesis: A First-Generation Tissue Valve With Excellent Long-Term Clinical Performance
Jamieson WRE, Allen P, Miyagishima RT, Gerein AN, Munro AI, Burr LH, Tyers GFO (Univ of British Columbia, Vancouver)
J Thorac Cardiovasc Surg 99:543–561, 1990   15–3

Porcine bioprostheses, which have been in use for more than 15 years, are satisfactory cardiac valvular substitutes. During the past 5 years the primary concern with bioprostheses has been altered durability. Data were reviewed on 1,190 patients in whom the Carpentier-Edwards prosthesis was implanted during a 13-year period. Although 3 design changes were implemented over the years, the last, an additional sterilant incorporated in 1982, was not evaluated because most of the implants were performed before 1982.

The mean age of the patients was 57 years and the mean length of follow-up was 5.6 years. Analyses included causes of early and late mortality, valve-related death, valve-related reoperation, valve-related complications, and structural and nonstructural valve dysfunction and deterioration.

The early mortality was 7.6% and the late mortality was 3.9% per patient-year overall. Valve-related causes of late mortality included thromboembolism (22), antithromboembolic therapy-related hemorrhage (8), prosthetic valve endocarditis (12), nonstructural dysfunction (8), and structural valve deterioration (12). There were 8 early and 62 late valve-related deaths and 136 valve-related operations.

The most significant valve-related complication was structural valve deterioration. Freedom from this complication was 97.5% at 5 years, 77% at 10 years, and 72.7% at 12 years. Freedom from structural valve deterioration was significantly greater for aortic valve replacement compared with mitral valve replacement and multiple valve replacement; mitral valve replacement was superior to multiple valve replacements in this regard. Freedom from all valve-related complications was superior for aortic valve replacement.

The improved anulus incorporated into the Carpentier-Edwards prosthesis in 1980 facilitated hemodynamic improvement. Whereas preoperatively almost 93% of these patients were in either New York Heart Association class III or IV, 92% were in classes I and II postoperatively. Overall, the Carpentier-Edwards porcine bioprosthesis delivers satisfactory clinical performance with a low incidence of valve-related complications and affords patients an excellent quality of life.

▶ This excellent report describes long-term results in 1,190 patients operated on between 1975 and 1986. The authors' institution in Vancouver has been a primary area of clinical investigation with porcine prostheses. Their total experience includes about 2,900 patients, with 1,300 prostheses of the type described in this report and about 1,700 supra-annular prostheses used since 1981. Hence, these data related to an earlier prosthesis.

Structural valve deterioration, of course, is the principal concern with porcine prostheses. At 5 years, more than 97% of prostheses were functioning satisfactorily, with a striking increase in deterioration in the next 5 years, at which time only 77% were all right. Aortic valves functioned significantly better than mitral valves, 83% vs. 72%. There was little difference between aortic and mitral prostheses regarding frequency of endocarditis or thromboembolism.—F.C. Spencer, M.D.

Long-Term Relative Survival Rates After Heart Valve Replacement
Lindblom D, Lindblom U, Qvist J, Lundström H (Karolinska Hosp; Statistics Stockholm, Sweden)
J Am Coll Cardiol 15:566–573, 1990   15–4

Actuarial analysis allows identification of high-risk patients scheduled for prosthetic heart valve replacement. Calculation of the relative survival rate, however, could be used to estimate the proportion of patients considered cured by the treatment. Long-term relative survival rates after valve replacement were assessed in 2,805 Swedish patients who underwent replacement of aortic valves (1,741), mitral valves (792), or both (272). Follow-up data available for all of the patients, extended over a mean of 6 years for operative survivors and over 7 years for current survivors. The observed survival rate was compared with the expected survival rate, which was derived from a control group of all Swedish inhabitants of the same gender and age as the patient and alive at the time of operation.

There were 156 early deaths (5.6%) and 700 (25%) that occurred later during the follow-up period. Valve-related causes accounted for 156 of the deaths (18%). The actuarial survival rate at 10 years was 63% and was significantly higher in the aortic valve group (66%) than in the mitral (57%) or double-valve (58%) group. Analysis of relative survival rates showed that, among patients undergoing aortic valve replacement, mortality was more than twice as high among those operated on for aortic regurgitation than for those operated on for aortic stenosis.

A normalized survival pattern was observed only from the second postoperative year in patients aged 65 years or older who underwent aortic valve replacement for pure aortic stenosis. Except in this group, valve replacement is not a "cure," and the relative survival rate was much lower than the actuarial freedom from valve-related death.

▶ The proper timing of valve replacement for aortic or mitral disease is uncertain, considering the morbidity from a prosthetic valve as opposed to the hazard of irreversible preoperative myocardial injury from the valvular disease. Hence, these data are particularly valuable.

A total of 2,800 patients undergoing aortic or mitral valve replacement over a period of 15 years had a 100% follow-up, with autopsy performed in 75% of deaths. Long-term survival was significantly better for patients with aortic valve disease than for those with mitral valve disease, whereas results with double-valve replacement were similar to those with simply mitral valve replacement alone. An unusual fact emerged that survival after replacement for aortic stenosis was much better than that for aortic insufficiency, emphasizing the importance of earlier operation in the latter group.

The authors make the cogent point that with an operative mortality of less than 3%, and a frequency of valve-related deaths in only 5% within 10 years, earlier operation for aortic valve replacement should be considered seriously.— F.C. Spencer, M.D.

Valve Repair With Carpentier Techniques: The Second Decade
Deloche A, Jebara VA, Relland JYM, Chauvaud S, Fabiani J-W, Perier P, Dreyfus G, Mihaileanu S, Carpentier A (Hôp Broussais, Paris)
J Thorac Cardiovasc Surg 99:990–1002   15–5

More than 6,000 mitral valve repairs have been done at the authors' center since 1968. A total of 206 patients had repair with a prosthetic ring in 1972–1979, when most modern technical procedures had been established and the "functional" approach introduced. Most of the 195 operative survivors had valve insufficiency caused by degenerative disease. Nearly all patients were in New York Heart Association functional class III or IV preoperatively.

A Carpentier ring annuloplasty was done in 95.5% of cases. Sixty-two percent of patients required resection of the posterior mitral leaflet, and 19% had resection of the anterior leaflet. Chordal shortening was necessary in 46% of the patients. Small numbers of patients had leaflet mobilization and commissurotomy.

The overall actuarial survival after 17 years was 72%. There were 20 valve-related deaths and 23 patients required reoperation, 10 of them within 2 years of primary valve repair. Ten patients had thromboembolic events and 6 had anticoagulant-related hemorrhage. Four patients had significant residual regurgitation but have not required reoperation. More patients with rheumatic disease had valve-related complications. Three fourths of the survivors were in functional class I or II at follow-up. Ventricular contractility was normal in 84% of the patients assessed. The low rate of reoperation and relatively infrequent complications in this series affirm the predictability and stability of results achieved by mitral valve repair.

▶ A series of 206 patients undergoing mitral valve repair before 1979 were evaluated. The findings represent the largest amount of data available concerning long-term results with the Carpentier method of reconstruction. Using the actuarial method, at 15 years, 94% of patients were free from thromboembolism, 97% were free from endocarditis, and 87% were free from reoperation.

Mitral regurgitation was absent in 74%, was trivial in 17%, and was significant in 2.5%.—F.C. Spencer, M.D.

Intraoperative Doppler Color Flow Mapping for Decision-Making in Valve Repair for Mitral Regurgitation: Technique and Results in 100 Patients

Stewart WJ, Currie PJ, Salcedo EE, Lytle BW, Gill CC, Schiavone WA, Agler DA, Cosgrove DM (Cleveland Clinic Found)
Circulation 81:556–566, 1990   15–6

Mitral valve repair has many advantages over valve replacement as a treatment for severe regurgitation, but it is necessary to accurately determine the adequacy of the repair before closing the chest. The usefulness of intraoperative epicardial Doppler color flow mapping was examined in 100 patients with pure mitral regurgitation, which was caused most frequently by myxomatous prolapse and ischemic heart disease. Transthoracic Doppler studies were done under standard ambulatory condition.

Intraoperative assessments of mitral regurgitation agreed well with both the preoperative left ventriculographic findings and findings of standard precordial Doppler echocardiography. Postrepair intraoperative Doppler studies indicated satisfactory surgical results in 92 patients. Four others had persistent significant regurgitation, 3 had systolic anterior motion of the valve with dynamic left ventricular outflow tract obstruction, and 1 had a persistent flail leaflet. Six of these patients had further procedures at the same thoracotomy. Intraoperative Doppler color flow mapping can help to ensure a successful outcome in patients undergoing mitral valve repair for regurgitation.

▶ Evaluation of the results of mitral valve reconstruction are primarily subjective from visual observations at operation. This experience from the Cleveland Clinic describes results in 100 patients with intraoperative epicardial Doppler color flow mapping immediately before and after repair. In 8 of the 100, significant persistent regurgitation was demonstrated in 5 and left ventricular outflow tract obstruction from systolic anterior motion of the mitral valve in 3. All 8 were successfully reoperated on, 6 at the time of the initial operation and 2 at a later date.—F.C. Spencer, M.D.

Comparative Assessment of Chordal Preservation Versus Chordal Resection During Mitral Valve Replacement

Hennein HA, Swain JA, McIntosh CL, Bonow RO, Stone CD, Clark RE (Natl Heart, Lung, and Blood Inst, Bethesda, Md)
J Thorac Cardiovasc Surg 99:828–837, 1990   15–7

Compared to other open cardiac procedures, mitral valve replacement (MVR) for mitral regurgitation is associated with a high rate of morbidity and mortality. Left ventricular function often deteriorates after MVR, possibly because of disruption of the mitral valve apparatus at operation. Whether chordal preservation results in more favorable left ventricular function was investigated in 69 patients who underwent MVR. They were evaluated before and 6 months after surgery by exercise testing, catheterization, echocardiography, and radionuclide angiography.

Fifty-five patients had MVR with complete excision of the native valve, 9 had preservation of the entire mitral apparatus, and 5 had preservation of the posterior leaflet and the attached chordae. Although disparate preoperative findings make direct comparison of the 2 preservation techniques difficult, both led to similar significant improvement in preserving the left ventricular ejection fraction. No operative or late deaths occurred in patients undergoing chordae-preserving MVR. The operative mortality of patients undergoing conventional MVR was 7% and the 5-year survival was approximately 82%. Patients having conventional MVR had deterioration of left ventricular function and showed no improvement in exercise capacity, cardiac index, and left ventricular systolic dimensions. Patients in the chordae-preserving group improved in all of these areas.

In both chordal preservation groups, postoperative survival, exercise capacity, and left ventricular ejection fraction and function, and cardiac index were better than in the group in which the chordae were excised. No statistically significant differences were found between the group undergoing posterior chordal resection only and the group with preservation of the entire apparatus.

▶ This important paper provides significant data supporting the concept that cardiac function is better preserved with prosthetic replacement when some chordae are preserved, at least those to the posterior leaflet. Among the group of 69 patients studied, 55 had replacement with no chordae preservation, 9 had all chordae preserved, and 5 had only the posterior leaflet. Subsequent detailed studies of cardiac function clearly demonstrated much better function in the group with preservation of some chordae. However, those with posterior chordae preservation only did as well as those in whom all of the chordae were preserved. These data strongly support the concept of preservation of as many chordae as possible when the mitral valve is replaced. The authors are to be congratulated on this important study.—F.C. Spencer, M.D.

Replacement of Chordae Tendineae With Expanded Polytetrafluoroethylene Sutures

David TE (Toronto Western Hosp)
J Cardiac Surg 4:286–290, 1989
15–8

Data were reviewed on the use of polytetrafluoroethylene (PTFE) sutures for replacement of ruptured chordae tendineae of the anterior leaflet.

Technique.—A double-armed suture is passed 2–3 times through the head of the papillary muscle that anchors the ruptured chorda and is then tied. The suture arms are passed twice at the point of the chorda attachment and tied together on the ventricular side of the leaflet. The lengths of the new chorda are approximated as in a chordal shortening procedure. In multiple chorda replacements the suture is brought up to the free margin of the anterior leaflet, passed 2–3 times, and advanced. It is passed through the papillary muscle head twice,

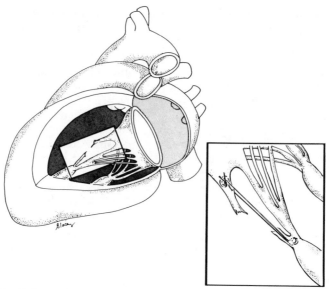

Fig 15–1.—Technique for replacement of ruptured chordae tendinae of the anterior leaflet of the mitral valve. (Courtesy of David TE: *J Cardiac Surg* 4:286–290, 1989.)

brought up to the free margin, passed, and advanced again. It is then passed through the papillary muscle head and tied. The technique is illustrated in Figure 15–1.

At least 1 primary chorda was replaced in 22 patients (mean age, 59 years) who were undergoing mitral valve reconstruction and 1 patient undergoing tricuspid valve repair. In patients with rheumatic mitral valve disease, calcified or excessively thickened chordae were resected and replaced with PTFE sutures. There were no operative deaths. All patients received adequate anticoagulation, but 1 had a transient ischemic attack on day 5 postoperatively. Patients were followed for a mean of 17 months. Of the 23 patients, 21 were in New York Heart Association functional class I and 2 in class II. Doppler echocardiography showed moderate tricuspid regurgitation in the patient who underwent tricuspid repair. There was no regurgitation in 18 patients who underwent mitral valve repair; 3 had mild and 1 had moderate regurgitation. The mean mitral orifice was 3 cm^2 in patients who had degenerative disease and 2.2 cm^2 in those who had rheumatic disease. The PTFE chordae seem to remain pliable.

Sutures with PTFE appear to be safe for replacement of diseased chordae tendineae when conventional techniques are impossible. Results of animal studies have shown that these synthetic chordae are completely covered by fibrous tissue within 3–24 months. No dehiscence was seen in the clinical study. The limited experience with PTFE replacement of fused and calcified chordae in rheumatic heart disease patients has been encouraging.

▶ In a period of 4 years, 1 or more primary chordae of the anterior leaflet of the mitral valve were replaced with PTFE sutures in 22 patients as part of a mitral valve reconstructive procedure. A 5–0 Goretex suture was used. All patients recovered and have been evaluated periodically with a mean follow-up of 17 months. No complications have been recognized. Eighteen of the 22 have no insufficiency, 3 have mild insufficiency, and 1 has moderate insufficiency.

As the author indicates, these encouraging results should lead to further use of the technique in selected patients in whom more conventional techniques of repair of ruptured chordae cannot be used.—F.C. Spencer, M.D.

Operation for Acute Postinfarction Mitral Insufficiency Using Continuous Oxygenated Blood Cardioplegia
Panos A, Christakis GT, Lichtenstein SV, Wittnich C, El-Dalati H, Salerno TA (St Michael's Hosp, Toronto; Univ of Toronto)
Ann Thorac Surg 48:816–819, 1989   15–9

Patients who require urgent operation for severe mitral regurgitation and cardiogenic shock after acute myocardial infarction are at high risk for operative and in-hospital death. The reported mortality rate in these patients ranges from 21% to 85%. Despite improvements in surgical techniques, acute pump failure continues to be a major problem. In a prospective trial, a new technique of continuous infusion of oxygenated cold blood cardioplegia was used during revascularization.

In a 4-year period, 13 men and 6 women (average age, 64 years) had acute-onset mitral regurgitation and cardiogenic shock within 4 weeks after myocardial infarction. They required urgent myocardial revascularization or mitral valve replacement, or both. Sixteen patients had a left ventricular ejection fraction of less than 40%. A continuous infusion of blood cardioplegia was instituted at aortic cross-clamping and continued throughout the cross-clamp period. Electromechanical arrest and cooling to septal temperatures of 10° required a mean of 1,200 mL of initial high-potassium cardioplegia, infused at a rate of 150 mL/min with an aortic root pressure of 80 mm Hg.

The mean pump time was 88.3 minutes and the mean cross-clamp time was 58.6 minutes. The mean serum level of potassium at the end of bypass was 5.90 mEq/L (range, 4.1–7.5 mEq/L). There were 2 in-hospital deaths (10.5%) and 10 patients (53%) experienced low-output syndrome. One patient had a transient stroke 2 days after operation. Another patient had renal failure and required hemodialysis but recovered renal function before discharge. After a mean follow-up of 2.5 years, there was 1 late death. Fourteen of the 16 remaining patients were in New York Heart Association functional class I or II.

Continuous infusion of cold blood cardioplegia is technically more demanding than traditional intermittent infusion. It may offer improved myocardial protection, however, in high-risk patients undergoing urgent operation for life-threatening complications after acute myocardial infarction.

▶ This impressive report from Toronto describes 19 consecutive patients operated on acutely for severe mitral regurgitation and shock after myocardial infarction. This condition has usually been associated with an operative mortality of between 30% and 70%. These results are quite remarkable: only 2 deaths, even though low cardiac output was present in nearly 50% of the survivors. With a subsequent follow-up of more than 2 years, 14 of 16 patients were in functional class I or II.

The technique of continuous cold blood cardioplegia described seems worthy of careful investigation by others. It has long been a puzzle why correction of a severe mechanical defect—rupture of the mitral valve apparatus after myocardial infarction—was nonetheless associated with such a high operative mortality. The experiences suggest that standard techniques of myocardial preservation are inadequate in these emergency circumstances. Hence, this method merits serious thought.—F.C. Spencer, M.D.

Ten-Year Experience With Aortic Valve Replacement in 482 Patients 70 Years of Age or Older: Operative Risk and Long-Term Results
Galloway AC, Colvin SB, Grossi EA, Baumann FG, Sabban YP, Esposito R, Ribakove GH, Culliford AT, Slater JN, Glassman E, Harty S, Spencer FC (New York Univ Med Ctr; City Univ of New York)
Ann Thorac Surg 49:84–93, 1990   15–10

Aortic balloon valvoplasty, rather than aortic valve replacement (AVR), has been widely used to correct aortic stenosis in the elderly, partly because of the high operative mortality associated with AVR. To verify this, a retrospective review was made of an institutional experience with AVR in patients 70 years or older during 1976–1987. Follow-up was 94% complete during a mean period of 34 months (range, 1–144 months).

During the 10-year period, 483 patients aged 70–89 years (mean, 75 years) underwent AVR, either as an isolated procedure (38%) or plus a concomitant operative procedure (62%). A porcine valve prosthesis was used in 83% of patients, whereas the remaining had mechanical prostheses. Preoperatively, 32% of patients were in New York Heart Association (NYHA) class III and 59% were in class IV.

Overall operative mortality was 12.4%. It was 5.6% after elective isolated AVR for pure aortic stenosis, 8.2% after all isolated AVR procedures, and 14.3% after AVR with concomitant coronary artery bypass grafting. Significant predictors of increased operative risk were emergency operation, isolated aortic regurgitation, and a previous cardiac surgical procedure. The incidence of perioperative complications was low and included stroke (2.7%), sternal infections (1.9%), myocardial infarction (2.7%), prolonged respiratory support (4.8%), and low cardiac output syndrome (7%).

The 5-year survival rate was 81%. The yearly risk of death in survivors aged 70 years or older who underwent AVR was 5.42%, which is similar to the 5.77%/year rate for age- and sex-matched controls from the general population. Hazard function analysis identified NYHA functional class as a predictor of diminished survival and peak aortic valve gradient of 75 mm Hg or higher as a predictor of improved survival.

The 5-year freedom from reoperation was 99%; from late thromboembolic complications, 91%; and from late anticoagulant-related complications, 94%. The 5-year rates of freedom from all valve-related morbidity and mortality were 83% and 61%, respectively. At follow-up, 22% of survivors were in NYHA class III and 2% were in NYHA class IV. In patients 70 years of age or older, AVR should remain the procedure of choice to correct substantial aortic valve disease.

▶ This report from my institution well indicates the excellent long-term results that can be obtained in patients older than 70 years of age. The report was prepared specifically because of the unsupported assertions that the high mortality and morbidity after operation in such patients was an indication for the use of palliative balloon valvuloplasty. Particularly significant aspects of the data reported include the operative mortality of 5.6% for elective isolated aortic valve replacements; the 5-year survival from late cardiac-related deaths of 81%; and the yearly hazard rate for late death of 5.4%, which is similar to a 5.7% annual rate for age-matched controls.—F.C. Spencer, M.D.

Aortic Valve Replacement With Stentless Porcine Aortic Bioprosthesis
David TE, Pollick C, Bos J (Toronto Western Hosp; Univ of Toronto)
J Thorac Cardiovasc Surg 99:113–118, 1990   15–11

After satisfactory functional results were obtained by replacing the sheep aortic valve with a stentless glutaraldehyde-fixed porcine aortic valve, use of this type of bioprosthesis was assessed in 29 patients who required aortic valve replacement. Eighteen patients had predominant stenosis, 10 had insufficiency, and 1 had a failed aortic bioprosthesis. In addition to replacing the aortic valve with the porcine valve, 4 patients had mitral valve repair, 2 had mitral valve replacement, and 10 had coronary artery bypass surgery.

There was 1 postoperative death and 2 patients had low cardiac output syndrome. During a mean follow-up of 1 year no thromboembolism or infective endocarditis occurred. Twenty-five patients improved to New York Heart Association class I and 3 improved to class II. Five patients had trivial or mild aortic insufficiency. Valve gradients were significantly lower than in patients who were given a Hancock II bioprosthesis. Effective aortic valve areas were larger in the patients given a stentless bioprosthesis.

The hemodynamic characteristics of a glutaraldehyde-fixed porcine aortic bioprosthesis are much improved when the aortic root is used as a stent for the valve. Durability probably will be enhanced as the aortic root may dampen the mechanical stress on the valve leaflets. It is reasonable to believe that the normal aortic valve anatomy reflects the optimal functional adaptation, and that an operation closely mimicking the anatomical and functional principles should give good clinical results.

▶ The influence of the stent on the durability of a bioprosthesis was investigated in this preliminary report. In 29 patients a stentless glutaraldehyde-fixed porcine valve was inserted, using the same technique as that used for inserting an aortic allograft.

As the authors indicate, this technique was used more than 20 years ago but was essentially discarded because of the technical advantages of insertion of a stent-mounted prosthesis. As indicated by Carpentier in the Discussion of this paper, the long-term question is whether the theoretical improved durability will outweigh the technical hazards of implantation.—F.C. Spencer, M.D.

Neonatal Critical Valvar Aortic Stenosis: A Comparison of Surgical and Balloon Dilation Therapy
Zeevi B, Keane JF, Castaneda AR, Perry SB, Lock JE (Harvard Med School; and Children's Hosp, Boston)
Circulation 80:831–839, 1989   15–12

Balloon dilatation is an attractive initial approach to neonates having critical valvar aortic stenosis. The procedure was performed in 16 consecutive neonates in 1985–1988, and the results were compared with those of surgical valvotomy in 16 patients operated on in 1978–1984. The groups were comparable in age, body weight, hemodynamic findings, and associated lesions. Left ventricular size also was similar in the 2 treatment groups.

There were 6 early deaths and 1 late death in the surgical group. Five of the 6 infants who required a second operation died. All 3 neonates with a small or hypoplastic left ventricle died after surgical valvotomy. There were 3 early deaths after balloon valvotomy, and 2 late deaths occurred. Patients with a normal-sized left ventricle had the best outlook. Five of 6 surgical patients followed for a mean of 26 months had mild aortic regurgitational and 1 had moderate aortic regurgitation. Three of 6 patients followed for 1½ years had mild aortic regurgitation. Six patients in the balloon valvotomy group required a second procedure.

Percutaneous balloon valvotomy may be as effective as surgical valvotomy in neonates with critical valvular aortic stenosis. The 2 procedures are comparable with regard to both relief of valvar stenosis and the later development of aortic regurgitation.

▶ This report from the Boston Children's Hospital compares the results of balloon aortic valvotomy in 16 neonates treated since 1985 and the results of surgical valvotomy in 16 patients treated in the 7 previous years. The outcome was a bit better with balloon valvotomy, although results naturally were poor in both series with a hypoplastic left ventricle. In the 9 survivors in the balloon group, the peak systolic gradient was 40–45 mm.

Although the results are acceptable, as the authors indicate, the series are not comparable. In the current era in which dramatic results are achieved with total correction of complex congenital malformations in neonates (e.g., transposition) with low operative mortality, it is difficult to believe that a blind balloon dilatation in a patient with a severely malformed aortic valve would be superior to a precise surgical incision. Hence, I would consider the issue by no means settled.—F.C. Spencer, M.D.

Aortic Root Replacement With Pulmonary Autograft
Stelzer P, Jones DJ, Elkins RC (Univ of Oklahoma)
Circulation 80 (Suppl III):III-209–III-213, 1989   15–13

The pulmonary valve has been successfully transferred to the aortic position. This concept has now been expanded to include patients with aortic root disease or a narrow anulus, or both. The main pulmonary artery with its valve is used as a conduit to replace the proximal ascending aorta, with reimplantation of the coronary ostia into the pulmonary trunk.

Technique.—Under cardiopulmonary bypass the distal main pulmonary artery is divided as far out as possible at the bifurcation. A cuff of muscle 3–4 mm wide is left below the lowest point of leaflet attachment as the night ventricular outflow tract is opened transversely (Fig 15–2). The aortic pathology is dealt with, and root enlargement is carried out if necessary. The proximal aortic suture line then is made (Fig 15–3). Aortic tissue about the left coronary ostium is trimmed

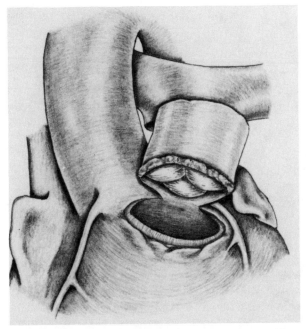

Fig 15–2.—Sketch detailing surgical technique. Pulmonary trunk is harvested from right ventricular outflow tract. There is close proximity of left coronary artery system. (Courtesy of Stelzer P, Jones DJ, Elkins RC: *Circulation* 80 (Suppl III):III-209–III-213, 1989.)

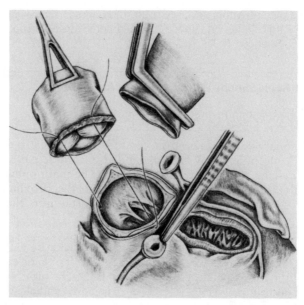

Fig 15–3.—Sketch detailing surgical technique. After coronary arteries have been mobilized away from aorta, autograft root is positioned as shown. (Courtesy of Stelzer P, Jones DJ, Elkins RC: *Circulation* 80 (Suppl III):III-209–III-213, 1989.)

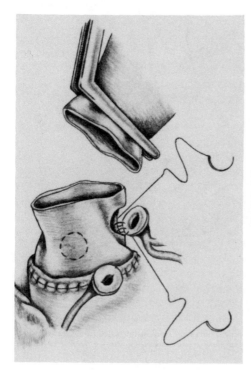

Fig 15–4.—Sketch detailing surgical technique. Coronary arteries are reimplanted with 6-0 sutures, avoiding underlying leaflets. (Courtesy of Stelzer P, Jones DJ, Elkins RC: *Circulation* 80 (Suppl) III):III-209–III-213, 1989.)

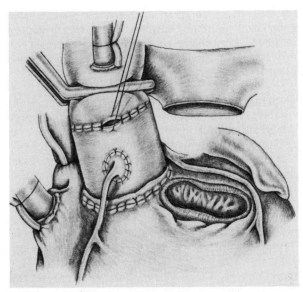

Fig 15–5.—Sketch detailing surgical procedure. Distal suture line of new aortic root is performed with 4-0 or 5-0 polypropylene sutures. (Courtesy of Stelzer P, Jones DJ, Elkins RC: *Circulation* 80 (Suppl III):III-209–III-213, 1989.)

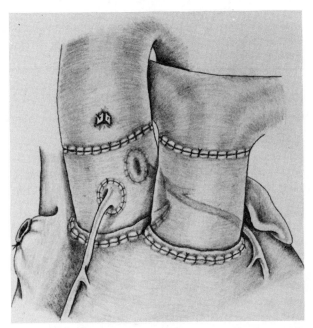

Fig 15–6.—Sketch showing completed operation demonstrates pulmonary autograft replacement of aortic root and pulmonary allograft in place of native pulmonary conduit. (Courtesy of Stelzer P, Jones DJ, Elkins RC: *Circulation* 80 (Suppl III):III-209–III-213, 1989.)

and an orifice is made in the autograft to receive the tissue button (Fig 15–4). After inserting the distal suture line, any size discrepancy is gathered evenly, as shown in Figure 15–5. A cryopreserved allograft is the preferred conduit. A pericardial strip may be used posteriorly to enhance hemostasis when completing graft insertion (Fig 15–6).

Seventeen patients aged 2–62 years received pulmonary autografts by using the root replacement technique. Five patients had previous aortic surgery and 4 had subacute bacterial endocarditis. Postoperative mortality was 18%; 2 of the 3 patients who died had endocarditis. There were no infectious or thromboembolic complications. All but 1 of the 14 survivors were in New York Heart Association class I a mean of 9 months after operation.

Although there is an increased risk of bleeding, the root replacement technique has potential advantages over intra-aortic methods. Pulmonary autograft replacement of the aortic valve now may be done when it is necessary to replace or enlarge the left ventricular outflow tract.

▶ This short report describes experiences at the University of Oklahoma with use of the pulmonary valve to replace the aortic valve, a technique developed by Donald Ross in London more than 20 years ago. Long-term data from this institution published in the past 2 or 3 years indicate continued adequate function of the pulmonary autograft after 20 years.

This report describes experiences in 17 patients, with 3 deaths. No late problems with the autograft were encountered. This seems to be a particularly useful technique in children with a hypoplastic annulus. The illustrations are excellent.—F.C. Spencer, M.D.

Valve Repair in Acute Endocarditis

Dreyfus G, Serraf A, Jebara VA, Deloche A, Chauvaud S, Couetil JP, Carpentier A (Hôp Broussais, Paris)
Ann Thorac Surg 49:706–713, 1990   15–14

Despite the wide use of antibiotics some patients still require surgery for acute bacterial endocarditis. Forty patients underwent surgery within

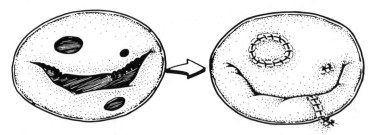

Fig 15–7.—Leaflet perforation treated by pericardial patch closure (anterior leaflet) and quadrangular resection (posterior leaflet). (Courtesy of Dreyfus G, Serraf A, Jebara VA, et al: *Ann Thorac Surg* 49:706–713. 1990.)

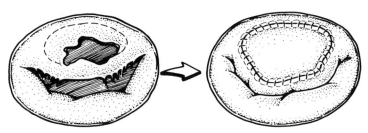

Fig 15–8.—Pericardial patch replacement of almost the entire anterior leaflet. (Courtesy of Dreyfus G, Serraf A, Jebara VA, et al: *Ann Thorac Surg* 49:706–713, 1990.)

the first 6 weeks after onset of symptoms and before completion of the initial full course of antibiotics. Indications for early surgery included hemodynamic deterioration in 37 patients, persistent sepsis in 4, and mobile vegetations (determined at echocardiography) with or without previous emboli in 6. Sixty percent of patients had underlying valve pathology. Time between onset of symptoms and surgery ranged from 12 days to 45 days (mean, 30 days). The mitral valve was involved in 28 patients, the aortic in 3, both mitral and aortic valves in 7, and the tricuspid valve in 2.

Autologous pericardial patching was used for cusp perforations of the aortic valve and for perforations of the anterior leaflet of the mitral valve (Fig 15–7). In 3 patients the entire anterior leaflet of the mitral valve was replaced with pericardium (Fig 15–8). Chordal transposition was used whenever marginal chordae of the anterior leaflet were ruptured (Fig 15–9). A sliding commisuroplasty was performed for prolapse of both anterior and posterior leaflets in the paracommissural area (Fig 15–10).

Seventeen patients had cusp perforations, 4 had annular abscesses, 13 had vegetation, and 22 had chordal rupture. Seventy-five percent of patients had positive cultures. Bacterial findings were *Staphylococcus* in 15 patients, *Streptococcus* in 12, gram-negative in 3, and unknown in 10. Criteria for performing valve repair included adequate antibiotic therapy for at least 1 week and extensive excision of all macroscopically involved tissues. The Carpentier reconstructive techniques were used in all cases; a prosthetic ring was required in only 19 patients.

There was 1 perioperative death and 1 late death. Doppler echocardi-

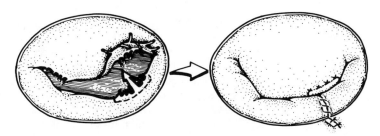

Fig 15–9.—Chordal transposition from posterior leaflet to free edge of anterior leaflet. (Courtesy of Dreyfus G, Serraf A, Jebara VA, et al: *Ann Thorac Surg* 49:706–713, 1990.)

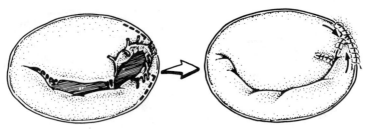

Fig 15–10.—Sliding commissuroplasty for prolapse of both anterior and posterior leaflets in paracommissural area. (Courtesy of Dreyfus G, Serraf A, Jebara VA, et al: *Ann Thorac Surg* 49:706–713, 1990.)

ography performed before discharge revealed no regurgitation in 32 patients. Seven had mild regurgitation. During mean follow-up of 30 months for all survivors there was no recurrence of endocarditis, and no reoperation has been required for valvular insufficiency. Surgical repair is possible in most patients with acute valve endocarditis who require early surgery for hemodynamic, bacteriologic, or echocardiographic reasons. Results seem to be superior to those of valve replacement.

▶ When operating for acute endocarditis, the safety of valve repair, as opposed to prosthetic valve replacement, is unknown. Hence, the experiences with 40 patients described in this report are of particular interest. Operations were performed in a period of 9 years. Endocarditis had been present between 12 and 45 days and involved the aortic and mitral valves of most patients. No underlying valve pathology was present in 40%. The severity of the pathology is impressive, with 17 cusp perforations, 4 annular abscesses, and 22 chordal ruptures.

Valve repair was performed when adequate antibiotic therapy had been instituted for the previous few days, and it was possible to excise all microscopically involved tissues. There was only 1 operative death; reoperation was necessary in 1 patient; there was no recurrence of endocarditis, an impressive fact. Several of the various Carpentier reconstructive techniques were used, implanting a prosthetic ring in 19 patients.—F.C. Spencer, M.D.

Surgery of Right-Sided Endocarditis: Valve Preservation Versus Replacement

Turley K (Univ of California, San Francisco)
J Cardiac Surg 4:317–320, 1989   15–15

Right-sided endocarditis is commonly treated by resection and replacement of the tricuspid valve. The more conservative approach of retaining and repairing the tricuspid valve when at all possible is preferred.

During the period 1981–1989, repair of the tricuspid valve was attempted in 19 patients aged 2–68 years with right-sided endocarditis. Six patients had congenital valve disease; 3 of these had Ebstein's anomaly. One patient had a traumatic ventricular septal defect, and 2 had pacemaker-induced endocarditis. Eight patients (40%) had endocarditis as a result of intravenous drug abuse. *Staphylococcus aureus* was the causative pathogen in 8 of the 19 patients. Treatment included débridement, leaflet resection, pericardial patching, annuloplasty in 3 patients, chordal resection and repair in 3 patients, and associated congenital repair in 6 patients. Intraoperative assessment was facilitated by transesophageal echo and use of a hand-held color Doppler unit.

Tricuspid valve repair was successful in 14 patients. The other 5 required valve replacement at the time of the original procedure. One patient (5%) died in the hospital of paradoxical embolus. Another patient (5%) with chronic renal failure who had a double valve replacement died 6 months after operation of a hypotensive arrest while on hemodialysis. Two patients had recurrences after valve repair. Repair of the tricuspid valve without prosthetic replacement in the treatment of right-sided endocarditis was successful in 75% of the patients in whom it was attempted.

▶ This paper is taken from a presentation at a workshop on surgery of endocarditis. It is not well written, but the data are quite significant.

In a period of 8 years, 19 patients with tricuspid valve endocarditis were treated. There was only 1 death. Repair, rather than replacement, was successful in 14 of the group. Recurrence of the endocarditis developed in 2. The various procedures used included débridement, pericardial patching, annuloplasty (3 patients), and chordal resection and repair (3 patients).

Detailed information is not given, but the basic information is important, indicating that some type of valve reconstruction, rather than replacement, can be performed safely despite active endocarditis.—F.C. Spencer, M.D.

Bioprosthetic Versus Mechanical Valve Replacement in Patients With Infective Endocarditis
Reul GJ, Sweeney MS (Texas Heart Inst, Houston; Univ of Texas, Houston)
J Cardiac Surg 4:348–351, 1989   15–16

Infective endocarditis can cause death, especially in patients with prosthetic cardiac valves. To determine whether patients with endocarditis who receive bioprosthetic or mechanical valves are more prone to recurrence of the infection, data on 4,598 patients who underwent valve replacement procedures over a 6-year period were retrospectively reviewed. Of these, 185 procedures were done for infective endocarditis. The patient's own valve was infected in 125 patients and a prosthetic valve was infected in 60. In 80% of patients, the infecting organism was *Staphylococcus* or *Streptococcus*. Congestive heart failure was the indication for surgery in 117 patients.

Patients were divided into 2 groups, 1 of which received Ionescu-Shiley bioprosthetic valves and the other, St. Jude Medical mechanical valves. In both groups, but particularly the mechanical valve group, the aortic valve was most commonly replaced. More patients in the bioprosthetic valve group had mitral valve replacement.

After 4 years, the mechanical valve group was 94.6% free from operation, compared with 75% in the bioprosthetic valve group. In the latter, 15 of 88 patients needed reoperation compared with 5 of 97 given mechanical valves. Patients with mechanical valves did better even though more had endocarditis of a previous replacement valve.

Mechanical valves are recommended as replacement valves in patients with acute infective endocarditis. These valves are probably less prone to reinfection because of their low-profile, highly polished pyrolitic carbon leaflets, which better resist infective processes. In addition, the double-velour Dacron sewing ring of the St. Jude Medical valve promotes rapid tissue growth; the annulus is usually completely covered with tissue within 3 months.

▶ In a 5-year period, 185 valve replacements were done for acute endocarditis. Until 1982, 88 patients received bioprosthetic valves, after which 92 patients received the metallic St. Jude prosthesis. The 30-day operative mortality was about 15% in both groups. Hence, the groups of patients were operated on at different periods of time.

A comparison of freedom from reoperation in the next 4 years showed a striking difference. Ninety-five percent of patients with a metallic prosthesis was free from reoperation as compared to only 75% of those receiving a bioprosthesis (Ionescu-Shiley).— F.C. Spencer, M.D.

16 Coronary Artery Disease

Saphenous Vein Graft Patency 1 Year After Coronary Artery Bypass Surgery and Effects of Antiplatelet Therapy: Results of a Veterans Administration Cooperative Study
Goldman S, Copeland J, Moritz T, Henderson W, Zadina K, Ovitt T, Doherty J, Read R, Chesler E, Sako Y, Lancaster L, Emery R, Sharma GVRK, Josa M, Pacold I, Montoya A, Parikh D, Sethi G, Holt J, Kirklin J, Shabetai R, Moores W, Aldridge J, Masud Z, DeMots H, Floten S, Haakenson C, Harker LA (VA Central Office, Washington, DC)
Circulation 80:1190–1197, 1989   16–1

Four antiplatelet regimens were compared with placebo in a series of about 500 men undergoing elective coronary bypass surgery at 12 centers between 1983 and 1986. Aspirin was given alone in a dose of 325 mg once or 3 times daily, or was combined with 75 mg of dipyridamole and given 3 times daily. Sulfinpyrazone was used in a dose of 267 mg 3 times daily. Aspirin was begun 12 hours before bypass surgery and the other medications 48 hours preoperatively. Postoperative treatment began 6 hours after surgery and continued for 1 year.

All regimens containing aspirin lowered the early graft occlusion rate compared with placebo. The respective occlusion rates at 1 year were 16% and 23%. Aspirin proved to be protective for vein grafts placed to vessels 2 mm or less in diameter, but no significant effect was noted at 1 year for grafts to larger vessels.

Aspirin probably inhibits acute platelet thrombus formation immediately after mechanical or surgical injury to vein grafts and anastomotic sites. It probably fails, however, to modify the occlusive process once the grafts and anastomoses are reendothelialized. It is possible that aspirin has an effect on graft patency after 1 year. In addition, stopping aspirin shortly after surgery could have a rebound effect.

▶ This broad cooperative study provides valuable data substantiating the routine use of antiplatelet therapy after bypass. The difference in patency with aspirin as opposed to a placebo was impressive. This was more marked in vessels smaller than 2 mm—20% thrombosis vs. 32%—whereas in vessels larger than 2 mm there was no significant difference. If a vein graft remained patent after bypass surgery, there were no data to indicate that aspirin would improve the likelihood of continued patency. Combining dipyridamole with aspirin did not provide additional benefit. The Medical Research Service of the Veterans Administration should be commended for organizing this significant

221

cooperative study. These valuable data can be used with any patient undergoing bypass.—F.C. Spencer, M.D.

Seventeen-Year Experience With Bilateral Internal Mammary Artery Grafts

Galbut DL, Traad EA, Dorman MJ, DeWitt PL, Larsen PB, Kurlansky PA, Button JH, Ally JM, Gentsch TO (Miami Heart Inst)
Ann Thorac Surg 49:195–201, 1990   16–2

Previous studies have shown that the internal mammary artery (IMA) graft has superior early and long-term patency as compared with the saphenous vein when used in myocardial revascularization. A retrospective analysis was carried out to assess the long-term results after myocardial revascularization with bilateral IMA and supplemental vein grafts.

During a 17-year period, 917 men and 170 women aged 29–84 years (mean, 62 years) received bilateral IMA and supplemental vein grafts. Of the 1,087 patients, 394 had unstable angina and 194 had left main coronary artery stenosis of more than 50%. A total of 3,741 coronary grafts were performed, or a mean of 3.4 per patient.

Twenty-nine patients died in the hospital, for a 2.7% in-hospital mortality rate. In-hospital complications included reoperation for bleeding in 19 patients, sternal infection in 16, respiratory failure in 35, perioperative myocardial infarction in 22, and stroke in 20. Fifty-three patients underwent follow-up arteriography at a mean of 53 months after operation, which revealed 92% patency for left IMA grafts and 85% patency for right IMA grafts.

Complete follow-up data were available for 1,058 hospital survivors. There were 82 late deaths, and 17 patients were subsequently lost to follow-up. The cumulative follow-up was 3,393.7 years. The linearized occurrence rate and number of late cardiac events in the 959 survivors were 1.18% per patient-year for nonfatal myocardial infarction, .27% per patient-year for reoperation for coronary artery disease, and .21% for patient-year for percutaneous transluminal coronary angioplasty. The actuarial survival rate for patients discharged from the hospital was 80% at 10 years and 56% at 17 years. The linearized late mortality rate was about 2.5% per patient-year. At follow-up, 90% of the patients were asymptomatic.

Internal mammary artery grafting in myocardial revascularization is associated with a low operative risk and provides excellent long-term functional improvement and survival. Bilateral IMA usage should be preferred for coronary revascularization.

▶ The Miami group has periodically reported impressive experiences with bilateral mammary grafts. The total series is now more than 1,000 patients. These data indicate a survival of 80% at 10 years and 60% at 15 years. A more informative analysis would be to present the data in comparison to normal survival curves and the matched population. The frequency of nonfatal infarction was 1% per patient per year. Reoperation was rarely necessary—.3% per year.

An important characteristic of the authors' data is that the mammary artery was used as an isolated artery, independent of fascia, veins, or lymphatics. An additional unique feature was the low rate of sternal infection—1.5%. The authors are to be complimented for this excellent report.—F.C. Spencer, M.D.

Bilateral Internal Mammary Grafts for Coronary Artery Bypass Operations in Children

Kitamura S, Kawachi K, Seki T, Morita R, Nishii T, Mizuguchi K, Fukutomi M, Hamada Y, Iioka S (Nara Med College, Nara, Japan)
J Thorac Cardiovasc Surg 99:708–715, 1990   16–3

The short- to middle-term clinical and angiographic follow-up data on 8 children who underwent coronary artery bypass grafting (CABG) with bilateral internal mammary artery (IMA) grafts were reviewed. The mean age of the 7 boys and 1 girl at the time of bilateral IMA grafting was 8 years. All had multiple vessel obstructions or stenoses as a result of Kawasaki disease; 3 had a previous myocardial infarction.

At surgery, the left IMA was anastomosed to the left anterior descending artery, and the right IMA was sutured to the right coronary artery. The children were followed for a mean of 23 months. All patients had an uneventful recovery and normal body structural development, including the sternum and thorax. None had recurrent angina or signs of myocardial ischemia. By the time of follow-up, 6 children no longer required medications. The IMA graft patency was 100% in both the early and late postoperative periods. Although there was no difference in patency between the right and left IMA grafts, the angiographic diameter of the IMA graft varied according to the diameter of the degree of stenosis of the recipient coronary arteries, or both.

The IMA, with its excellent long-term patency and growth potential, is the graft of choice for myocardial revascularization in pediatric patients. Because bilateral IMAs had no adverse effects on sternal development, this approach is recommended in children whenever indicated.

▶ This fascinating report describes the use of bilateral internal mammary grafts in 8 children with coronary problems caused by Kawasaki disease. The average age at operation was 8 years. In the operative procedure, 8-0 prolene was used. An excellent result was obtained in all, with 100% patency of both mammary arteries. There was no evidence of an adverse influence on chest wall development. The authors are to be congratulated on a significant accomplishment and excellent report.—F.C. Spencer, M.D.

Surgical Standby for Percutaneous Transluminal Coronary Angioplasty: A Survey of Patterns of Practice

Cameron DE, Stinson DC, Greene PS, Gardner TJ (Johns Hopkins Med Insts)
Ann Thorac Surg 50:35–39, 1990   16–4

Surgical standby is generally provided for elective percutaneous transluminal coronary angioplasty (PTCA). As the number of procedures has grown, this practice has become burdensome, and a consensus is lacking on the optimal standby arrangement. To determine patterns of surgical standby, 196 United States institutions were surveyed in which PTCA and coronary artery bypass grafting (CABG) are performed routinely. Of these, 89 institutions responded.

The mean number of hospital beds in responding institutions was 615. Physicians in these institutions performed a mean 337 PTCAs and 558 CABGs in 1987. There was a 4.4% rate of complications with PTCA that required emergency CABG. The rate of urgent CABG for PTCA failure was 3.7%. The incidence of urgent CABG for PTCA complications was higher at low-volume PTCA institutions than for those that treated more than 250 cases per year. Further, 64% of institutions maintained an open operating room on standby; 24% made the next open operating room available; i.e., they allowed operating room access within 1–3 hours; 29% maintained a flexible standby arrangement based on PTCA risk.

Thirty-eight percent of patients were routinely evaluated by the surgeon and/or anesthesiologist before PTCA. Fifty-one percent of surgical teams charged fees for standby services, as did 39% of anesthesia teams and 38% of operating room facilities. Present standby arrangements were unsatisfactory to 37% of the surgeons. Reasons included poor communication with cardiologists about high-risk or possibly inappropriate candidates for PTCA, waste of operating room resources, and inadequate fee structure.

Today, PTCA seldom requires emergent surgical revascularization. Nevertheless, many institutions still keep an open operating room on standby. The cost of this support is often not reimbursed. Current practices for surgical standby for PTCA should be further examined in the light of their cost.

▶ This report addresses the significant problem of surgical standby while PTCA is performed. The data described in the report were tabulated from a questionnaire survey, with 89 responses.

In general, 4% to 5% of patients undergoing coronary angioplasty will require urgent operation. Whether an operating room is kept available during the procedure or whether some alternative arrangement is used varies among different programs. The unsolved nature of the problem is indicated by the fact that more than one third of the surgeons were dissatisfied with their present arrangements.

As operation is needed for no more than 1 in 20 patients undergoing angioplasty, maintaining an operating room and staff on full standby is almost surely economically impractical. Using the next available operating room is clearly feasible when a center performs a substantial number of cardiac operations daily. An alternative mechanism, not discussed in this report, is the timing of the angioplasty. Cases in which there is a greater than usual risk of needing operation could either be done in the early morning, before the surgical procedures commenced, or be scheduled during the day, starting when an operative procedure is being completed but before the next patient has been anesthetized.— F.C. Spencer, M.D.

Myocardial Salvage After Failed Coronary Angioplasty
Stark KS, Satler LF, Krucoff MW, Rackley CE, Kent KM (Georgetown Univ Hosp)
J Am Coll Cardiol 15:78–82, 1990   16–5

Patients who have complications of percutaneous transluminal coronary angioplasty (PTCA) and require urgent coronary artery bypass grafting (CABG) provide a unique opportunity for study of the effects of early reperfusion for impending infarction. A retrospective study reviewed the effects of early reperfusion on preservation of left ventricular function in this situation.

Between 1981 and 1985, 859 patients underwent elective PTCA, of whom 42 required emergency CABG for objective evidence of impending myocardial infarction. Patients were contacted by telephone at a mean of 36 months after operation to determine current functional class, employment status, and any cardiac event since operation. Follow-up radionuclide ventriculography was performed at a mean of 39 months after operation.

Five patients (average age, 62 years) died and 1 was lost to follow-up. The average age of the remaining 36 patients was 57 years. Before CABG, 33 patients had Canadian Heart Association Class 3 or 4 unstable angina. At follow-up, 34 patients were asymptomatic or had class 1 angina, and 25 reported their activity level as moderate or strenuous. Twenty-one of the 36 patients underwent follow-up radionuclide ventriculography that was normal in 11 patients. Of the remaining 20 patients, 5 had a depressed ejection fraction with wall motion abnormalities that were unchanged from preangioplasty studies, 4 had a significant decrease in ejection fraction over baseline with new wall motion abnormalities, and 1 had myocardial infarction 3 years after CABG. There is an 80% chance that left ventricular function will be unchanged after 3 years of follow-up in patients surviving emergency CABG for failed PTCA, suggesting that early CABG for impending myocardial infarction in this setting has a good late outcome.

▶ During a period lasting between 4 and 5 years, 42 of 859 patients undergoing coronary angioplasty required emergency grafting. Five of these died. Subsequent long-term follow-up found that about 80% of the group had left ventricular function unchanged from that existing beforehand, well documenting the high salvage rate with early revascularization.—F.C. Spencer, M.D.

Failed Elective Percutaneous Transluminal Coronary Angioplasty Requiring Coronary Artery Bypass Surgery: In-Hospital and Late Clinical Outcome at 5 Years
Talley JD, Weintraub WS, Roubin GS, Douglas JS Jr, Anderson HV, Jones EL, Morris DC, Liberman HA, Craver JM, Guyton RA, King SB III (Emory Univ; Crawford W, Long Hosps, Atlanta)
Circulation 82:1203–1213, 1990   16–6

The outcome of coronary bypass surgery was examined in a series of 430 patients in whom attempted percutaneous transluminal coronary angioplasty failed. They represented 5.9% of all patients having elective angioplasty in 1980–1986. More than two thirds of the patients had single-vessel disease. The mean left ventricular ejection fraction at the time of surgery was 59%. Patients received an average of 1.9 bypass grafts.

One fourth of the patients with ischemia and 3.6% of the others had a new nonfatal postprocedure Q wave infarct. The in-hospital mortality rate was 1.4%. Sixteen cardiac deaths occurred in the subsequent 5 years. The overall rate of freedom from death and nonfatal infarction at 5 years was 71%. Preoperative myocardial ischemia and multivessel disease correlated with cardiac death or nonfatal infarction, as did preangioplasty stenosis of less than 90%.

Efforts in patients with failed angioplasty should focus on preventing or reducing myocardial ischemia and infarction. Effectively stabilizing or reversing ischemia before bypass surgery may well improve the immediate and long-term outcome, especially in elderly patients, women, and those with compromised myocardial function.

▶ This extensive report from Emory University evalutes the important clinical decision about how much long-term results are influenced by a percutaneous angioplasty that fails and is followed by myocardial revascularization.

There were 430 such patients treated over a period of 5 years, 346 of whom had ongoing myocardial ischemia. The severity of the coronary disease was not great in most patients, for 72% had single-vessel disease; the average ejection fraction was normal—near 59% percent. The frequency of myocardial infarction was high, similar to that reported by other groups—25% in the ischemic groups. However, 5 years later the long-term results were excellent, with a similar survival in both groups—near 95%. Hence, in this group of patients with moderate coronary disease, failure of angioplasty did not significantly complicate long-term survival despite the high frequency of perioperative myocardial infarction. It should be emphasized that these data are derived principally from patients with single-vessel disease. Whether or not the conclusions are applicable to patients with severe triple-vessel disease is unknown.—F.C. Spencer, M.D.

True Emergency Coronary Artery Bypass Surgery

Edwards FH, Bellamy RF, Burge JR, Cohen A, Thompson L, Barry MJ, Weston L (Walter Reed Army Med Ctr, Washington, DC, Uniformed Services Univ of Health Sciences, Bethesda, Md)
Ann Thorac Surg 49:603–611, 1990   16–7

Recent reports suggest that the operative mortality rate associated with emergency coronary artery bypass grafting (CABG) is approximately 5%. Some of these studies, however, included patients who were not true surgical emergencies; thus patient selection may result in underestimation of the actual operative risks associated with CABG. Data were analyzed on 117 patients (mean age, 59 years) who underwent true emergency bypass grafting for acute coronary artery ischemia refractory to other therapies.

Emergency CABG was performed in 50 patients when their condition deteriorated in the catheterization suite after percutaneous transfemoral coronary angioplasty or diagnostic catheterization. The other 67 patients were taken to the operating room from the intensive care unit or ward. Most operations were performed within an hour of surgical consultation. A statistical analysis of 18 preoperative risk factors was conducted to determine those variables predictive of an adverse outcome.

The operative mortality was 14.5%. In 13 of 17 patients the cause of death was cardiac related. Operative mortality was lowest (2.7%) in the 37 patients taken directly to the operating room after a percutaneous transfemoral coronary angioplasty misadventure. Most operative deaths occurred in patients taken to surgery from the ward or intensive care unit (15 of 67). The postoperative morbidity was 35.9%.

Univariate analysis demonstrated that the significant risk factors for operative mortality were ejection fraction, number of coronary arteries involved, previous myocardial infarction, hypertension, need for inotropic support, need for an intra-aortic balloon pump, and cardiopulmonary resuscitation. Independent risk factors identified by stepwise multivariate logistic regression were previous myocardial infarction, cardiopulmonary resuscitation, hypertension, and reoperation. Although 21.2% of patients with triple-vessel disease died, none of those with single-vessel coronary artery disease died.

True emergency CABG carries a high risk, with an operative mortality in the range of 15%. Using a logistic risk equation developed from this patient group, operative mortality could be accurately modeled. This realistic estimate of operative risk must be considered in therapeutic decisions concerning patients who need emergency CABG.

▶ This significant report addresses the peculiarity of the nomenclature defining "emergency coronary artery surgery" as that requiring operation more urgently than would usually be scheduled. This broad definition includes a wide range of severity of disease, ranging from cardiac arrest or cardiogenic shock to refractory unstable angina.

Experiences with 117 patients treated in a 5-year period are described. The overall mortality was 15%, although operations were performed within 4 hours of surgical consultation, most within an hour. Quite significant is the fact that among the 50 patients taken directly from the catheterization laboratory there was only a 4% operative mortality, whereas those taken from the intensive care unit or the ward had a mortality rate of almost 22%. Obviously, the 2 groups of patients are not comparable. The overall high mortality inherent in emergency operation, however, is evident from these data.—F.C. Spencer, M.D.

Long-Term Survival After Postinfarction Bypass Operation: Early Versus Late Operation

Floten HS, Ahmad A, Swanson JS, Wood JA, Chapman RD, Fessler CL, Starr A (St Vincent Hosp, Portland, Ore; Oregon Health Sciences Univ, Portland)
Ann Thorac Surg 48:757–763, 1989
16–8

It is controversial whether postinfarction bypass operations should be performed on an urgent basis to avoid infarct extension or should be delayed at least 1 month to permit the patient to stabilize medically. The outcome of patients who had coronary artery bypass grafting (CABG) operations within 30 days after acute myocardial infarction was compared with the outcome in those who had a CABG operation more than 30 days after infarction and those who had no history of infarction.

There were 832 patients in the first group (11%), 2,844 in the second (36%), and 4,162 in the last (53%). With the exception of 74 patients who were operated on to treat cardiogenic shock, this retrospective review included all patients who had a CABG operation from 1974 to 1987 at St. Vincent Hospital.

Operative mortality for patients who had a CABG procedure within 30 days after acute infarction was 4.7%. Among patients operated on within 24 hours mortality was 7.6%, compared with 4.1% for those operated on between 2 days and 30 days after infarct, but this difference in mortality was not statistically significant. Operative mortality was affected by the extent of anatomical disease and the presence of postinfarction angina.

Timing of operation was not a significant predictor of long-term survival, which was affected only by patient age and left ventricular end-diastolic pressure. Five-year survival for patients who were operated on within 30 days of infarct and for those who were operated on remotely was 84% and 85%, respectively. Ten-year survival was 71% and 68%, respectively, compared with 78% for those with no previous infarction.

Operative mortality for patients who undergo CABG procedures within 30 days of acute infarction is low. Delaying such procedures may increase the risk of recurrent infarction or extension of the infarct if ischemia or threatening coronary anatomy is present after acute infarction.

▶ These data from Oregon indicate the relative safety of prompt operation, when indicated, within the first 30 days after myocardial infarction. The authors report experiences with 832 patients operated on within 30 days of an infarction in a period of 13 years. This experience represents 11% of the nearly 8,000 patients operated on during this time. Patients with cardiogenic shock were excluded. Operative mortality was almost 8% for patients operated on within 24 hours, but decreased to only 4% for those operated on between 2 days and 30 days.

Of particular importance was the fact that the 5- and 10-year survival rates were not significantly different between those who had a recent infarction and those who had a remote infarction; the 5- and 10-year survival rates were slightly better, however, in those who had never had an infarction before bypass.—F.C. Spencer, M.D.

Surgical Coronary Revascularization in Survivors of Prehospital Cardiac Arrest: Its Effect on Inducible Ventricular Arrhythmias and Long-Term Survival
Kelly P, Ruskin JN, Vlahakes GJ, Buckley MJ Jr, Freeman CS, Garan H (Massachusetts Gen Hosp, Boston)
J Am Coll Cardiol 15:267–273, 1990   16–9

The role of coronary revascularization in the treatment and prevention of recurrent ventricular arrhythmias was examined in a subgroup of patients with cardiac arrest. The effects of several clinical, angiographic, and electrophysiologic variables on arrhythmia recurrence and survival were analyzed.

The patients included 41 men and 9 women, none of whom had an acute myocardial infarction at the time of the arrest, although 24 had a clinical history of myocardial infarction. Most patients (42) had triple-vessel coronary artery disease with greater than 70% reduction of the luminal diameter of the involved vessels. The mean follow-up was 39 months. Of the 41 patients who underwent preoperative electrophysiologic study, 33 had inducible ventricular arrhythmias. Of 42 patients not taking antiarrhythmic drug therapy postoperatively, 19 had inducible ventricular arrhythmias. Arrhythmias induction was suppressed in 14 of 30 patients with preoperative inducible arrhythmias who underwent postoperative testing while not receiving antiarrhythmic drug therapy.

The only significant predictor of induced ventricular arrhythmia suppression by coronary surgery was the induction of ventricular fibrillation at preoperative electrophysiologic study. Although inducible ventricular fibrillation was not present postoperatively in any of the 11 patients who manifested this arrhythmia preoperatively, inducible ventricular tachycardia persisted in 80% of the patients in whom preoperative testing induced this arrhythmia.

During the follow-up period, 4 arrhythmias recurred and 1 was fatal. There were 3 noncardiac and 3 nonsudden cardiac deaths. The 5-year survival rate determined by life-table analysis, was 88%, cardiac survival was 98%, and arrhythmia free-survival was 88%. In a substantial proportion of patients in this selected subgroup of survivors of cardiac arrest, coronary revascularization succeeded in abolishing inducible ventricular arrhythmias, especially when the induced arrhythmia was ventricular fibrillation and ventricular function was well preserved. The long-term prognosis for these patients is excellent.

▶ With the availability of implantable defibrillator electrodes, although expensive, a particularly important question is the ability of revascularization alone to control arrhythmias. Hence, this report of experiences with 50 patients treated at the Massachusetts General Hospital over a period of 8 years is of particular interest. Fifty patients who survived cardiac arrest were revascularized. Eighty percent had inducible arrhythmias beforehand. Postoperatively, about half of these still had inducible arrhythmias. Hence, revascularization was about 50% effective. Inducible ventricular fibrillation preoperatively in 11 patients could not be induced after revascularization; however, inducible ventricular tachycardia persisted in 80%.

In an average follow-up of slightly more than 3 years, there were 4 arrhythmia recurrences, 1 of which was fatal.—F.C. Spencer, M.D.

Reoperation for Coronary Atherosclerosis: Changing Practice in 2509 Consecutive Patients

Loop FD, Lytle BW, Cosgrove DM, Woods EL, Stewart RW, Golding LAR, Goormastic M, Taylor PC (Cleveland Clinic Found)
Ann Surg 212:378–386, 1990   16–10

Data were reviewed on 2,509 consecutive patients having reoperation for myocardial revascularization at the Cleveland Clinic between 1967 and 1987. Left ventricular performance worsened over the years. The operative mortality rate ranged from 2% to 5% and was 2.9% in the most recent cohort. New Q wave perioperative infarction occurred in 7% to 8% of the first 3 cohorts and in 4% of the last cohort (1985–1987). Vein graft atherosclerosis now is the leading indication for reoperation. Both patient age and time between operations continue to increase. Use of the internal thoracic artery has increased from 27% in 1967–1978 to 67% in 1985–1987.

Advanced age and left main coronary artery disease affected late survival adversely. Patients operated on in 1967–1978 had relatively few risk factors, explaining their higher survival rate when compared with more recent cohorts. Factors associated with better actuarial 10-year survival include age under 65 years, mild angina, the lack of major comorbidity, the absence of left main coronary disease, good left ventricular performance, and use of an internal thoracic artery graft.

Vein graft atherosclerosis now is a more prominent cause of reoperation than progressive coronary atherosclerosis per se. The interval to reoperation continues to increase. Improved techniques of reentry, myocardial protection, and blood conservation now allow more time for exposure and complete revascularization. A higher-risk population undergoes reoperation now compared with past years. The chief risk factors are age and left main coronary artery disease.

▶ This extensive experience with 2,509 reoperations for myocardial revascularization is almost surely the largest in the world. Particularly significant aspects in the data presented include the fact that vein graft atherosclerosis is the leading indication for reoperation; also, operative mortality has gradually decreased to 2.9% in the most recent group. New Q wave myocardial infarction also decreased in frequency from 8% earlier to about 4%, probably reflecting better techniques of myocardial preservation.—F.C. Spencer, M.D.

17 Miscellaneous Cardiac Conditions and the Great Vessels

Does the Addition of Albumin to the Prime Solution in Cardiopulmonary Bypass Affect Clinical Outcome? A Prospective Randomized Study
Marelli D, Paul A, Samson R, Edgell D, Angood P, Chiu RC-J (McGill Univ)
J Thorac Cardiovasc Surg 98:751–756, 1989   17–1

Nonblood colloid priming solutions are used routinely in cardiopulmonary bypass to decrease plasma oncotic pressure that occurs during extracorporeal circulation. The effectiveness of that practice was assessed in 100 adults undergoing cardiac operations. Forty-nine patients (mean age, 63 years) were randomly allocated to receive Ringer's lactate solution plus 50 g of albumin; 51 patients (mean age, 57 years) did not receive any colloid in the prime solution. Patients were evaluated on 40 clinical parameters of preoperative, intraoperative, and postoperative status.

The mean volume of crystalloid solution used during operation was 2,620 mL in the albumin group and 3,052 mL in the control group. Controls had a lower mean cardiac filling pressure and a higher hematocrit value in the immediate postoperative period compared with those who received albumin in the prime solution. However, all mean values in both groups were within the normal range. There were no differences between the 2 groups with respect to any of the postoperative clinical parameters measured, and outcome was not affected by the addition of albumin to the prime solution. Nor was the incidence of postoperative complications affected by the addition of albumin to the priming solution. Both groups were discharged from the surgical intensive care unit at similar rates.

The addition of albumin to prime solution used in cardiac bypass procedure provides no clinically relevant benefit. Adding albumin to the prime solution routinely in adults undergoing cardiopulmonary bypass is not cost effective.

▶ The significance of the oncotic pressure of the perfusate during cardiopulmonary bypass remains unknown. This short paper reports a randomized study of 100 patients, half of whom had 50 g of albumin added to the crystalloid prime. No clinical difference could be measured. Unfortunately, oncotic pressures were not measured during perfusion. The critical question seems to be: "Are low oncotic pressures in the perfusate (less than 10 mm Hg) during bypass hazardous?"—F.C. Spencer, M.D.

Low Activated Coagulation Time During Cardiopulmonary Bypass Does Not Increase Postoperative Bleeding

Metz S, Keats AS (Texas Heart Inst, Houston; Univ of Texas Health Science Ctr, Houston)
Ann Thorac Surg 49:440–444, 1990   17–2

Many institutions use the activated coagulation time (ACT) to monitor the adequacy of anticoagulation during cardiopulmonary bypass (CPB). An ACT of at least 400 seconds is widely accepted as ensuring adequate heparinization during CPB. However, the ACT value below which adverse outcomes are likely to occur has not been defined. The relationship was assessed between heparinized ACT values during CPB and clot formation in the CPB circuit or excessive postoperative blood loss.

Of 202 patients scheduled for elective cardiac operations requiring CPB, 126 underwent coronary artery bypass operations and 76 had open cardiac chamber operations with or without coronary artery bypass grafting. Each patient was given heparin, 300 units per kg intravenously, before aortic cannulation. Activated coagulation time was measured before heparin administration and at 3 predetermined sampling times thereafter. Heparin levels were measured simultaneously with ACT levels in 117 patients. The CPB circuits were examined for blood clots. The postoperative blood loss was measured as cumulative chest tube output during the first 24 hours after arrival in the intensive care unit. Complete data sets were available for 193 patients.

Cardiopulmonary bypass averaged 59 minutes and ranged from 30 to 138 minutes. The ACT values showed a normal distribution at each sampling period. Fifty-one patients (26.4%) had ACT values of less than 400 seconds and 4 of them had ACT values of less than 300 seconds at some sampling time after heparinization. Three patients died within 24 hours of operation but the causes were unrelated to blood loss. Six patients required reexploration for control of postoperative bleeding, but all 6 patients had surgical causes for the bleeding. Patients with low ACT values did not bleed more than those with high ACT values, nor was bleeding related to heparin levels. No blood clots were found in any of the perfusion circuits. The minimal ACT value that would ensure adequate heparinization during CPB lies somewhere below the 400-second ACT value that is presently regarded as safe for avoiding complications during and after CPB.

▶ This short paper emphasizes the paucity of data defining the minimum safe level of ACT during bypass. In a series of 193 patients, a single dose of heparin, 300 units per kg, was given. The average bypass time was nearly 1 hour. Serial measurements of both ACT and heparin units were done. In about 25% of the patients, the ACT was below 400 seconds at some time, but abnormal bleeding was not recognized from postoperative drainage. Similarly, heparin concentrations were usually above 2 units per mL and did not correlate closely with ACT.

Although the measures of effective anticoagulation were somewhat broad—simply measuring the amount of postoperative bleeding—the information does reemphasize the point that the precise minimum safe level of ACT is not well defined.—F.C. Spencer, M.D.

Heparin Dosing and Monitoring for Cardiopulmonary Bypass: A Comparison of Techniques With Measurement of Subclinical Plasma Coagulation
Gravlee GP, Haddon WS, Rothberger HK, Mills SA, Rogers AT, Bean VE, Buss DH, Prough DS, Cordell AR (Wake Forest Univ)
J Thorac Cardiovasc Surg 99:518–527, 1990   17–3

Prolongation of the activated coagulation time (ACT) is thought to be more important than heparinization, hypothermia, or hemodilution during cardiopulmonary bypass (CPB). Published recommendations of appropriate ACTs have been empirical and vary widely. The different methods of heparin administration were compared using plasma fibrinopeptide A (FPA) concentrations to measure subclinical coagulation activity.

The study involved 21 patients: In group 1, 10 patients were given heparin, 300 units per kg, or more if the ACT decreased to less than 400 seconds; in group 2, 6 patients were given heparin, 250 units per kg, or more if the ACT decreased; in group 3, 5 patients were given heparin, 350–400 units per kg, or more if whole blood heparin concentration was 4.1 units per mL or less. During CPB, the FPA levels showed a marked increase, but not as great as before and after CPB. Levels of FPA were inversely correlated with the heparin concentration during CPB, but increased FPA levels showed no correlation with coagulopathy after CPB. Patients in group 3 received the most heparin and lost the most blood.

Postoperative mediastinal drainage showed the best correlation with protamine dose and heparin concentration during CPB. Because protamine does not neutralize all of the anticoagulant actions of heparin, particularly on factor X, higher doses of heparin should increase the amount of circulating heparin that cannot be pharmacologically neutralized, although traditional methods do not detect this effect. Some tissue distribution of heparin does occur; this reservoir should enlarge proportionately to the blood concentration, predisposing to postoperative heparin rebound.

Plasma coagulation activity is normal during CPB, but it is compensated and shows no correlation with bleeding after CPB. Excessive heparin should be avoided during CPB; an ACT in the range of 350–500 seconds is recommended. There appears to be no heparin concentration threshold that protects against clotting factor consumption, and heparin dosing during CPB cannot be guided by monitoring heparin concentrations.

▶ These studies of the adequacy of heparin anticoagulation during CPB measured plasma FPA, the ACT, and the heparin concentration. This careful study and its conclusions should be examined in detail by investigators studying coagulation indices during bypass. The somewhat surprising conclusions reached from these studies need confirmation by others.

Three different types of heparin management were studied; 1 group given 300 units of heparin per kilogram, another given 250 per kilogram, and a third given an initial dose of 350–400 per kilogram. Supplemental heparin was given in all 3 groups for an ACT below 400 seconds or a blood heparin concentration of less than 4 units.

Coagulation activity was measured by plasma FPA concentrations. Some subclinical plasma coagulation activity continued during bypass in all 3 groups, although it was less with higher doses of heparin. An activated clotting time between 350 and 400 seconds produced acceptable results. Surprisingly enough, the higher heparin dosage group, which had lower plasma coagulation activity, was associated with a significantly higher degree of postoperative bleeding in 24 hours—1,100 mL vs. about 700 mL. This challenges the time-honored concepts that excessive heparin is harmless. The authors carefully point out that not all heparin is effectively neutralized by protamine. These studies indicate that the proper range of anticoagulation is produced with an ACT between 350 and 400 seconds, with the possibility of less benefit with either higher or lower levels.—F.C. Spencer, M.D.

Protection of the Immature Myocardium During Ischemic Arrest: Dose Dependent Effects of Glucose and Mannitol When Added to St Thomas' Cardioplegic Solution

Yang SS, Hearse DJ (Rayne Inst; St Thomas' Hosp, London)
Can J Cardiol 5:401–407, 1989   17–4

Advances in cardioplegia have led to better preservation of the myocardium and improved outcome in adults undergoing cardiac surgery. Recovery in children, however, may be poor because of inadequate myocardial protection. Although the adult myocardium makes use primarily of fatty acids as energy sources, cardiac metabolism in infants depends on glucose. The addition of glucose or mannitol might improve the protective ability of cardioplegic solution in immature hearts.

Experiments were performed on hearts from Wistar rats aged 3–5 days. The hearts were perfused as Langendorff preparations with an indwelling left ventricular balloon. Animals received the St Thomas' Hospital cardioplegic solution to which had been added various concentrations of glucose or mannitol. Postischemic recovery was assessed after various periods of ischemia.

Increasing durations of ischemia were, as expected, associated with decreasing postischemic functional recoveries. Overall, glucose actually reduced the protective properties of the cardioplegic solution. Mannitol had relatively little effect or tended to offer some degree of protection. Neither addition to the solution significantly affected tissue water content except at high concentrations when a small protective effect was observed. This study of the immature rat heart does not support the addition of glucose to cardioplegic solutions given as a bolus at the start of a period of global ischemia.

▶ The senior investigator in this report, David Hearse, pioneered the development of the St Thomas' cardioplegia solution through a series of investigations over a period of years. This short report evaluated myocardial preservation in immature rat hearts. The striking vulnerability was confirmed, as recovery of preischemic function was only 48% after 60 minutes of ischemia, decreasing to 15% after 90 minutes. The authors theorize that this may be attributable to basic metabolic differences, as the immature heart depends primarily on glucose for oxidation, whereas the adult heart can also use fatty acids. Surprisingly, however, the addition of glucose in increasing amounts was clearly harmful rather than helpful. Mannitol, designed to decrease the tissue accumulation of water, had a slightly beneficial effect.— F.C. Spencer, M.D.

Reoperation After Pericardial Closure With Bovine Pericardium
Eng J, Ravichandran PS, Abbott CR, Kay PH, Murday AJ, Shreiti I (Leeds Gen Infirmary, England)
Ann Thorac Surg 48:813–815, 1989   17–5

Bovine pericardium has been used increasingly as a pericardial substitute to shield the anterior surface of the heart from direct adhesion to the sternum. In all, 113 bovine pericardial patches were used to reconstruct the pericardium after a second repeat valve operation. Three men and 1 woman aged 34–53 years underwent resternotomy for the third time 3–8 years after valve replacement and closure of the pericardial cavity with glutaraldehyde-preserved bovine pericardium.

At resternotomy, with use of an oscillating saw, dense adhesions to the posterior surface of the sternum and epicardium were revealed. Careful, sharp dissection permitted the freeing of the heart of all 4 patients. Intracardiac procedures were uneventful, and all patients had successful postoperative recoveries.

Histologic examination of samples of the previously implanted bovine pericardium showed that although the pericardium itself was well preserved, it was surrounded by dense, poorly vascularlized fibrous connective tissue, with foreign body giant cell reaction and chronic inflammatory cell infiltrates. The tissue reaction was stronger in a patch that had been implanted for 8 years than in a patch that had been in place for 3 years.

The use of bovine pericardium should be discontinued, because it seems to increase the difficulty of repeat cardiac operations. If a careful technique is used, resternotomy is possible if the pericardium has been left open after a previous cardiac operation. Even when reoperation appears likely, it is recommended that pericardial substitutes be used cautiously; instead, primary pericardial closure should be attempted, perhaps aided by methods of traction to prevent pericardial contraction after its incision.

▶ This report cautions about the use of bovine pericardium for pericardial closure after open-heart operations. This institution in Leeds, England, used pericardium in about 113 patients over a period of several years. Four required reoperation after 3–8 years because of dense adhesions between the pericardium, the heart, and the sternum. For this reason, the use of bovine pericardium was abandoned. If other institutions report similar experiences, its continued use needs reassessment.—F.C. Spencer, M.D.

A Randomized Study of Carbon Dioxide Management During Hypothermic Cardiopulmonary Bypass

Bashein G, Townes BD, Nessly ML, Bledsoe SW, Hornbein TF, Davis KB, Goldstein DE, Coppel DB (Univ of Washington)
Anesthesiology 72:7–15, 1990   17–6

There are 2 approaches to the optimal management of blood gas during deliberate hypothermia. The methods were compared to determine whether the known physiologic responses to carbon dioxide management during cardiopulmonary bypass (CPB) with moderate hypothermia affect the cerebral or cardiac outcome of patients.

Eighty-six patients undergoing coronary artery bypass grafting were randomly assigned to 1 of 2 groups according to the target value for arterial carbon dioxide pressure ($PaCO_2$) during bypass. In 44 patients, the target $PaCO_2$ was 40 mm Hg, measured at the electrode temperature of 37° C. In 42 patients, the target $PaCO_2$ was 40 mm Hg, corrected to the patient's rectal temperature. Perfusion was maintained during CPB using a bubble oxygenator without arterial filtration. Other parameters included mean hematocrit of 23% and a mean arterial blood pressure of 70 mm Hg that was achieved by infusion of phenylephrine or sodium nitroprusside. Neuropsychological function was assessed before surgery, just before discharge, and at 7 months postoperatively.

Neuropsychological scores at 8 days varied widely and showed generalized impairment unrelated to the $PaCO_2$ group or to hypotension during CPB. At 7 months there was no significant difference in neuropsychological performance between the $PaCO_2$ groups. Nor was there any significant difference in the appearance of new Q waves on ECG, need for inotropic or intra-aortic balloon pump support, postoperative creatine kinase-MB fractions, or length of either postoperative ventilation or stay in intensive care.

Carbon dioxide management during CPB at moderate hypothermia has no significant effect on cardiac outcome or neurobehavior. Because moderate hypothermia is widely used in adult cardiac surgery, these results should have extensive applicability; they cannot be extrapolated to deeper hypothermia, however. Further research is required to determine whether carbon dioxide management affects outcome when lower temperatures are used.

▶ This carefully done randomized study compared 2 forms of $PaCO_2$ management during bypass, keeping the $PaCO_2$ near 40 mm (measured at room temperature) in 44 patients and comparing results with another 42 patients with a $PaCO_2$ corrected to moderate hypothermia (near 30° C). Subsequent evaluation included assessment of both hemodynamic function and neurologic function. No significant differences were found in the 2 groups. Various neuropsychological abnormalities were observed 8 days after operation, but 7 months later there was no significant difference between the 2 groups.—F.C. Spencer, M.D.

Effect of Intraoperative Intervention on Neurological Outcome Based on Electroencephalographic Monitoring During Cardiopulmonary Bypass
Arom KV, Cohen DE, Strobl FT (Minneapolis Heart Inst)
Ann Thorac Surg 48:476–483, 1989   17–7

Intact neurons have predictable electrical patterns. Neuronal electrical activity is a direct reflection of cerebral perfusion under appropriate anesthesia. Inadequate cerebral perfusion pressure is immediately reflected by suppressed electroencephalographic (EEG) activity. Whether online computerized EEG changes correlated with neurologic outcome in patients undergoing cardiopulmonary bypass (CPB) was determined. Neurologic outcomes were compared with those in a second group of patients who received intraoperative interventions based on EEG data.

Ninety-one unselected patients undergoing heart surgery were studied. Part 1 involved 50 patients who were monitored by computerized EEG during surgery. These patients also served as controls for part 2. In part 1, a power-drop index was developed to correlate with new global neurologic deficits. Neurologic examinations were performed preoperatively and postoperatively. Station and gait were included when possible. In part 2, criteria for intraoperative intervention included any drop in power to 25% of baseline activity during the pump run. Interventions included increasing the cerebral perfusion pressure to 60–65 mm Hg, increasing CPB pump flow, and increasing blood carbon dioxide.

There were no intraoperative deaths. In part 1 statistically significant difference was observed between diagnostic groups—normal vs. global deficits—and in their respective drop in global EEG power averaged over the entire head. There was also a significant difference relative to cerebral perfusion pressure and outcome. Because of a decrease in the number of global complications, the neurologic outcome was considerably improved in patients who received interventions.

Applying digital computer techniques to the analysis of EEG increases the sensitivity for detection of EEG changes associated with ischemia. In this study, global neurologic deficits were reduced to 5% in patients who received interventions. Computerized EEG can reduce global neurologic deficits in patients undergoing CPB procedures.

▶ Neurologic injury is the most serious complication with CPB, the estimated frequency ranging from 2% to 5% or higher. The causes are usually unknown. Emboli of gas or particulate matter from either the heart, the oxygenator, or aortic arch are the most common hypotheses, but this remains speculative. Hence, this report of using computerized EEG monitoring as an index of cerebral blood flow is of particular interest. Although the findings are preliminary, the potential significance seems large.

Preliminary studies in 50 patients established a baseline, constructing a "power index" based on the intensity of the electrical signals recorded in the EEG from the brain. The frequency of postoperative neurologic abnormalities was astonishing, being present in nearly one third of 50 patients operated on. Details are not given.

In a subsequent study of 41 patients, techniques of perfusion were altered if a significant decrease appeared in the "power index." Details are not given, but, in general, perfusion pressure or flow rate was increased, possibly by changes in blood carbon dioxide. These adjustments resulted, in the next group, in a decreased frequency of global deficits from 20% a few days after operation to 2%. This was particularly noteworthy the first day after operation.

There was no correlation with either duration of perfusion or mean arterial pressure, averaging about 60 mm. Hence, the cause of the problem, as well as the changes in technique that corrected it, are unclear. However, the technique seems feasible and clearly merits further analysis.—F.C. Spencer, M.D.

Influence of Oxygenator Type on the Prevalence and Extent of Microembolic Retinal Ischemia During Cardiopulmonary Bypass: Assessment by Digital Image Analysis

Blauth CI, Smith PL, Arnold JV, Jagoe JR, Wootton R, Taylor KM (Hammersmith Hosp, London)
J Thorac Cardiovasc Surg 99:61–69, 1990   17–8

Fluorescein angiography has been used to document the occurrence of microembolic ischemia in the retina during cardiopulmonary bypass (CPB). This approach has been extended to include computer-assisted digital image analysis to provide a measure of the extent of microembolic ischemia in the retina. The combined technique was applied to a comparative study of perfusion with a bubble oxygenator and with a flat sheet-membrane oxygenator.

Sixty-four patients undergoing elective first-time coronary surgery were studied. In 30 patients, perfusion was maintained with a bubble oxygenator during CPB surgery. A flat sheet-membrane oxygenator was used in the remaining 34. Bypass procedures were standardized with pulsatile flow and a 40-μm arterial line filter. All patients underwent preoperative fluorescein angiography of the right eye (Fig 17–1). Retinal angiography was also performed 5 minutes before the end of the bypass period (Fig 17–2). Angiograms underwent digital image analysis. Microembolic perfusion defects were identified by digital subtraction of preoperative and end-bypass angiograms (Figs 17–3 and 17–4); their total area was computed.

All 30 patients in the bubble-oxygenator group had perfusion defects indicative of microembolism. In contrast, more than half the patients in the sheet-membrane group had normal retinal perfusion. The prevalence of perfusion defects was significantly less in the sheet-membrane group

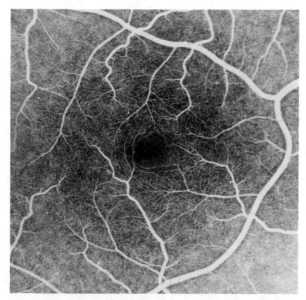

Fig 17–1.—Fluorescein angiogram of normal right optic fundus, taken before operation, that shows a central area of 31 mm² of the retina centered on the macula. (Courtesy of Blauth CI, Smith PL, Arnold JV, et al: *J Thorac Cardiovasc Surg* 99:61–69, 1990.)

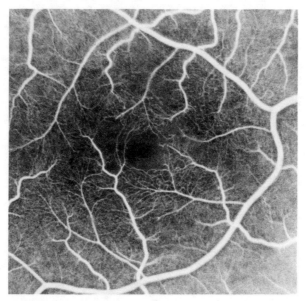

Fig 17–2.—Retinal fluorescein angiogram from the same patient, taken 5 minutes before CPB was discontinued, that shows several perfusion defects. (Courtesy of Blauth CI, Smith PL, Arnold JV, et al: *J Thorac Cardiovasc Surg* 99:61–69, 1990.)

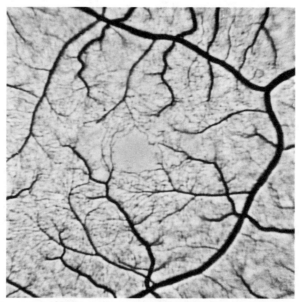

Fig 17–3.—Computer digitized image of retinal angiogram. (Courtesy of Blauth CI, Smith PL, Arnold JV, et al: *J Thorac Cardiovasc Surg* 99:61–69, 1990.)

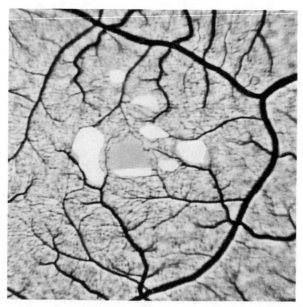

Fig 17–4.—Computer digitized image of retinal angiogram with the areas of retinal ischemia highlighted. (Courtesy of Blauth CI, Smith PL, Arnold JV, et al: *J Thorac Cardiovasc Surg* 99:61–69, 1990.)

than in the bubble group. Patients in the sheet membrane group also had significantly smaller total areas of retinal ischemia and significantly fewer lesions. There was no correlation between the extent of retinal ischemia and bypass time, volume of cardiotomy suction or donor blood returned to the pump, arterial blood-gas concentrations, or recent treatment with aspirin.

Digital image analysis of retinal fluorescein angiograms might provide a procedure for quantifying microembolic ischemia in the CNS during CPB. Flat sheet-membrane oxygenation apparently provides significantly better protection against microembolic ischemia than bubble oxygenation.

▶ The significance of microemboli during CPB remains uncertain. An arterial filter in the circuit is frequently used for this reason. This report from England by Blauth et al. supplements a previous report. Fluorescein retinal angiograms were performed preoperatively and 5 minutes before the end of perfusion, and then processed with a digital image analyzer. Microembolic defects were found in all 30 patients perfused with a bubble oxygenator but in less than half of a similar group perfused with a membrane oxygenator. A 40-μ Pall filter was used in the arterial line routinely. The vessels occluded by microemboli were estimated to be about 20 μ in diameter. Further studies are awaited with much interest as the clinical significance of these observations remains unknown.— F.C. Spencer, M.D.

Four Years' Experience With Fibrin Sealant in Thoracic and Cardiovascular Surgery
Matthew TL, Spotnitz WD, Kron IL, Daniel TM, Tribble CG, Nolan SP (Univ of Virginia)
Ann Thorac Surg 50:40–44, 1990   17–9

Fibrin sealant or glue is an established surgical material in Europe and Canada where it is available as a commercially manufactured system, but fibrin sealant products are not yet commercially available in the United States because of the potential risk of blood-borne disease transmission when fibrinogen is obtained from pooled human plasma. However, fibrin sealant using single-donor fibrinogen in combination with bovine thrombin is available. Fibrin sealant can be used in surgical procedures for hemostasis and to reduce air and body fluid leakage.

During a 4-year study, a single-donor fibrin sealant system was used in 689 thoracic and cardiovascular surgical procedures. The concentrated fibrinogen was prepared in the blood bank from single-donor human plasma that had been tested for hepatitis B surface antigen and HIV-I antibody. The fibrinogen was applied either from individual syringes, from a spray bottle, or via a fiberoptic bronchoscope to seal staple lines, suture lines, anastomoses, conduits, fistulas, and raw surfaces.

Success rates ranged from a low of 60% when the sealant was used for bronchopleural fistulas to a high of 100% when used to seal esophageal anastomoses. The overall success rate was 94%, and the overall infection rate was 2%. No complications secondary to blood-borne disease were documented. Fibrin sealant has application in a wide variety of thoracic and cardiovascular procedures in which it can be used to control the leakage of air, blood, and fluid.

▶ This report describes experiences with fibrin glue in a period of 4 years at the University of Virginia, during which time it was used in nearly 700 procedures. No major complications occurred. Uniform effectiveness was reported, although obviously this is principally a subjective consideration.

Several important technical maneuvers are described. A particularly attractive one is using concentrated fibrinogen from single-donor human plasma, thus minimizing the risk of infectious disease transmission by using conventional cryoprecipitate. Another attractive technique is the use of spray bottles to simultaneously cover a large bleeding surface.—F.C. Spencer, M.D.

Protein C Deficiency Associated With Massive Cerebral Thrombosis Following Open Heart Surgery
Ridley PD, Ledingham SJM, Lennox SC, Burman JF, Chung HI, Sheffield EA, Talbot S, Bevan D (Brompton Hosp; St Georges Hosp Med School, London)
J Cardiovasc Surg 31:249–251, 1990   17–10

Congenital protein C deficiency is an inherited condition associated with thrombotic disorders. A patient with protein C deficiency died of massive cerebral venous thrombosis after routine open-heart surgery.

Woman, 75, underwent routine cardiopulmonary bypass (CPB) to correct symptomatic severe aortic stenosis. She had no personal or family history suggestive of thromboembolic disorders, and she had not received anticoagulant therapy. At operation, a moderately stenosed calcific valve was replaced with a xenograft via an aortotomy. Cross-clamp time was 88 minutes. The patient was returned to the intensive care unit in apparently stable condition. However, within 8 hours after operation she had no movement in the left arm. Her neurologic condition rapidly deteriorated, and she died 48 hours after operation. Postmortem examination revealed thrombosis of the superior vena cava tracking up the right brachiocephalic vein, the right internal jugular vein, and both transverse intracranial venous sinuses and part of the superior sagittal sinus. There was no evidence of gross trauma at the site of central line insertion. Retrospective assay of a stored citrated blood sample for 5 clotting factors revealed a reduced protein C level of 40%.

The occurrence of massive cerebral venous thrombosis after routine CPB in a patient with a reduced protein C level suggests that CPB exacerbated the existing protein C deficiency.

▶ This case report describing fatal thrombosis of the superior vena cava and jugular vein after routine CPB is said to be the first reported case of this event associated with protein C deficiency. This is an uncommon syndrome. This interesting case report is included to alert others to investigate the possibility of protein C deficiency when massive thrombotic phenomena occur without obvious explanation.—F.C. Spencer, M.D.

Pericardial Window: Mechanisms of Efficacy
Sugimoto JT, Little AG, Ferguson MK, Borow KM, Vallera D, Staszak VM, Weinert L (Univ of Chicago)
Ann Thorac Surg 50:442–445, 1990   17–11

A pericardial window can be created by several approaches and with varying results. This discrepancy in results implies that not all techniques achieve equivalent outcomes. It was postulated that the mechanism of success is not a window but, rather, fusion of the epicardium to the pericardium with obliteration of the potential space. This theory was examined in 28 patients who had undergone a subxiphoid pericardial window procedure.

Twenty-six patients had symptomatic pericardial effusions; the other 2 had no symptoms directly related to the presence of fluid. The underlying diagnosis was carcinoma in 24 patients and renal failure in 4. Tube drainage was maintained until output was minimal, usually within 3–5 days after surgery. Results were assessed by pre- and postoperative echocardiograms. Autopsies were performed on 4 patients who died between 6 weeks and 8 months after the operation.

All patients with malignancy eventually died of their underlying disease, but the patients with uremic effusions were alive at the end of the study. The operation resulted in permanent relief in 26 patients. Autopsy findings showed no free pericardial fluid. Postoperative echocardiograms revealed a thickened, fused epicardium/pericardium in all patients. Histologic examination showed fusion of the epicardium and pericardium into a single tissue plane.

The subxiphoid pericardial window is a procedure that can be performed quickly and safely, providing definitive diagnostic and therapeutic results in all forms of effusive disease. Success depends on achieving initial complete drainage of the pericardial fluid and continued decompression of the pericardial space until adherence of the epicardium and pericardium begins. This technique will, in most patients, yield results comparable with those obtained by total pericardiectomy.

▶ This clinical study analyzed the mechanisms by which surgical drainage of pericardial effusion is effective. The authors concluded that fusion of the epicardium to the pericardium, obliterating the pericardial space, is the basic mechanism, rather than maintaining an open "window." If this conclusion is correct, maintenance of adequate tube drainage is the most important point, rather than the extent of the pericardium resected.—F.C. Spencer, M.D.

Vocal Dysfunction Following Cricothyroidotomy: A Prospective Study
Holst M, Hertegård S, Persson A (Huddinge Univ Hosp, Huddinge, Sweden)
Laryngoscope 100:749–755, 1990   17–12

Cricothyroid muscle function was evaluated on the basis of pitch, vocal strength, and ability to sing and to produce falsetto in 19 patients who underwent cricothyroidotomy. They were among 54 patients operated on in a 1-year period and 29 who survived the primary disease or injury. The follow-up interval was about 6 months. The mean endotracheal intubation time was 2½ days.

Twelve patients reported some vocal dysfunction at follow-up and 3 of them described changes consistent with cricothyroid muscle dysfunction. Ten patients had a normal larynx; several others had bowed vocal folds or slightly swollen vocal folds. Only 1 patient had a subnormal speaking fundmental frequency analysis. Five patients had a pathologic phonetogram. The voices of 4 patients were considered to be monotonous. In all, 4 of the 19 patients had signs of a decreased external tensor effect on the vocal folds and 5 had other vocal disorders. Elective cricothyroidotomy should be avoided in patients who have heavy demands placed on their voices.

▶ This unusual report from the Karolinska Institute in Sweden describes detailed analyses of vocal cord function and voice in 19 patients after cricothyroidotomy. The analyses performed, including electromyography of the cricothyroid muscle, are beyond my capacity to evaluate, but the significant finding is that only 10 of the 19 patients, about 50%, had a normal voice. No dysfunction of the cricothyroid muscle was detected, so the tentative conclusion reached was that the abnormalities may be related to formation of scar tissue. If correct, this conclusion is even more alarming, indicating that voice changes may be inevitable in a certain percentage of patients if a cricothyroidotomy is used for a long period of time. The changes were minor and apparently not troublesome in most patients, but 3 of the 19 had problems that led them to seek therapy. The authors advise avoiding cricothyroidotomy in patients who are particularly dependent on their voice for their vocation, such as professional singers.

I studied this article in detail, because cricothyroidotomy has been widely employed at NYU for more than a decade. Careful review of the report is recommended for those performing this procedure.— F.C. Spencer, M.D.

Is Diaphragmatic Elevation a Serious Complication of Open-Heart Surgery?
Bogers AJJC, Nierop G, Bakker W, Huysmans HA (Univ of Leiden)
Scand J Thorac Cardiovasc Surg 23:271–274, 1989   7–13

The reported incidence and severity of elevation or paralysis of the diaphragm after open-heart surgery vary among authorities. This complication was analyzed, in 370 consecutive operations performed on 365 adults who underwent open-heart surgery without the use of ice in any form as a topical cardiac coolant.

The incidence of diaphragmatic elevation was 7.2%. The condition was unilateral in all cases. The complication was significantly correlated with ipsilateral pleural effusion and lower-lobe atelectsis; however, no predisposing or causal factors were determined. Diaphragmatic elevation did not result in a prolonged hospital stay. When data from follow-up chest radiograms were analyzed actuarily, the diaphragmatic position was found to be normalized within 6 months in 44% of the patients. By the end of the first year it had normalized in 90%.

Other studies have reported serious, and even fatal, problems arising from diaphragmatic paralysis, but such problems were not encountered in these cases, suggesting that the problem is rare. The incidence of diaphragmatic elevation after open-heart surgery is low and, at least when unilateral, the condition seldom leads to clinical problems. Diaphragmatic elevation usually resolves spontaneously.

▶ This interesting report describes a frequency of diaphragmatic elevation or paralysis of 7% in a consecutive series of 370 operations. No specific predisposing causes could be identified. Topical iced slush was not used.

The clinical significance seemed small as the associated pleural effusion did not prolong hospitalization.

Quite important is the fact that subsequent chest radiographs found that the diaphragm returned to normal position within 6 months in 44% of the patients, and within a year in 90%.—F.C. Spencer, M.D.

Diaphragmatic Plication for Unilateral Diaphragmatic Paralysis: A 10-Year Experience
Graham DR, Kaplan D, Evans CC, Hind CRK, Donnelly RJ (Broadgreen Hosp, Liverpool, England)
Ann Thorac Surg 49:248–252, 1990   17–14

Unilateral diaphragmatic paralysis is infrequent in patients without malignant disease, but it may sometimes produce troublesome dyspnea and orthopnea. Seventeen patients with this disorder underwent diaphragmatic plication in 1979–1989. The cause of diaphragmatic paralysis was unknown in 8 patients. Eleven patients had medical problems such as chronic obstructive lung disease or asthma. The mean time from onset of symptoms to surgery was 1.8 years.

The elevated hemidiaphragm was plicated in layers until it became taut. Breathlessness and orthopnea lessened subjectively in all patients after plication, and siprometric values and lung volumes improved significantly. Arterial oxygen tension improved from a mean of 73 mm Hg to 86 mm Hg after surgery. On radiographs, the plicated diaphragm was almost in a normal position. There were no serious operative complications.

Plication of the elevated hemidiaphragm provides lasting symptomatic improvement. It is a safe procedure in adults who have dyspnea from unilateral diaphragmatic paralysis not associated with malignant disease.

▶ This valuable report describes long-term results in 17 patients after unilateral diaphragmatic plication. The respiratory function data indicate a significant statistical improvement in the majority of patients. A particularly important point is that 6 patients were studied more than 5 years after plication; improvement was maintained in all of them. The pre- and postoperative radiographs from 1 patient, published in the full-length article, are quite impressive.—F.C. Spencer, M.D.

Sternal Wound Complications After Isolated Coronary Artery Bypass Grafting: Early and Late Mortality, Morbidity, and Cost of Care
Loop FD, Lytle BW, Cosgrove DM, Mahfood S, McHenry MC, Goormastic M, Stewart RW, Golding LAR, Taylor PC (Cleveland Clinic Found)
Ann Thorac Surg 49:179–187, 1990   17–15

The records of 6,504 consecutive patients who underwent isolated coronary artery bypass grafting from January 1, 1985 through December 1987 were reviewed to determine the incidence of wound complications. Among 5,369 patients who had a first-time coronary bypass 15 women and 40 men (median age, 62 years) had wound complications. Among 1,135 patients who underwent reoperation 3 women and 14 men (median age, 59 years) experienced wound complications. All 72 patients with sternal wound complications (1.1%) were followed.

When grouped by type of conduit used in grafting, wound complication rates were 1% for vein grafts only, .9% for 1 internal thoracic artery graft, and 1.6% for bilateral internal thoracic artery grafts. There were no significant differences in wound complication rates between patients having primary and reoperation procedures. The mean interval between operation and wound complication was 11 days. Wound cultures were negative in 11 patients and positive in 61. Forty-one cultures grew *Staphlococcus* species and 17 grew *Enterobacteriaceae*. Ten patients (14%) with wound infections died in the hospital of multisystem failure. Two additional patients died in the first postoperative year of renal failure.

Univariate analysis identified 12 variables that achieved significance in the calculation of risk factors for sternal wound complications. Subsequent multivariate analysis identified 4 clinical factors that were predictive of an increased risk of wound complication after isolated coronary bypass grafting: operating time, bilateral internal thoracic artery grafting in the presence of diabetes, obesity, and number of blood units used.

▶ This extensive report from the Cleveland Clinic describes the frequency of sternal infections among more than 6,500 patients undergoing operation between 1965 and 1987. Sternal wound complications developed in 72, about 1.1%. There was no difference in frequency between primary operations and reoperations. The greatest risk of infection was in patients with diabetes and bilateral mammary grafts—a relative risk of 5. Less significant factors were duration of operation, obesity, and units of blood used. Bilateral mammary grafting, however, in the nondiabetic patient was not associated with a great increase in the frequency of infection, although others have found contrary results.—F.C. Spencer, M.D.

Sternal Wire-Induced Persistent Chest Pain: A Possible Hypersensitivity Reaction
Fine PG, Karwande SV (Univ of Utah)
Ann Thorac Surg 49:135–136, 1990   17–16

Persistent chest pain after median sternotomy for open-heart operations is a common complaint that is often attributed to nonspecific anxiety-related or muscular pain disorders. In 1 case the sternal pain may have resulted from sensitivity to nickel in the stainless steel sternal wires.

Woman, 47, underwent successful ablative surgery through a midline sternotomy incision as therapy for Wolff-Parkinson-White syndrome. She then had persistent, disabling peri-incisional pain. Computed tomography of the chest showed partial nonunion of the lower aspect of the anterior table of the sternum, although no clinical instability was apparent. Because of the patient's continuing pain, the sternum was split and surgically rewired. Disabling pain again developed that was refractory to nonsteroidal anti-inflammatory drugs, nortriptyline, and clonazepam. Topical capsaicin cream was discontinued when a severe rash developed after the first application. A more detailed history revealed multiple allergic reactions, including skin sensitivity to jewelry. A skin patch test showed a 4+ reaction to nickel. Because the stainless steel sutures used to close the patient's sternum in both operations contained 8% nickel, the wires were removed. The patient returned to work without pain and was asymptomatic at 3-month follow-up.

The overall incidence of nickel sensitivity has recently been reported to be 7.3%, and it is possible that, in some cases, postoperative sternal pain is caused by nickel hypersensitivity. Such cases can be cured or prevented by the use of a suture material that does not contain nickel.

▶ This fascinating case report describes experiences with poststernotomy pain in a patient who did not respond to reoperation, nonsteroidal agents, or topical capsaicin (Zostrix) cream. After skin hypersensitivity was demonstrated to nickle, the wires were removed, with prompt relief of the discomfort.

The authors state that the stainless steel wires used contain about 8% nickle. In the general population, nickle hypersensitivity is present in about 10% of females but in only about 2% of males. It will be of particular interest to see whether others recognize this unusual syndrome. The authors are to be complimented for this unusual and potentially significant case report.—F.C. Spencer, M.D.

A Plea for Sensible Management of Myocardial Contusion

Baxter BT, Moore EE, Moore FA, McCroskey BL, Ammons LA (Univ of Colorado)
Am J Surg 158:557–562, 1989   17–17

Cardiac evaluation of blunt myocardial injury in patients with nonpenetrating chest trauma from motor vehicle accidents commonly consists of the same diagnostic procedures as used in the evaluation of patients with atherosclerotic coronary artery disease. However, unlike acute myocardial infarction, cardiac muscle ischemia from blunt chest trauma causes only a transient decrease in ventricular function, after which coronary perfusion is rapidly normalized. A prospective study was done to evaluate the clinical course in patients with nonpenetrating cardiac trauma to delineate a safe but more cost-effective policy.

During a 3-year study period, 280 patients (mean age, 39 years) were evaluated to exclude myocardial contusion after they sustained blunt chest trauma. During the initial 48 hours after trauma, serial determinations of creatinine phosphokinase (CPK) and lactate dehydrogenase and their isoenzymes were determined at baseline and at 8-hour intervals thereafter for a minimal total of 48 hours. All patients underwent continuous cardiac monitoring for 24 hours.

Myocardial contusion was diagnosed in 35 (13%) of the 280 patients. The diagnosis was based on ECG abnormalities in 30 patients, an increase in CPK isoenzymes in 9 patients, and on both in 4 patients. The increase in CPK isoenzyme levels always occurred within the first 24 hours after admission, and it remained abnormal for more than 24 hours in only 2 patients. Total lactate dehydrogenase levels were elevated in only 2 patients and appeared to be a false positive finding in 1 of these 2 patients. Two patients died of cardiac decompensation at 4 hours and 12 hours post injury. Seven patients required treatment of arrhythmias or myocardial failure. None of the remaining 271 patients had cardiac symptoms.

Patients who sustain blunt chest trauma in motor vehicle accidents are at low risk for myocardial contusion. The clinical diagnosis of myocardial contusion can safely be excluded in the presence of a normal ECG with normal cardiac enzyme levels during the initial 24-hour period of observation.

▶ With the mounting concern about the sharp rise in the cost of medical care, much of which is attributable to use of intensive care units and expensive technology, this article is especially pertinent. The data, based on 280 patients with blunt chest trauma, clearly indicate that significant myocardial contusion can be detected reliably within 12 hours after injury, relying on the ECG and the CPK-MB studies. More sophisticated studies, or longer periods of observation, do not seem warranted.—F.C. Spencer, M.D.

Cardiac Missiles: A Review of the Literature and Personal Experience
Symbas PN, Picone AL, Hatcher CR Jr, Vlasis-Hale SE (Emory Univ; Grady Hosp, Atlanta)
Ann Surg 211:639–648, 1990   17–18

There is controversy as to the proper management of retained missiles in the heart and pericardium. A 48-year literature review and a 20-year experience were carried out to shed more light on the subject.

Group 1 comprised cases from the literature review, and group 2 the experience at 1 hospital. In group 1, 222 missiles were retained in 201 patients: 45 bullets in 45 patients, 109 shrapnel in 99, 18 pellets in 7, and 50 unidentified missiles in 50. Missiles were completely embedded in the myocardium in 13 cases, partially embedded in 122, free in a cardiac chamber in 47, and within the pericardium in 40. Management consisted of removal of 104 missiles; 118 were left in place.

In group 2, 24 missiles, 18 bullets, 1 bullet fragment, and 5 pellets were retained in 24 patients. Of these, 10 missiles were removed and 13 were left undisturbed; there was 1 unsuccessful attempt to remove a missile.

Six group 1 patients died, including 1 in whom removal was unsuccessful and 5 others in whom removal was not attempted. These 6 fatalities were caused by 3 partially intramyocardial missiles, 2 intracavitary missiles, and 1 intrapericardial missile. Symptoms occurred in 27 patients, in 25 of whom attempts to remove the missile were unsuccessful or were not made. All group 2 patients did well and were free of symptoms.

Treatment for retained missiles should be individualized. Those that are completely embedded in myocardium and those in the pericardium or pericardial space are well tolerated. All but completely embedded shrapnel should be removed. Management of intracavitary missiles may depend on the time since injury and which side the missile is on. Missiles may enter the heart directly or embolize from a vein. Missiles in the left side of the heart usually enter an artery soon after injury; those in the right side may embolize or be entrapped and subsequently become encysted with fibrous tissue.

► This report from Dr. Symbas' group at Emory summarizes the available information in the English literature, as well as their personal experience with 24 patients treated in a period of 20 years. Hence, the report is a valuable reference source when this unusual problem is encountered. As the data indicate, a decision about elective removal of an intracardiac missile must be individualized. In a significant percentage of patients, an intracardiac missile remains asymptomatic.—F.C. Spencer, M.D.

Blunt Injuries to the Aortic Arch Vessels
Rosenberg JM, Bredenberg CE, Marvasti MA, Bucknam C, Conti C, Parker FB Jr (State Univ of New York Health Science Ctr, Syracuse; Hartford Hosp, Conn)
Ann Thorac Surg 48:508–513, 1989   17–19

Because blunt trauma that involves the major arterial branches of the aortic arch are uncommon, the literature contains only few reports of extensive experience with this type of injury. The combined experience of 2 institutions with patients who sustained blunt trauma to the brachiocephalic branches of the aortic arch was reviewed.

Between 1978 and 1985, 22 males and 8 females aged 16–60 years sustained 33 injuries to the brachiocephalic artery from blunt trauma. Twenty-seven patients had acute injuries and 3 had false aneurysms from previous injuries. Three patients were injured in industrial accidents (crush injuries) and 27 were involved in motor vehicle accidents. The mechanism of injury was deceleration in 19, traction in 8, and crush in 3. There were 17 injuries of the innominate artery, 8 of the subclavian artery, and 8 of the common carotid artery. Four patients had aortic rupture concomitant with their brachiocephalic arterial injury.

Associated injuries included head injuries in 14 patients, long bone fractures in 19, tracheal or bronchial injury in 3, facial injuries in 14, brachial plexus injury in 6, and abdominal trauma in 7. The chest radiographs of 28 patients showed a widened mediastinum or extrapleural hematoma, or both. All patients underwent angiography to identify the nature and site of injury.

One patient died of head injury before operation and 2 died during operation. The remaining 27 patients were alive 6 months to 10 years after injury. Of the 27 survivors, 18 had a total of 20 arterial reconstructions, 4 underwent ligation of a subclavian artery, and 5 with injuries of the intimal artery were observed and did well without operation. Twenty-two patients underwent transsternal exploration. Ten patients had posterolateral thoracotomies for left subclavian injury. Several patients required more than 1 approach to accomplish reconstruction. After up to 10 years of follow-up, 18 of the 20 arterial reconstructions were patent. However, none of the 6 patients with brachial plexus injuries regained neurologic function.

Prompt and precise diagnosis, combined with early operation and optimal surgical exposure for control of hemorrhage, are important to the successful management of patients with injuries of the aortic arch vessels caused by blunt trauma. Angiography facilitates operative planning in these patients.

▶ Experiences with 30 patients who sustained blunt vascular injuries to the brachiocephalic branches of the aortic arch are described in this report, said to be the largest series reported at this time. Injuries occurred from either deceleration, traction, or crush injuries, and were divided among the innominate, common carotid, and subclavian arteries. Angiography established the diagnosis; otherwise, the clinical picture was similar to that occurring with aortic rupture. Twenty-seven of the 30 patients were alive more than 6 months later. It is sobering that no patient with a brachial plexus injury had a return of neurologic function.—F.C. Spencer, M.D.

Surgical Excision of Intracardiac Myxomas: A 20-Year Follow-Up
Bortolotti U, Maraglino G, Rubino M, Santini F, Mazzucco A, Milano A, Fasoli G,
Livi U, Thiene G, Gallucci V (Univ of Padova, Italy)
Ann Thorac Surg 49:449–453, 1990   17–20

The most frequent benign tumors involving the cardiovascular system
are myxomas. Although the management of myxomas has often been
studied, the long-term outcome has seldom been evaluated. Fifty-four patients who underwent excision of intracardiac myxomas were studied.
Myxomas were located in the left atrium in 85% of the patients, the right
atrium in 11%, and the right ventricle in 4%. The 19 male and 35 female
patients had a mean age of 48 years (range, 7–68 years). Four patients
were asymptomatic. The remainder had exertional dyspnea, palpitation,
signs of systemic illness, and/or syncopal episodes. Before surgery, 13 patients with left atrial myxomas had embolic episodes. The mean follow-up was 6.5 years, but some patients were followed for 20 years.

There were 2 operative deaths, both of patients with left atrial myxomas; there were also 2 late deaths from myocardial infarction and bowel
carcinoma. Eleven patients had major early postoperative complications.
Actuarial survival was 91% both at 10 years and 20 years. Of 47 current
survivors contacted, 45 are in functional class I, 2 are in class II; 42 are
in sinus rhythm, and 4—all of whom had excision of a left atrial
myxoma—are in atrial fibrillation. No patients have had tumor recurrence.

Excision of intracardiac myxomas is curative, and long-term survival is
excellent. A transseptal approach provides adequate exposure; tumors
can be removed completely regardless of their location.

▶ The likelihood of recurrence of an atrial myxoma after excision is an unlikely
but troublesome consideration. Hence, this report of long-term results in 54 patients undergoing excision of an intracardiac myxoma over a period of 20 years
is of particular interest. The tumor was routinely excised with a small amount
of adjacent tissue at the stalk. The mean length of follow-up is now near 7
years, with actuarial survival at 20 years of 91%. There were no instances of
tumor recurrence. Of 47 current survivors, 45 are functional class I, with 42 in
sinus rhythm and 4 in atrial fibrillation.—F.C. Spencer, M.D.

**Surgical Treatment of Aneurysm and/or Dissection of the Ascending
Aorta, Transverse Aortic Arch, and Ascending Aorta and Transverse Aor-
tic Arch: Factors Influencing Survival in 717 Patients**
Crawford ES, Svensson LG, Coselli JS, Safi HJ, Hess KR (Baylor College of
Medicine; The Methodist Hosp, Houston)
J Thorac Cardiovasc Surg 98:659–674, 1989   17–21

To be successful, treatment of disease of the ascending aorta and arch
may require extensive graft replacement up to and including the entire
aorta. Data were analyzed on 717 patients treated in a 9-year period for

aneurysm or dissection involving the ascending aorta and transverse aortic arch.

The study population consisted of 445 males and 272 females aged 10–88 years (median, 61 years). Causes of aortic disease included trauma in 6 patients, infection in 20, aortitis in 46, acute dissection in 72, chronic dissection in 189, and medial degeneration in 384. Patients with long-standing disease and older patients often had atherosclerosis superimposed on the basic mural lesions. Of 717 patients, 150 had undergone 173 previous cardiac or aortic operations. Concurrent distal aneurysmal disease was present or developed in 37% of the patients, and was most prevalent in patients with aortic arch involvement. Aneurysm symptoms were absent or mild in 593 and severe in 124 patients. Atriofemoral cannulation was used in 597 patients. Treatment included ascending aorta or aortic arch reconstruction, or both, by composite valve graft in 281, separate valve graft in 117, graft only in 256, and other procedures in 63 patients.

The 30-day survival rate was 91%. Independent determinants predictive of early death were increasing age, severe aneurysm symptoms, diabetes, previous proximal aortic operation, need for cardiac support, postoperative tracheostomy, postoperative heart dysfunction, and stroke. Survival among 319 patients with none of the 4 preoperative factors was 97%. Survival decreased to 74% among patients with 2 or more of these factors. The entire aorta was replaced in 53 and near-total aorta in 35; the entire thoracic artery was replaced in 78; and the total aorta except for the arch was replaced in 27 patients.

The 5-year survival rate was 66% and the 7-year survival rate, 57%. Independent predictors of death were severe aneurysm symptoms, preoperative angina, extent of proximal replacement, associated residual distal aneurysm, balloon pump, renal dysfunction, cardiac dysfunction, and stroke. The 5-year survival rates varied with the incidence of the 4 preoperative variables and age present in a single patient: 78% in 413 who had up to 1 variable, 57% in 193 with 2 or 3 variables, and 39% in 111 with 3 or 4 variables. The introduction of profound hypothermic circulatory arrest, composite valve grafting, and other technical improvements have led to more favorable results in the treatment of ascending aorta and arch disease.

▶ This monumental report from Stanley Crawford and his group in Houston describes their experiences with 717 patients who had aneurysmal disease in the ascending and transverse aortic arch, treated in a period of 9 years. The 30-day survival rate was 91% and the 5-year survival rate, 66%.

The manuscript contains a wealth of technical information. With composite grafts the original technique of direct attachment of the coronary ostia to side openings in the aortic prosthesis was used until about 1985 (135 patients). Technical problems led to gradual abandonment of this technique with the use of an aortic button method. However, since 1986, the preferred method in 94 patients has been to use a 10-mm Dacron graft. The manuscript should be studied in detail by surgeons treating these complex problems.—F.C. Spencer, M.D.

Sutureless Ring Graft Replacement of Ascending Aorta and Aortic Arch

Oz MC, Ashton RC Jr, McNicholas KW, Lemole GM (Med Ctr of Delaware, Wilmington; Columbia-Presbyterian Med Ctr, New York)
Ann Thorac Surg 50:74–79, 1990   17–22

Surgically managed diseases of the ascending aorta and aortic arch have a high attendant morbidity and mortality. Complications, including suture line hemorrhage through friable tissue, often arise from technical difficulties with the use of conventional tube grafts.

Between 1978 and 1989 the ascending aorta or aortic arch was replaced with a sutureless intraluminal ring graft in 49 patients (Figs 17–5 and 17–6). Twenty-six patients underwent aortic valve replacement; 20

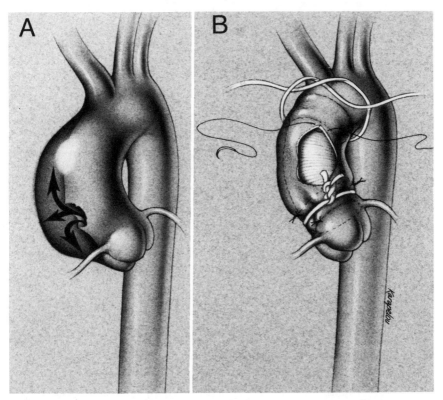

Fig 17–5.—**A,** pathology encountered in acute aortic dissection. Aortic valve is competent. **B,** repair is accomplished with sutureless device secured above aortic valve with several nylon sutures above commissures, followed by Dacron tape ties around spools and aortic wall. (Courtesy of Oz MC, Ashton RC Jr, McNicholas KW, et al: *Ann Thorac Surg* 50:74–79, 1990.)

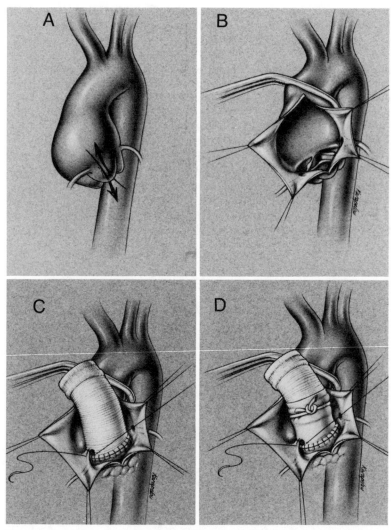

Fig 17–6.—A, aortic aneurysm with aortic insufficiency. **B,** anterior aortic wall is incised to show aortic valve anulus. **C,** proximal spool of sutureless graft has been removed, and free cuff is attached to aortic prosthetic valve and sutured in place in usual fashion, including reanastomosis of coronary arteries. **D,** alternatively, prosthetic valve attached to polytetrafluoroethylene material is inserted and proximal spool of sutureless device is secured within free end of polytetrafluoroethylene graft with Dacron tie.

of the 26 had aneurysmal disease. Eight patients required concomitant coronary artery bypass grafting. At completion of the procedure, 4 patients received an aortoatrial polytetrafluoroethylene shunt. Most patients underwent digital subtraction angiography before hospital discharge. Some patients were later followed with digital subtraction angiography, CT, or MRI to evaluate ring graft function.

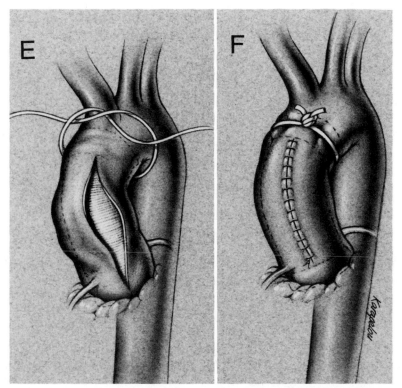

Fig 17-6 *cont.* **E,** no matter how proximal anastomosis is accomplished, distal spool is inserted and secured with Dacron tape. **F,** aortic wall is closed over ascending aortic graft. (Courtesy of Oz MC, Ashton RC Jr, McNicholas KW, et al: *Ann Thorac Surg* 50:74–79, 1990.)

In no case was it impossible to place a sutureless graft during a procedure. Operative mortality for ascending aortic aneurysm repairs was 4%, and operative mortality for dissections was 18%. Five of 8 patients who required aortic arch replacement survived. There were no complications related to anastomotic hemorrhage, graft migration, formation of pseudoaneurysm, or thromboemboli. Complications included phrenic nerve palsy, transient ischemic attack, and acute tubular necrosis. All these resolved completely. The actuarial 5-year survival was 64%.

Sutureless intraluminal devices are particularly useful in aortic dissections, but they may also be used in aortic aneurysms and infected aortitis. Although the advantages over sutured anastomoses are not as great for these procedures, the reduction in operating time warrants their use, especially in patients with unstable conditions.

▶ This report describes a decade of experience with replacing the ascending aorta or aortic arch with a sutureless intraluminal ring graft, a device developed and investigated by Dr. LeMole for several years. Among the series of 49 patients the operative mortality associated with ascending aortic aneurysms was 4%, and for dissections, 18%; 5 of 8 patients requiring aortic arch replacement survived.

Apart from the operative technique, the report is noteworthy in that late complications did not occur. It was of particular interest that the tape ligating the spool of the prosthesis in position did not erode and cause hemorrhage, nor did the prosthesis migrate from insufficient fixation.

Although the concept is attractive in terms of simplicity, the mortality results are not convincing. The operative mortality for ascending aneurysms was 4%, similar to that reported by other groups. However, the mortality for dissection of 18% is considerably higher than has been reported by several groups using conventional suture techniques; certainly, the mortality rate—5 of 8 patients requiring aortic arch replacement—is much too high.—F.C. Spencer, M.D.

An Analysis of the Cost Effectiveness of the Implantable Defibrillator
Kuppermann M, Luce BR, McGovern B, Podrid PJ, Bigger JT Jr, Ruskin JN (Battelle Human Affairs Research Ctrs Washington, DC; Massachusetts Gen Hosp, Boston; Columbia Univ)
Circulation 81:91–100, 1990   17–23

The automatic implantable defibrillator reduces mortality in patients surviving cardiac arrest caused by ventricular tachycardia or fibrillation who are at high risk for recurrence. A cost-effectiveness analysis was conducted using data from the 1984 Medicare database, the medical literature, Medicare carriers, individual pharmacies and hospitals, and expert opinion.

Combinations of principal and secondary discharge diagnoses across 18 diagnosis-related groups were used to estimate the cost of hospitalization for a comparison group of patients. Hospitalization costs for the patients with a defibrillator obtained from reported empirical data were considered. Rehospitalization rates and other health-care use estimates were obtained. Using a decision-analytic model, the net cost-effectiveness of the defibrillator used in a high-risk patient was about $17,100 per life-year saved. Sensitivity analyses suggested that the true cost is between $15,000 and $25,000. The cost effectiveness of the defibrillator in a 1991 scenario when the device would have greater longevity, would be programmable, and would not require a thoracotomy was $7,400 per life-year saved. The true value was between an amount less than that of pharmacologic therapy and $19,600 per life-year saved. The cost of the implantable defibrillator is well within the range of currently accepted life-saving technologies. As the technology develops, the defibrillator may actually become cost saving.

▶ This socioeconomic report from the Battelle Research Center analyzes the cost effectiveness of the implantable defibrillator. The initial hospitalization cost for defibrillator implantation, obtained from the Health Care Financing Administration, based on data collected from 138 patients, was nearly $50,000.

A detailed analysis of the benefit ratio, comparing the cost of recurrent hospitalizations for treatment of arrhythmias, indicates a significant cost saving of between $5,000 and $15,000 per life-year saved. Although the methodology of this analysis is beyond my competence, the conclusions seem strongly applicable to the economic analysis of any institution considering wider use of the implantable defibrillator.—F.C. Spencer, M.D.

18 The Arteries, the Veins, and the Lymphatics

Prospective Study of the Effectiveness and Durability of Carotid Endarterectomy
Sundt TM Jr, Whisnant JP, Houser OW, Fode NC (Mayo Clinic and Found, Rochester, Minn)
Mayo Clin Proc 65:625–635, 1990   18–1

In the past several years the medical community has expressed justifiable concern about the frequency, indications, and results of carotid endarterectomy. Some wonder whether the treatment is worse than the disease. A study was begun in 1982 when digital subtraction angiography (DSA) became available in an effort to correlate postoperative and follow-up DSA findings with clinical results in 252 patients undergoing 282 carotid endarterectomies. Angiographic follow-up was done for 2–6 years.

Digital subtraction angiography was performed after surgery in 95% of the cases; DSA follow-up was possible in 66%. Overall, the operative minor morbidity was 1% and mortality, .7%. There was no major morbidity. Complications were well correlated with the patient's preoperative risk category. Ten major strokes occurred during follow-up, only 1 of which was attributable to the reconstructed artery. There were also 10 transient ischemic attacks, 3 of which were presumably related to recurrent stenosis.

Asymptomatic mild to moderate restenosis of the internal carotid or common carotid artery was found in 10% of follow-up DSAs. Severe stenosis or occlusion occurred in 3%. Stenosis in the opposite common carotid or internal carotid artery progressed in 48 patients, 10 of whom became symptomatic. According to actuarial analysis of patients with endarterectomy, the cumulative probability of ipsilateral stroke was 1.5% at 1 month and 2% at 5 years. The cumulative probability of ipsilateral stroke, transient ischemic attack, or reversible ischemic neurologic deficit was 4% at 1 month and 8% at 5 years. This was less than 1% per year after the first month, with censoring at the time of the second surgery.

Digital subtraction angiography is an excellent method of visualizing the carotid bifurcation and assessing the adequacy of endarterectomy after surgery. In this series, the durability of an endarterectomized vessel appeared to compare favorably with the natural history of an asymptomatic stenosis identified by ultrasonography.

▶ The issue of recurrent carotid stenosis was addressed by Shumway et al. (1). Fifty-four patients underwent a second carotid endarterectomy or reconstructive procedure, with a complication incidence of 9%. Further, 67% of the patients remained asymptomatic, and about 17% died between 1 month and 33 months after the operation. Bernstein et al. (2) analyzed 507 patients with Doppler examination. Life-table analysis to 10 years revealed a significantly greater life expectancy among those patients with restenosis. Stroke was also less likely to occur in patients with restenosis. The likelihood of patients with more than 50% restenosis remaining alive and stroke free was greater than in the less than 20% stenotic group.—S.I. Schwartz, M.D.

References

1. Shumway, SJ et al: *Am Surg* 53:61, 1987.
2. Bernstein EF, et al: *Ann Surg* 212:629, 1990.

Carotid Endarterectomy Contralateral to an Occluded Carotid Artery: Perioperative Risk and Late Results
Mackey WC, O'Donnell TF Jr, Callow AD (Tufts Univ-New England Med Ctr, Boston)
J Vasc Surg 11:778–785, 1990   18–2

To clarify the short-term risk and long-term benefit of carotid endarterectomy opposite an occluded carotid artery, angiographic data available for 598 of 670 patients entered in a carotid registry since 1961 were reviewed. In 63 (10.5%) patients, the internal or common carotid artery on the side opposite the endarterectomy was occluded. Surgery was performed under general anesthesia with shunting based on electroencephalographic criteria. Shunting was necessary in 29 (46%) of 63 patients with contralateral occlusion and in 72 (13.5%) of 535 control patients. Perioperative strokes occurred in 3 (4.8%) of 68 patients with contralateral occlusion and 6 (2.6%) of 535 controls. None of the patients with contralateral occlusion and 1.1% of the control patients died during surgery.

Patients with contralateral occlusion had life-table cumulative stroke-free rates of 95.2% at 1 year, 91% at 5 years, and 76.2% at 10 years; the rates for control patients were 96% at 1 year, 89.4% at 5 years, and 84.1% at 10 years. Life-table cumulative survival rates in patients with contralateral occlusion were 93.1% at 1 year, 80.8% at 5 years, and 75.4% at 10 years; in controls, the rates were 94.8% at 1 year, 77% at 5 years, and 57.9% at 10 years. Carotid endarterectomy contralateral to an occluded carotid artery can be performed with an acceptable short-term risk. The late stroke-free rates and survival rates in these patients were comparable to those among patients undergoing carotid endarterectomy.

▶ The conclusions run counter to those of previous articles suggesting that the stroke rate in patients undergoing carotid endarterectomy with contralateral occluded carotid artery is prohibitive. As is pointed out in the discussion by Whittemore, his group achieved results similar to those reported in the present article. The discussants stress that in this subset of patients undergoing carotid artery surgery, the need for a shunt is significantly increased; using continuous electroencephalographic monitoring, approximately 40% of patients will require interluminal shunting. McKittrick et al. (1) recently reported on 27 patients with complete occlusion of the carotid artery. Eight of the 27 were asymptomatic and 16 had a transient ischemic attack before surgery. All were operated on under general anesthesia, and only 3 had intraoperative shunting. There is no increase in the risk of stroke after endarterectomy in these patients when compared to those without contralateral occlusion.—S.I. Schwartz, M.D.

Reference

1. McKittrick, JE et al: *Ann Vasc Surg* 3:324, 1989.

Coeliac Artery Compression Syndrome: The Effect of Decompression
Geelkerken RH, van Bockel JH, de Roos WK, Hermans J (Univ Hosp, Leiden; Red Cross Hosp, The Hague, The Netherlands)
Br J Surg 77:807–809, 1990   18–3

To determine the long-term results of celiac decompression, data were reviewed on 11 consecutive patients with celiac artery compression syndrome who were treated with decompression. All patients were symptom free immediately after the surgery. Abdominal pain recurred 3 months postoperatively in 3 patients. Symptoms similar to those before surgery returned in all 8 patients for whom long-term (15–23 years) follow-up data were available.

These data indicate that the long-term results of such treatment were unsatisfactory in these patients who were followed for almost 20 years. Surgery should not be performed in patients with vague upper abdominal complaints and compression of the celiac artery by the median arcuate ligament who do not otherwise have pathologic conditions to explain their symptoms.

▶ Every several years an article appears emphasizing the unsatisfactory results associated with attempted surgical correction of celiac artery compression. Perhaps the most definitive article on the subject is that of Szilagyi et al. (1). They reviewed the entire literature and could find no patient with proved abnormality of intestinal structural function caused by extraluminal compression of the celiac artery. They suggested that the relief experienced after operation was a placebo effect. But despite all of this literature, cases continue to be done even in my own institution.—S.I. Schwartz, M.D.

Reference

1. Szilagyi, DE, et al: *Surgery* 6:849, 1972.

Variables That Affect the Expansion Rate and Outcome of Small Abdominal Aortic Aneurysms

Cronenwett JL, Sargent SK, Wall MH, Hawkes ML, Freeman DH, Dain BJ, Curé JK, Walsh DB, Zwolak RM, McDaniel MD, Schneider JR (Dartmouth-Hitchcock Med Ctr, Hanover, NH)
J Vasc Surg 11:260–269, 1990
18–4

Nonoperative management with observation is often advised for patients with small abdominal aortic aneurysms (AAAs). Even small (4 cm) AAAs, however, may have a high rupture rate in patients with hypertension or chronic obstructive pulmonary disease. In addition, there is considerable variation among individual patients in aneurysm expansion rates.

The influence of various clinical parameters on aneurysm expansion and subsequent outcome was examined in 54 men and 19 women (mean age, 70 years). All had small (≤6 cm in diameter) AAAs, and most (72%) were symptom free. More than half (59%) had overt cardiac disease; common conditions included coronary artery disease (45%), hypertension (45%), and chronic obstructive pulmonary disease (37%). All patients had at least 2 ultrasound measurements separated by at least 1 month, and 38% had 5 or more studies.

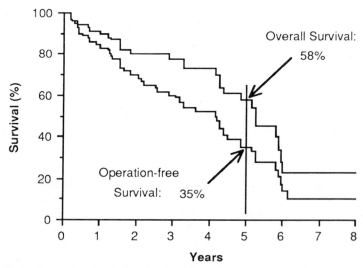

Fig 18–1.—Actuarial analysis indicated a 5-year survival of 58% in patients who did not undergo aneurysm surgery and a probability of surviving 5 years without requiring aneurysm repair of only 35%. (Courtesy of Cronenwett JL, Sargent SK, Wall MH, et al: *J Vasc Surg* 11:260–269, 1990.)

The mean initial AAA size was 4 cm in diameter. The AAA area increased by 20% per year during a mean follow-up of 3 years. There was a 10% per year increase in the diameter of the aneurysm. The expansion rate was not affected by the initial aneurysm size. The 3 aneurysms that required urgent repair during the observation period had each been larger than 5.5 cm in diameter at the last measurement. One of those aneurysms ruptured freely and the patient died.

Patients who did not undergo surgery had a 5-year life-table survival of 58%; operation-free survival was 35% (Fig 18–1). Only increased age and larger aneurysm size at the time of the initial evaluation predicted the probability of subsequent elective aneurysm surgery. Final aneurysm area, however, was predicted by initial area, duration of follow-up, and both diastolic and systolic blood pressure. Because the rate of expansion could not be predicted by any clinical parameter, AAAs less than 5 cm in diameter should be measured by ultrasound at 6-month intervals.

▶ The article discusses new data about the selection of patients for elective surgery for small aneurysms. It does seem reasonable to follow the patients for sequential ultrasound and not operate on them until the aneurysm reaches 5–6 cm. The data will have to be compared with the mortality rate in asymptomatic patients undergoing elective surgery. Mutirangura et al. (1) recently reported the mortality rate to be 1.1% in this group of patients.—S.I. Schwartz, M.D.

Reference

1. Mutirangura P, et al: *Br J Surg* 76:1251, 1989.

Transperitoneal Versus Retroperitoneal Approach for Aortic Reconstruction: A Randomized Prospective Study
Cambria RP, Brewster DC, Abbott WM, Freehan M, Megerman J, LaMuraglia G, Wilson R, Wilson D, Teplick R, Davison JK (Massachusetts Gen Hosp, Boston; Harvard Med School)
J Vasc Surg 11:314–325, 1990   18–5

Most studies recommending use of the retroperitoneal approach for aortic reconstruction suffer from the limitations of retrospective review. The merits of the retroperitoneal approach for aortic reconstruction were compared with those of the midline transperitoneal approach in a randomized, prospective study of 113 patients admitted for elective, infrarenal aortic reconstruction between March 1987 and October 1988. In addition, the records of 56 patients who underwent this procedure via a transperitoneal approach performed by the same surgeons in 1984 to 1985 were reviewed retrospectively.

Clinical and demographic features, such as age, male to female ratio, smoking history, incidence and severity of cardiopulmonary disease, indication for operation, and use of epidural anesthetics, did not differ among randomized patients undergoing transperitoneal or retroperitoneal operations. Similarly, operative details such as operative and aortic cross-clamp times, crystalloid and transfusion requirements, degree of hypothermia on arrival at the intensive care unit, and perioperative fluid and blood requirements, did not differ between groups. The postoperative course, defined in terms of recovery of gastrointestinal function, requirements for narcotics, metabolic parameters of operative stress, incidence of major and minor complications, and duration of hospital stay, was also similar in both groups. However, when compared with the retrospectively reviewed patients, randomized patients undergoing either transperitoneal or retroperitoneal operations experienced highly significant reductions in postoperative ventilation, transfusion requirements, resumption of oral alimentation, and duration of hospital stay. Adoption of the retroperitoneal approach as the preferred technique for aortic reconstruction is not supported.

▶ Chang et al. (1) indicated that the group from Albany has used the extended retroperitoneal approach preferentially for ruptured abdominal aneurysms. In a 6-year period, 25 patients operated on by the left retroperitoneal incision were compared with 38 operated on by standard transperitoneal celiotomy. Operative mortality was lower in the retroperitoneal group, and these patients required less ventilatory support and tolerated enteral feedings quickly. Those authors have also indicated that there is a distinct advantage to the retroperitoneal approach as far as postoperative care is concerned. This finding obviously contradicts the present paper.—S.I. Schwartz, M.D.

Reference

1. Chang, et al: *J Vasc Surg* 11:326, 1990.

False Aneurysms After Prosthetic Reconstructions for Aortoiliac Obstructive Disease
van der Akker PJ, Brand R, van Schilfgaarde R, van Bockel JH, Terpstra JL
(Univ Hosp Leiden; Univ Hosp Groningen, The Netherlands)
Ann Surg 210:658–666, 1989   18–6

The development of an anastomotic or false aneurysm after prosthetic vascular reconstruction is considered a rare late complication. However, its exact incidence is not known, as previous studies have reported widely divergent incidence rates. A long-term follow-up study was conducted to calculate the cumulative incidence rate and chance for a false aneurysm developing after prosthetic vascular insertions. In addition, an attempt was made to identify risk factors that may be associated with the late development of false aneurysms.

In 1958–1980, 518 patients (median age, 55.9 years) underwent prosthetic reconstruction for aortoiliac obstructive disease (AIOD). Completeness of follow-up data was 91.3% at 5 years after operation, 87.8%

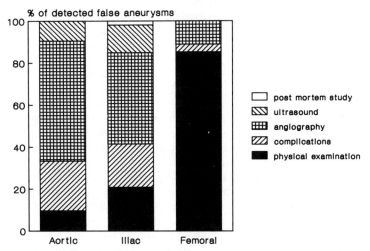

Fig 18–2.—Contribution of several ways of clinical presentation to the detection of false aneurysms at specific locations. (Courtesy of van den Akker PJ, Brand R, van Schilfgaarde R, et al: *Ann Surg* 201:658–666, 1989.)

at 10 years, 83.2% at 15 years, and 72% at 20 years. Because the number of patients available for evaluation at 20 years was too small for meaningful results, only the 15-year data were analyzed.

A total of 101 false aneurysms were detected in 69 patients, for an incidence rate of 13.3%. All false aneurysms were verified by operation. There were 21 aortic, 53 iliac, and 27 femoral false aneurysms (Fig 18–2). The interval between prosthesis insertion and detection of the first false aneurysm ranged from 1 to 238 months, with a median interval of 92 months. Only 36 false aneurysms were detected by physical examination, 17 were detected during emergency operation for complications, and 48 were detected during routine follow-up ultrasound examination. At 15 years the chance of being free of a false aneurysm was 77.2% for any anastomotic site, 92.3% for an aortic anastomotic site, 84.5% for an iliac anastomotic site, and 76.2% for a femoral anastomotic site.

Analysis of risk factors that could contribute to anastomotic disruption included the use of silk suture and end-to-side anastomoses. In all, 4 factors were identified as correlating significantly with the development of a false aneurysm after prosthetic vascular reconstruction, including the presence of multilevel disease, presence of hypertension, suture material used, and type of anastomosis constructed. Patients with prosthetic arterial reconstructions should be included in a life-long recall program with periodic ultrasound and angiographic evaluation.

▶ The unexpectedly high chances of a false aneurysm developing after aortoiliac or femoral prosthetic reconstruction suggests that in these patients routine surveillance with ultrasonography be continued for the rest of their lives. As the authors point out, the incidence of false aneurysm varies from .5% to almost 24%, and much of this can be explained by the length of follow-up.—S.I. Schwartz, M.D.

Popliteal Artery Entrapment: An Evolving Syndrome

Collins PS, McDonald PT, Lim RC (Uniformed Services Univ of the Health Sciences, San Francisco and Oakland; Univ of California, San Francisco)
J Vasc Surg 10:484–490, 1989   18–7

Popliteal artery entrapment can result in calf and foot claudication and limb-threatening ischemi in otherwise healthy young adults. Preestablished noninvasive and arteriographic criteria were used to establish the diagnosis of popliteal artery entrapment in symptomatic patients.

All patients were examined by Doppler ultrasonography of the posterior tibial artery and the dorsal artery of the foot at the ankle. An ankle/brachial index (ABI) was established for each patient. Patients who had normal ABIs performed a treadmill test of increasing difficulty until symptoms recurred and ABIs decreased. Patients with diminished ABIs at rest and with exercise underwent standard aortic, pelvic, and run-off arteriography. If the x-ray films showed no lesion to account for the symptoms, contrast-enhanced biplanar arteriography was obtained with the feet in a neutral position, passively dorsiflexed, and actively plantar flexed. Both legs were imaged to determine the incidence of bilateral disease.

Ten men and 2 women had popliteal artery entrapment. Eleven were younger than 40 years of age. All patients complained of calf pain, and 2 had foot pain on ambulation. One patient had acute occlusion of the popliteal artery with limb-threatening ischemia. In 10 patients the ankle pulse decreased with exercise. Four patients had ankle/brachial indexes of less than 1. All had diminished ankle/brachial indexes after performing a treadmill test at 4.2 mph at a 10% grade for 10 minutes.

Arteriography showed abnormal extrinsic compression or occlusion of the popliteal artery in all 12 patients; 8 patients had bilateral entrapment. Thirty-seven percent of lesions were type IV, 32% were type II, and 26% were type III. There was 1 type I lesion and no type V lesions.

Popliteal artery entrapment should be suspected in young, otherwise healthy adults with claudication. A treadmill test followed by biplanar arteriography can establish the diagnosis. Bilateral entrapment may be more common than has been thought.

▶ As Dr. Whelan, who contributed so significantly to this subject, indicated in his discussion, it is interesting to note increasing recognition of the bilateral nature of this disorder. This has been related to the use of noninvasive Doppler pressure determinations. He also called attention to the entity described as "functional" popliteal entrapment syndrome, in which hypertrophy of the gastrocnemius muscle in a highly trained athlete causes compression of the artery and claudication.—S.I. Schwartz, M.D.

Comparison of Infrainguinal Graft Surveillance Techniques

Green RM, McNamara J, Ouriel K, DeWeese JA (Univ of Rochester, NY)
J Vasc Surg 11:207–215, 1990   18–8

The fate of hemodynamically compromised but patent grafts in asymptomatic patients who have undergone infrainguinal bypass grafting is unknown. Consequently, there is still controversy over the role of periodic postoperative noninvasive graft surveillance and graft revision in asymptomatic patients. To learn more about the natural history of hemodynamic abnormalities in asymptomatic patients with patent infrainguinal bypass grafts, data on 300 patients who underwent successful infrainguinal bypass procedures and were followed on a standardized graft surveillance protocol during a 5-year period were reviewed.

All patients underwent noninvasive duplex scanning at 1 month, then every 6 months for the first 2 years, and yearly thereafter. A duplex scan was considered abnormal if the peak systolic flow velocity was more than 120 cm/sec or less than 40 cm/sec. Ankle systolic pressures were determined by a transcutaneous Doppler ultrasonographic flow detection technique. A decrease in the ankle/brachial pressure ratio (ABI) of at least 10% was considered abnormal. A total of 177 asymptomatic patients met the criteria for this analysis.

During the 5-year observation period, 18 graft thromboses (10%) occurred, of which 9 were successfully revised. Graft revision was necessary in 20 patients because of recurrent symptoms; 18 of these underwent successful secondary operations. Of the 38 revisions, 29 became necessary within the first 18 months of surveillance, and 17 were performed as early as 6–12 months after operation.

The 1-year primary cumulative patency rate (CPR) was 86%, compared with a secondary CPR of 91%. The 5-year primary CPR was 66%, compared with a secondary CPR of 80%. Sudden graft occlusion occurred in 5 patients after a finding of a normal ABI. Usually, abnormal

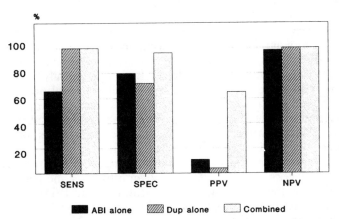

Fig 18–3.—Conditional probabilities for the tests with stated norms. The sensitivity *(SENS)* or the probability that a graft is about to occlude will yield a positive test result was highest for the duplex scan with or without the ABI. The specificity *(SPEC)* or the probability that a nonthreatened graft will test normally was highest when both the duplex and the ABI were normal. The predictive value of an abnormal test result *(PPV)* was highest for the combination of an abnormal duplex and ABI. The predictive value of a negative test result *(NPV)* was similar for all the tests. (Courtesy of Green RM, McNamara J, Ouriel K, et al: *J Vasc Surg* 11:207–215, 1990.)

ABIs found at a follow-up examination spontaneously reverted to normal by the next visit. Of the 26 patients whose ABIs had not reverted to normal by the next visit, 19 had significant graft problems; only 8 of them had operable conditions, however, and 5 of these 8 patients already had occluded grafts. None of the patients with a normal ABI and a normal duplex scan had graft occlusion before the next surveillance visit.

The incidence of sudden graft occlusion with an abnormal duplex scan but a normal ABI was 4%. In contrast, the risk of graft occlusion with an abnormal duplex scan and a reduced ABI was 66% (Fig 18–3). These findings support the recommendation of prophylactic revision of an infrainguinal bypass graft in any asymptomatic patient who has a reduced ABI and an abnormal duplex scan.

▶ Cohen et al. (1) demonstrated the importance of recognition in the management of impending vein graft failure. Late failure of a bypass vein graft may result from progressive atherosclerosis or from intrinsic lesions in the graft. Those authors demonstrated an ability to detect impending graft failure by Doppler study, and they did intravenous angiography. They focused on 29 patent grafts with stenoses identified by a decreased Doppler ABI.—S.I. Schwartz, M.D.

Reference

1. Cohen, JR, et al: *Arch Surg* 121:758, 1986.

Graft Stenosis: Justification for 1-Year Surveillance
Taylor PR, Wolfe JHN, Tyrrell MR, Mansfield AO, Nicolaides AN, Houston RE (St Mary's Hosp and Med School, London)
Br J Surg 77:1125–1128, 1990   18–9

Most authors agree that stenoses occur in about 25% of femorodistal grafts. Many patients with graft stenoses are asymptomatic. Clinical assessment alone cannot reliably detect hemodynamically compromised grafts that remain patent in these cases. Doppler arterial pressure assessment at the ankle is the simplest method. However, many times this may be inadequate. Duplex scanning and intravenous digital subtraction angiography (IVDSA) are more sensitive in detecting stenoses, but their expense and time requirements necessitate justification.

A total of 412 femorodistal grafts done between 1984 and 1988 were studied at 6 weeks and 3, 6, 9, and 12 months after the procedure and every 6 months thereafter with duplex scanning and IVDSA. Nonhemodynamically significant stenoses were observed, but no intervention was undertaken. Stenoses that were significant hemodynamically were repaired. In 16% of the grafts a stenosis developed at a mean of 22 months. Twenty-four of the 66 stenoses were not hemodynamically significant and 42 were. Twenty-two occurred next to the distal anastomosis, 13 next to the proximal anastomosis, and 31 in the body of the graft.

The incidence of stenosis in femorocrural grafts was higher than that in femoropopliteal grafts, but the difference was not significant. Stenoses were more likely to be detected in vein conduits than in synthetic grafts. The incidence of stenoses in 214 femoropopliteal vein grafts was 16%, compared with only 9% in 76 polytetrafluoroethylene femoropopliteal grafts. The highest incidence of stenoses—26%—was found in femoro-crural vein grafts. Two of the 42 grafts with hemodynamically significant stenoses occluded. Fifteen balloon dilations and 22 operations were done on 30 grafts to date.

Duplex examination of femorodistal grafts is an effective screening tool for detecting stenoses, which occur in about 20% of such grafts. Although routine IVDSA is not necessary, it is mandatory before reconstruction to confirm the presence of a stenosis and to provide anatomical information for possible reconstructive procedures.

▶ There is increasing literature emphasizing the need for duplex scanning to provide a sensitive method of detecting restenosis. Mills et al. (1) demonstrated that duplex surveillance is significantly more reliable in identifying a failing vein graft than is determination of the ankle-brachial index. Only 29% of grafts identified as failing by duplex scan were associated with reduction of the ankle-brachial index by more than .15. Secondary reconstructions were performed on 48 grafts based on detection. All reconstructions were patent after a mean follow-up of 5 months.—S.I. Schwartz, M.D.

Reference

1. Mills JL, et al: *J Vasc Surg* 12:379, 1990.

Present Status of Reversed Vein Bypass Grafting: Five-Year Results of a Modern Series
Taylor LM Jr, Edwards JM, Porter JM (Oregon Health Sciences Univ, Portland)
J Vasc Surg 11:193–206, 1990   18–10

Autogenous greater saphenous vein is thought to be the best conduit for infrainguinal bypass, but there is no consensus on the best technique to be used. Of 564 limbs in 434 patients with infrainguinal arterial ischemia treated from January 1, 1980, through mid-December 1988, 516 limbs in 387 patients were subjected to autogenous reversed vein bypass grafting. In 285 grafts the ipsilateral greater saphenous vein was adequate; the remaining 231 operations used distal graft origins in 151 grafts or alternate venous sources or phlebophlebostomy. The distal anastomosis was to the below-knee popliteal artery in 199, the infrapopliteal artery in 241, and the above-knee popliteal artery in 76.

At 5 years the primary patency rate for all grafts was 75% and the secondary patency rate, 81% (Fig 18–4). The primary patency rate for grafts to infrapopliteal arteries was 69%, significantly worse than that for grafts to the popliteal artery, which was 77% for those above the

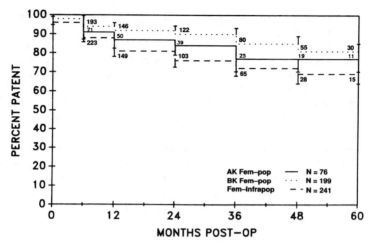

Fig 18–4.—Life-table primary patency for grafts grouped according to site of distal anastomosis. *AK,* above knee; *BK,* below knee; *bars,* standard error. (Courtesy of Taylor LM Jr, Edwards JM, Porter JM: *J Vasc Surg* 11:193–206, 1990.)

knee and 80% for those below. The primary patency rate was 80% for grafts of adequate ipsilateral greater saphenous vein and 68% for all other grafts. The secondary patency rates, whatever the source of conduit or site of graft origin or distal anastomosis, ranged from 76% to 85%.

Reversed vein bypass grafting is a preferred procedure for infrainguinal revascularization. It yields excellent patency rates and is applicable to the many patients without intact ipsilateral greater saphenous vein.

▶ The VA Cooperative Study Group (1) carried out a study of vascular grafts at 18 medical centers. The patency was similar for in situ and reverse saphenous vein bypass for both femoropopliteal below-knee and femorotibial reconstructions. Leather et al. (2) reported on 1,000 cases of in situ saphenous vein bypasses with a 1-year patency rate of 90% and a 5-year patency rate of 76%. Fogel et al. (3) also compared in situ and reverse saphenous vein grafts for infrainguinal reconstruction; their findings support the contention that in situ grafts provide significantly better cumulative patency rates. At the institutions where those authors practiced, the reverse graft was no longer used when an ipsilateral saphenous vein was available.—S.I. Schwartz, M.D.

References

1. Veterans' Administration Cooperative Study Group: *Arch Surg* 123:434, 1988.
2. Leather, RP, et al: *Ann Surg* 208:435, 1988.
3. Fogle MA, et al: *J Vasc Surg* 5:46, 1987.

Remote Distal Arteriovenous Fistula to Improve Infrapopliteal Bypass Patency

Paty PSK, Shah DM, Saifi J, Chang BB, Feustel PJ, Kaufman JL, Leather RP,

Wengerter KR, Ascer E, Gupta SK, Veith FJ (Albany Med College, NY; Monte-fiore Med Ctr, New York)
J Vasc Surg 11:171–178, 1990   18–11

The patency rate with use of autologous saphenous vein grafts in in-frapopliteal bypass grafting is far superior to that obtained with polytet-rafluoroethylene (PTFE) grafts. Construction of an adjunctive anasto-motic arteriovenous fistula (AVF) to augment blood flow and velocity through the graft to extend the duration of synthetic graft patency ap-pears to be feasible. However, the AVF may create turbulence at the anastomosis and cause steal syndrome. An AVF constructed remote from the distal anastomosis of a femorotibial PTFE bypass graft was evaluated for its effect on graft patency and distal arterial hemodynamics.

During a 2-year period, 10 men and 5 women underwent 16 infrapo-pliteal bypass procedures. All had undergone several failed infrainguinal bypass operations, and all had limb-threatening ischemia. None of the patients had a usable length of autogenous vein. After femorotibial by-pass graft reconstruction with PTFE, an autogenous distal side-to-side AVF was created 5–15 cm below the distal anastomosis in the same ar-tery and accompanying veins (Fig 18–5, p 274).

During the immediate postoperative period, 15 of the 16 PTFE grafts were patent and ischemic symptoms were improved. One patient whose graft occluded 3 days after operation underwent graft thrombectomy, but despite continued graft patency, below-knee amputation was performed 2 weeks later for relief of continuing rest pain. During a mean follow-up period of 9 months, 11 (67%) grafts remained patent; 3 limbs required amputation during late follow-up, yielding a limb salvage rate of 75%.

Serial measurements of blood flow and blood velocity were performed in the immediate postoperative period. The mean estimated blood flow through the PTFE graft was 264 mL/min, through the AVF, 157 mL/min, and through the distal artery, 19 mL/min. The remote distal AVF not only increased blood flow through the synthetic graft, it also augmented native arterial blood flow between the distal anastomosis and the AVF, which improved limb perfusion in these patients.

▶ In the discussion of this presentation, Dr. Dardik pointed out that the animal model may not be appropriate because there is no obliterative disease and there is significant collateral inflow. The need to perform a distal fistula is small and, in Dardik's experience, enhanced graft patency and lymph salvage rate did occur. Another discussant, Dr. Maurer, also noted that femorodistal bypass grafting with an adjunct AVF may be a useful procedure for lymph cell salvage in cases with poor runoff and/or nonopacifying or poorly opacifying plantar arches.—S.I. Schwartz, M.D.

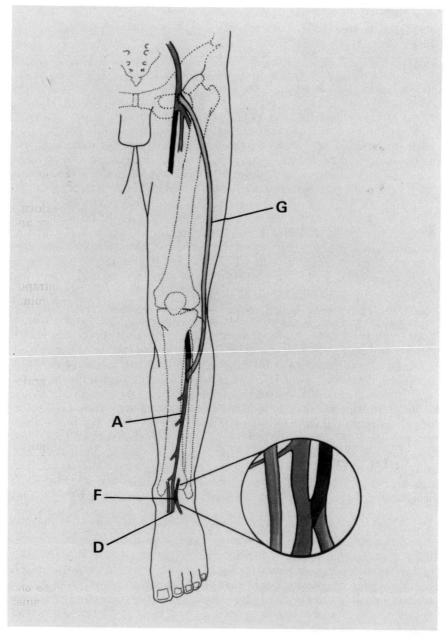

Fig 18–5.—Diagram of the lower extremity with femorotibial bypass graft and remote distal AVF. *G* indicates the PFTE graft; *A*, the intervening arterial segment; *F*, the fistula; and *D*, the distal artery. *Inset* shows details of the fistula constructed with the tibial artery and its accompanying veins. (Courtesy of Paty PSK, Shah DM, Saifi J, et al: *J Vasc Surg* 11:171–178, 1990.)

A Comparative Study of Intraoperative Angioscopy and Completion Arteriography Following Femorodistal Bypass

Baxter BT, Rizzo RJ, Flinn WR, Almgren CN, McCarthy WJ, Pearce WH, Yao JST (Northwestern Univ)

Arch Surg 125:997–1002, 1990   18–12

Technical problems are a significant cause of early graft failure after "femorodistal" bypass. Techniques have been developed for the detection and correction of technical problems such as intimal flaps, anastomotic narrowing, intraluminal thrombus, or kinking of the graft before completion of the primary surgical procedure.

In 49 femorodistal bypass grafting procedures in 47 patients standard completion arteriography and videoangioscopy were compared for their detection of technical defects, impact on operative decisions at time of primary procedure, early graft patency, and postoperative complications. Completion arteriography had a specificity of 95% but a sensitivity of only 67% in detection of technical problems. After angioscopy significant changes in surgical procedure occurred in 5 cases. Three patients had early graft failure, but none was attributable to technical problems. Four patients had postoperative myocardial infarctions, 2 of which were fatal. No patient had contrast-induced allergies or renal failure. Although angioscopy was more accurate in detecting technical problems than completion arteriography, it offered few data on distal arterial anatomy that may affect graft patency or the use of antithrombotic therapy.

Angioscopy undeniably contributes to clarification of questionable defects on completion arteriography and identification of technical defects not seen on arteriography. Intraoperative completion arteriography is a useful way to assess infrainguinal bypass grafting procedures. Although it lacks the sensitivity and specificity of angioscopy, it provides valuable information on distal anatomy that can aid in clinical decision making.

▶ Advances in technology are providing an increasing number of tools. The refinement of angioscopy has been significant. The applicability of angioscopy has not been defined because it remains difficult to evaluate the significance of the defects that are visualized. Karacagil et al. (1) analyzed a new grading system based on intraoperative postreconstruction serial angiography. Good runoff was defined as integrity of the anterior and/or posterior foot arch of the proximal femorodistal grafts and integrity of both arches in the low bypasses. In the proximal group, runoff was classified as poor when the arches were deficient or occluded and in the low group, when only 1 arch was intact. There is a good correlation between the 6-month patency rate with an 81% rate in the good run-off group; all grafts in the patients with poor run-off were occluded.—S.I. Schwartz, M.D.

Reference

1. Karacagil, S et al: *Arch Surg* 125:1055, 1990.

Efficacy of the Dorsal Pedal Bypass for Limb Salvage in Diabetic Patients: Short-Term Observations

Pomposelli FB Jr, Jepsen SJ, Gibbons GW, Campbell DR, Freeman DV, Miller A, LoGerfo FW (New England Deaconess Hosp, Boston)
J Vasc Surg 11:745–752, 1990   18–13

Occlusive disease in diabetic patients often involves the tibial and peroneal vessels. Recent advances in angiographic technology and surgical techniques have made limb salvage possible, even in those patients whose tibial vessels are extensively diseased.

Ninety-six patients (94% with diabetes) underwent 104 attempted dorsal pedal bypass grafts. Nearly half (42.3%) had associated secondary infection in addition to ischemia. All affected extremities were studied preoperatively with intra-arterial digital subtraction angiography (DSA). The dorsal pedal artery was visualized in 92 cases and 91 bypasses were

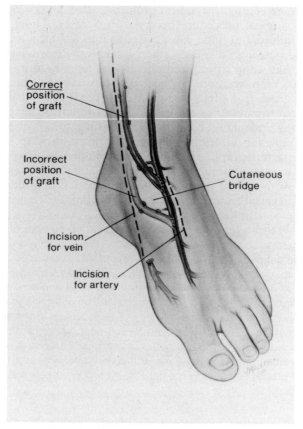

Fig 18–6.—Sketch of the correct and incorrect pathways for tunneling the saphenous vein for in situ dorsal pedal bypass. Tunneling through the skin bridge may result in necrosis. (Courtesy of Pomposelli FB Jr, Jepsen SJ, Gibbons GW, et al: *J Vasc Surg* 11:745–752, 1990.)

placed. In the remaining 12 cases, the artery was located with continuous-wave Doppler analyses and bypasses were completed successfully in 6.

Inflow was taken from the femoral artery in 48 cases, the popliteal artery in 45, and the tibial artery in 2; in 2 others a femoral tibial graft was used. The dorsal pedal artery is exposed as the initial step in the operative procedure. Proximally, the artery gives off its lateral tarsal branch. Distally, at the level of the proximal first metatarsal, it bifurcates into the deep plantar artery and the first dorsal metatarsal artery. The artery between the branches is usually suitable for bypass grafting. Undermining of the skin bridge to tunnel the graft should be avoided to prevent necrosis (Fig 18–6).

Perioperative mortality was 1.92%. Six bypasses (6.1%) failed during this period. Thirty-three of the 89 patients whose limbs were salvaged required additional surgery to achieve a healed foot. At 18 months, graft patency was 81.8%; limb salvage, 86.9%; and patient survival, 80%. The short-term results of dorsal pedal bypass are favorable. Intra-arterial DSA, especially in diabetic patients, often reveals a patent dorsal pedal artery that will permit arterial reconstruction and limb salvage.

▶ These results are excellent and parallel the experience reported by Harris et al. (1) In that series, foot salvage was achieved in 83% of patients. In situ saphenous vein graft from the common femoral artery were used in those patients. Ascer et al. (2) reported success with bypasses to the plantar arteries distal to the arch.—S.I. Schwartz, M.D.

References

1. Harris, et al: *Arch Surg* 124:1232, 1989.
2. Ascer E, et al: *J Vasc Surg* 8:434, 1988.

Role of Revascularization to Treat Chronic Nonhealing Fractures in Ischemic Limbs

Deitz DM, Taylor LM Jr, Beals RK, Porter JM (Oregon Health Sciences Univ, Portland)

J Vasc Surg 10:535–541, 1989   18–14

Although the importance of blood supply for healing of fractures is well documented, the literature contains only a single case report describing the healing of a previously nonunited fracture by correction of limb ischemia. In that patient, and the 3 additional patients described here, revascularization was successful in stimulating healing after nonunion. Nonunion because of limb ischemia is more common in older patients because of the increased prevalence of atherosclerotic occlusive disease.

During a 10-year period, 5% of tibial fractures seen in patients older than 50 failed to unite. Four patients in whom ischemia was suspected as a cause of nonunion were referred to the vascular service. The patients, all women, had a mean age of 63 years. The duration of nonunion in the 3 tibial fractures and 1 femur fracture ranged from 1 to 12 months. All patients had a history of claudication.

Angiography revealed multilevel disease in 3 patients and single-level

Clinical Data for 4 Patients With Nonunion of Lower Extremity Fractures Treated With Adjunctive Arterial Reconstruction

Patient	Age	Fracture site	Initial orthopedic treatment	Duration of nonunion	Preexisting ischemic symptoms (ABI)	Angiographic findings	Vascular surgical procedure	Time from vascular repair to fracture healing	Status
1	59	Distal left tibia	Cast immobilization	12 mo	Stable claudication (0.48)	Bilateral common iliac and external iliac stenosis	Prosthetic aortobifemoral bypass	5 mo	Alive and well at 3 years
2	58	Distal left tibia	Cast immobilization	7 mo	Left foot ischemic rest pain and ischemia ulceration (0.32)	Left external iliac stenosis and left superficial femoral occlusion	Left external iliac endarterectomy and left femoral popliteal vein bypass	7 mo	Graft stenosis successfully repaired at 2 years, alive and well at 3 years
3	67	Supracondylar right femur	Cast brace immobilization	1 mo	Right foot ischemic rest pain (0.24)	Bilateral common iliac occlusion, bilateral superficial femoral occlusion right profunda stenosis	Axillary bilateral femoral goretex-bypass, right femoroprofunda endarterectomy	5 mo	Alive and well at 2 years
4	57	Distal left tibia	Cast immobilization	5 mo	Left calf claudication 0.50	Left superficial femoral occlusion	Left femoral popliteal vein bypass	4 mo	Alive and well at 2 years

(Courtesy of Deitz DM, Taylor LM Jr, Beals RK, et al: *J Vasc Surg* 10:535–541, 1989.)

disease in the fourth. Each underwent surgical revascularization (table). The fractures healed completely within a mean of 5.3 months after revascularization. At a mean follow-up of 26 months, 3 patients were fully ambulatory. The fourth woman was nonambulatory because of an unrelated problem involving the contralateral knee, but she had a patent vascular reconstruction and healed fracture.

The importance of local blood supply in healing of fractures is confirmed in these cases. Although this appears to be the only reported series of patients undergoing elective limb revascularization to stimulate fracture healing, such a procedure should be considered more often in severely ischemic limbs.

▶ This represents a new concept, although it is true that 4 cases represent an anecdotol experience and 1 of these 4 patients had nonunion for only 1 month. The paper should serve as a stimulus for further investigation of this application of vascular reconstructive procedures.— S.I. Schwartz, M.D.

Experience With Cardiopulmonary Bypass and Deep Hypothermic Circulatory Arrest in the Management of Retroperitoneal Tumors With Large Vena Caval Thrombi

Novick AC, Kaye MC, Cosgrove DM, Angermeier K, Pontes JE, Montie JE, Streem SB, Klein E, Stewart R, Goormastic M (Cleveland Clinic Found)
Ann Surg 212:472–477, 1990   18–15

Cardiopulmonary bypass (CPB) with deep hypothermic circulatory arrest (DHCA) is a useful adjunct in the surgical treatment of patients with renal cell carcinoma and large inferior vena caval tumor thrombi. These techniques were used in management of a group of 43 patients with retroperitoneal tumors and large caval thrombi.

The primary malignancies were renal cell carcinoma in 39 cases. In these patients the entire kidney was mobilized and left attached by only the main renal vein with the tumor thrombus. After maximum tumor mobilization, a median sternotomy was done, the patients were heparinized, and the aorta and right atrium were cannulated. Bypass was initiated with systemic cooling, augmented by the use of topical cold solution in the abdomen and chest. After a core temperature of 18° to 20° C was attained, CPB was terminated and the blood volume drained into the pump. Circulatory arrest required 10–44 minutes.

There were 2 operative deaths, for a mortality of 4.7%. Neither died from the use of DHCA. Thirteen patients (30.2%) had major postoperative complications. However, there were no ischemic or neurologic complications or perioperative tumor embolization. The median hospital stay after surgery was 9 days. Twenty-two patients (51%) were alive with a good quality of life at follow-up. The 3-year survival rates in patients with localized compared with metastatic renal cell carcinoma were 63.9% and 10.9%, respectively.

For patients with an intrahepatic or suprahepatic inferior vena caval thrombus from retroperitoneal malignancy, CPB with DHCA is the preferred procedure. This approach appears to be effective and safe. Also, it allows extensive inferior vena caval thrombi to be removed completely with excellent exposure in a controlled operative setting.

▶ The management of renal cell carcinoma extending into the vena cava was reviewed by Pritchett et al. (1). Of 25 patients, 88% survived to be discharged from the hospital. Those authors did not use CPB in the circulatory lists routinely, nearly occluding the inferior vena cava distal to the thrombus and proximal at its entrance to the atrium. The presently described technique adds an element of safety.—S.I. Schwartz, M.D.

Reference

1. Pritchett, TR, et al: *J Urol* 135:460, 1986.

Reconstruction of the Vena Cava and of Its Primary Tributaries: A Preliminary Report

Gloviczki P, Pairolero PC, Cherry KJ, Hallett JW Jr (Mayo Clinic and Found, Rochester, Minn)
J Vasc Surg 11:373–381, 1990
18–6

The vena cava and/or its major branches were reconstructed in 16 patients in 1981–1989; ages ranged from 8 to 81 years. Eight patients had superior vena cava syndrome, in 2 because of malignant neoplasms. Two others had membranous occlusion of the inferior vena cava, and 4 had iliocaval venous thrombosis. One patient had undergone iliac vein excision for pelvic neurilemmoma, and 1 sustained an inferior caval injury during liver transplantation.

The superior cava was reconstructed with a spiral saphenous vein graft in 5 patients (Fig 18–7) and with expanded polytetrafluoroethylene (PTFE) in 3. One graft of each kind had to be revised, but 7 of the 8 superior caval grafts were patent at follow-up. A bifurcated spiral saphenous vein graft was occluded at 3 months.

The inferior cava and its tributaries were reconstructed with expanded PTFE in 5 cases, a spiral saphenous vein graft in 2, and Dacron in 1. Four PTFE grafts were patent at follow-up. Two of the 3 grafts with a concomitant temporary arteriovenous fistula at the groin were patent. One spiral saphenous vein graft was occluded and the other was not evaluable. The Dacron graft occluded, but the patient had only minimal symptoms.

The spiral saphenous vein graft is preferred for reconstructing the superior vena cava. Expanded PTFE grafts give better results in the abdomen. Caval grafting is appropriate for patients who have significant symptoms of venous stasis despite other forms of treatment.

▶ This is a large series undergoing an unusual operation. The selection of patients for whom this operation is indicated is critical. The results with the spiral

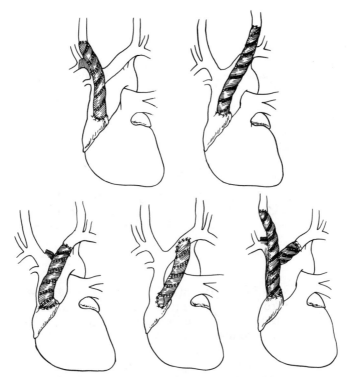

Fig 18–7.—Illustrations of different spiral saphenous vein grafts used for superior vena cava reconstruction. (Courtesy of Gloviczki P, Pairolero PC, Cherry KJ, et al: *J Vasc Surg* 11:373–381, 1990.)

saphenous vein graft in the superior vena cava are in keeping with those previously reported by Doty (1). The use of a temporary arterial venous fistula at the groin to enhance the patency rate of graft space in the inferior vena cava is appropriate. A femoral arteriovenous fistula should be maintained for several months to provide for a good endothelial covering.—S.I. Schwartz, M.D.

Reference

1. Doty DB: *J Thorac Cardiovasc Surg* 83:326, 1982.

Long-Term Results of Venous Thrombectomy Combined With a Temporary Arterio-venous Fistula
Plate G, Åkesson H, Einarsson E, Ohlin P, Eklöf B (Central Hosp, Helsingborg, Sweden; Univ of Lund, Sweden; Univ of Kuwait)
Eur J Vasc Surg 4:483–489, 1990   18–17

Although surgical thrombectomy is the most effective way to remove deep thrombi, particularly in the iliofemoral veins with a thrombus duration of less than 5–7 days, rethrombosis has been frequent, resulting in chronic venous obstruction, valvular incompetence, and late complica-

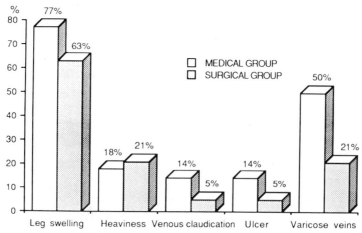

Fig 18–8.—Postthrombotic sequelae in 22 medical and 19 surgical patients at 5 years after acute iliofemoral venous thrombosis. (Courtesy of Plate G, Åkesson H, Einersson E, et al: *Eur J Vasc Surg* 4:483–489, 1990.)

tions in 70% to 80% of the patients. This has caused many surgeons to abandon venous thrombectomy. Further advances in surgical technique, however, have been made in some institutions. The long-term results of venous thrombectomy combined with a temporary arteriovenous fistula (AVF) were assessed in 41 patients.

The patients were randomly assigned to receive conventional anticoagulation, or acute thrombectomy combined with AVF and anticoagulation. There were 22 medical and 19 surgical patients. The 5-year follow-up showed slightly more asymptomatic patients and less frequent severe postthrombotic complications in the surgical group. Those values were 37% vs. 18%, and 16% vs. 27%, in the surgical and medical groups, respectively. The iliac vein was more often normal after thrombectomy as demonstrated by radionuclide angiography, but occlusion plethysmography showed an outflow capacity that was not significantly better. No obvious differences could be found in muscle pump function and reflux assessed by foot volumetry. The ambulatory venous pressure was significantly lower, however, in the surgical group (Fig 18–8).

Thrombectomy combined with a temporary AVF appears to improve the long-term outcome after acute iliofemoral venous thrombosis. However, the difference between the outcomes of this and anticoagulation treatment is not very striking. Thus anticoagulation therapy is still an acceptable alternative.

► The article is meaningful in that it comes from the group that introduced the concept of concomitant AVF to augment the patency associated with venous thrombectomy. Lansing and Davis (1) indicated that incidence of rethrombosis and venous incompetence followed venous thrombectomy in 70% to 80% of patients and that the procedure should be abandoned. The present authors demonstrated previously that construction of an AVF prevented rethrombosis of the ileofemoral segment, providing continued patency in about 66% of the patients. Swedenborg et al. (2) reported a group of 19 patients treated for ileofemoral venous thrombosis by thrombectomy and a temporary AVF; success was achieved in 17. At follow-up, 8 patients had complete patency and 8 had partial patency.—S.I. Schwartz, M.D.

References

1. Lansing, AM, Davis JM: *Ann Surg* 168:620, 1968.
2. Swedenborg J, et al: *Br J Surg* 73:871, 1986.

19 The Esophagus

Esophagectomy for Esophageal Disruption
Orringer MB, Stirling MC (Univ of Michigan)
Ann Thorac Surg 49:35–43, 1990   19–1

Disruption of the intrathoracic esophagus results in a high mortality rate, particularly when treatment is delayed or when established hydropneumothorax and mediastinal sepsis are present. Aggressive and definitive therapy individualized to the patient's needs may offer the only chance for survival. A retrospective review of 24 adult patients suggested that esophagectomy and either primary or delayed esophageal reconstruction offer less risk than more conservative therapy.

The average age of the 12 men and 12 women was 59 years. Twenty had preexisting esophageal disease. Causes of esophageal disruption included instrumentation (9 patients), emesis (2), and reoperation on the esophagus (3). The average interval between diagnosis and esophagectomy was 6.6 days. Thirteen patients were operated on within 24 hours after the injury. Fifteen underwent transhiatal esophagectomy without thoracotomy and 9 had a transthoracic esophagectomy.

In 13 patients restoration of alimentary continuity was accomplished with an immediate cervical esophagogastrostomy. The stomach was positioned in the posterior mediastinum in the original esophageal bed, and a pyloromyotomy and feeding jejunostomy were performed routinely. Eleven patients were thought to be too ill to undergo esophageal reconstruction at the time of esophagectomy. In these cases, care was taken to preserve the maximum amount of remaining esophageal length. Reconstruction was delayed for an average of 8.6 weeks.

Esophagectomy was well tolerated. Three hospital deaths occurred; 2 patients with chronic renal failure died of continuing sepsis and an 86-year-old woman died of a pulmonary embolus. Two hospital survivors died without being able to resume eating. Four patients died of other causes. Of the remaining 15 patients, 14 continued to do well at an average follow-up of 31 months. This surgical option, although radical, may be the safest and most effective approach in certain gravely ill patients.

▶ The plea for what some would regard as a more aggressive approach is analogous to the recommendation for an aggressive surgical approach to corrosive burns of the esophagus and stomach (1,2). In the discussion, Dr. McLaughlin indicates that in his institutional series of 65 patients, 8 underwent esophagectomies for perforation. In 6 of these patients the problem was related to lye stricture or perforation. The survival rate was 75%.—S.I. Schwartz, M.D.

References

1. Estrera A, et al; *Ann Thorac Surg* 41:276, 1986.
2. Gossot D, et al: *J Thorac Cardiovasc Surg* 94:188, 1987.

Surgical Management of 100 Consecutive Esophageal Strictures
Henderson RD, Henderson RF, Marryatt GV (Women's College Hosp, Toronto)
J Thorac Cardiovasc Surg 99:1–7, 1990   19–2

In this study of 100 consecutive patients with reflux-induced esophageal strictures, the advantages of treatment by a conservative antireflux procedure were weighed against those of esophageal resection. The results of preoperative investigation were analyzed to define those factors that negatively affected outcome.

Patients included in the study were treated over a period of 10 years 8 months. Preoperative factors found to predict eventual outcome were the presence of scleroderma, a previous esophageal or gastric operation, and severity of the esophageal stricture. Severe strictures were defined as those associated with marked ulceration. In such cases the esophagus is notably thickened and has a woody consistency.

Ninety-eight patients were treated by total fundoplication gastroplasty (TFG). Twenty-eight had a transabdominal incision, 30 were treated via a transthoracic approach, and 40 underwent a thoracoabdominal approach. The success of the operation depends on fundoplication. Two patients required esophageal resection. One had no remaining lumen endoscopically or radiologically, making dilatation impossible. The other patient's preoperative complications included destruction of a segment of esophageal wall.

There were 7 complications, all in the group having TFG. None necessitated further operation. At an average follow-up of 6.7 years, in 82 of the 87 TFG patients who had radiologic studies there was no evidence of recurrence or reflux. Postoperative dilatation was required in 98 patients, including 48.2% of those with severe stricture and 45% of those with scleroderma.

Excellent results can be obtained with TFG in patients with no complicating factors or with only 1 such factor. Patients with 2 or 3 complicating factors or preoperative disease may do better with esophageal resection. Total fundoplication gastroplasty with pre-and postoperative dilatation can replace surgical resection in selected patients.

▶

This article also indicates that, although most of the patients do well with gastroplasty and dilatation, a subset requires esophageal resection. Stirling and Orringer (1) reported excellent results in patients undergoing combined Collis-Nissen operation for esophageal reflux strictures. Waters et al. (2), like the authors of the present article, also identify patients who benefitted from esophagectomy for severe esophagitis and strictures.—S.I. Schwartz, M.D.

References

1. Stirling MC, Orringer MB: *Ann Thorac Surg* 45:148, 1988.
2. Waters PF, et al: *J Thorac Cardiovasc Surg* 95:378, 1988.

Indications for Esophagectomy in Nonmalignant Barrett's Esophagus: A 10-Year Experience

Altorki NK, Skinner DB, Segalin A, Stephens JK, Ferguson MK, Little AG (Cornell Univ, Univ of Chicago; Univ of Nevada, Las Vegas)
Ann Thorac Surg 49:724–727, 1990   19–3

The columnar-lined esophagus described by Barrett in 1950 is still a matter of controversy. There is confusion about its definition, pathogenesis, treatment, and follow-up. The indications for esophagectomy were investigated in 88 patients who were referred for surgical treatment of benign Barrett's esophagus between 1978 and 1988. Nineteen patients required esophageal resection. The male–female ratio was 13:6 and the age range was 13 to 84 years.

Eleven patients had strictures and 7 had ulcers on preoperative studies. In 5 cases the indication for resection was penetrating Barrett's ulcer resistant to treatment. Ulcers penetrated to the pericardium in 1 case, the pulmonary vein in 1, the lung in 1, and the mediastinum in 2. Strictures that could not be dilated, previous surgery, high-grade dysplasia, parietal cells that lined the esophagus, patient refusal of long-term surveillance, and inability to exclude adenocarcinoma before operation were other indications. Colon interposition or esophagogastrostomy was done for reconstruction in 19 patients.

One patient died after surgery. All patients were followed for a mean of 41 months. Three of the 18 patients who survived reconstructive surgery subsequently had occasional regurgitation, but none had dysphagia or weight loss.

Esophageal resection for Barrett's esophagus is indicated in selected patients. Absolute indications for esophageal resection are a deep penetrating ulcer confirmed at operation, high-grade dysplasia, a strong suspicion of cancer, and multiple previous operations. Relative indications for surgery include strictures that do not respond to dilation and the refusal of young patients to have long-term surveillance.

▶ Progression of Barrett's epithelium after antireflux operation remains a controversial topic. Williamson et al. (1) assessed 37 patients with Barrett's esophagus who had undergone an antireflux operation. In more than 70%, proven lower esophageal sphincter pressure was demonstrated and more than 90% had symptomatic relief. Cancer developed in 8%. The authors concluded that the indications for the antireflux operation in patients with Barrett's esophagus should remain the same as for other patients, but yearly endoscopic surveillance should be carried out.—S.I. Schwartz, M.D.

Reference

1. Williamson WA, et al: *Ann Thorac Surg* 49:537, 1990.

Reconstruction of the Cervical Esophagus: Free Jejunal Transfer Versus Gastric Pull-Up

Schusterman MA, Shestak K, deVries EJ, Swartz W, Jones N, Johnson J, Myers E, Reilly J Jr (Univ of Pittsburgh; Tulane Univ, New Orleans)
Plast Reconstr Surg 85:16–21, 1990   19–4

Use of enteric grafts is a popular technique for reconstructing the cervical esophagus and hypopharynx. Free jejunal transfer (FJT) and gastric pull-up (GP) are used most often. A retrospective review was made of experience with FJT and GP.

Fifty FJTs and 15 GPs were performed (Figs 19–1 and 19–2). The graft survival rate was 94% for FJTs and 87% for GPs. Eighty-eight percent of the patients undergoing FJT and 87% undergoing GP achieved successful swallowing. Patients with FJTs could swallow and leave the hospital sooner than those with GPs. Fistulas occurred in 16% of FJTs. Six of 8 healed spontaneously. Fistulas occurred in 20% of GPs; only 1 of these 3 fistulas healed spontaneously. Stricture was the most common late complication of FJTs, occurring in 22%. Reflux was the most common in GPs, occurring in 20%.

Extensive esophageal resection into the chest is often needed in patients with advanced cancer. Gastric pull-up seems to be an easier, more direct form of reconstruction. In limited resection of the hypopharynx and esophagus, particularly with proximal lesions, FJT is simpler and obviates the need for mediastinal dissection.

▶ Wright and Cuschieri (1) have reported excellent results with jejunal interposition. The present article parallels the experience reported by Jurkiewicz (2)

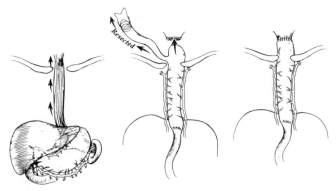

Fig 19–1.—Technique of gastric pull-up. (Courtesy of Schusterman MA, Shestak K, deVries EJ, et al: *Plast Reconstr Surg* 85:16–21, 1990.)

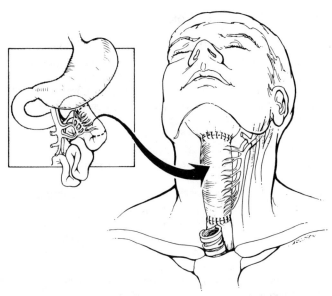

Fig 19–2.—Technique of free jejunal transfer. (Courtesy of Schusterman MA, Shestak K, deVries EJ, et al: *Plast Reconstr Surg* 85:16–21, 1990.)

using the free graft of the jejunum. Results achieved by this technique were superior to those of colon interposition. Curet-Scott et al. (3) reported that colon interposition for benign esophageal disease has a 30% major complication rate and a 37% reoperation rate. But those authors concluded that because of low mortality and high patient satisfaction, it is a procedure that can be recommended for benign esophageal disease.—S.I. Schwartz, M.D.

References

1. Wright C, Cuschieri A: *Am Surg* 205:54, 1987.
2. Jurkiewicz MJ: *J Thorac Cardiovasc Surg* 88:893, 1984.
3. Curet-Scott MJ, et al: *Surgery* 102:568, 1987

Free Jejunal Interposition Graft for Reconstruction of the Esophagus
Fisher SR, Cameron R, Hoyt DJ, Cole TB, Seigler HF, Meyers WC (Duke Univ)
Head Neck 12:126–130, 1990   19–5

Since the free jejunal interposition graft (FJIG) was used for pharyngoesophageal reconstruction in animal studies, varying degrees of success have been achieved in patients. Forty-seven patients who received FJIG transplants for reconstruction of the pharyngoesophagus in 1978–1988 were studied. Twenty-one patients with primary squamous cell cancer had not been treated previously, whereas 20 others had recurrent disease after initial surgery or radiotherapy. Six patients had an obstructing pharyngoesophageal stricture, 5 of them after laryngectomy and 1 after lye ingestion.

The overall median survival was 10 months, but 11% of the patients were alive more than 5 years after surgery. Patients operated on for recurrent cancer had a median survival of 20 months. Four patients died perioperatively. Swallowing function was adequate in 86% of 32 patients who were evaluable. The most frequent complications were graft failure, stricture formation, and hypoparathyroidism.

The FJIG is the most physiologic approach to pharyngoesophageal reconstruction. The graft tolerates irradiation without losing the ability to produce mucus. An oral diet generally can be continued until death.

▶ This technique is a 1-stage procedure that is most appropriate in those patients who have an anticipated low cure rate and relatively short survival. Rehabilitation of these patients as far as swallowing is concerned requires less time than other reconstructive techniques. Jurkiewicz (1) reported an impressive series of patients undergoing reconstructive surgery of the cervical esophagus using free revascularized jejunum. Six graft failures occurred among a total of 55 cases. Most patients took a regular diet within 10 days. The author concluded that the free jejunal graft procedure is the method of choice for reconstructing the cervical esophagus.—S.I. Schwartz, M.D.

Reference

1. Jurkiewicz MJ: *J Thorac Cardiovasc Surg* 88:893, 1984.

101-Oesophageal Cancers: A Surgeon Uses Radiotherapy
Earlam RJ, Johnson L (London Hosp, England; Karolinska Inst, Stockholm)
Ann Coll Surg Engl 72:32–40, 1990   19–6

There long has been uncertainty about the efficacy of radiotherapy in squamous cell esophageal carcinoma. A review was made of experience with 101 patients who had esophageal or gastroesophageal cancer; they were seen consecutively from 1979 to 1985. Fifty-eight of the patients received radiotherapy; 22 of them received radical radiotherapy for operative cancer. Twenty-five patients with inoperable esophageal cancer and 11 with unresectable gastric cancer spreading to the esophagus, or esophageal oat cell adenocarcinoma, were treated palliatively. Thirty-five patients were operated on and 10 received no treatment.

Twenty-eight percent of the patients lived for 1 year, 15% for 2 years, and 5% for 5 years or longer. Of the 22 patients given radical radiotherapy for operable squamous cell cancer of the esophagus, 10 (46%) lived for 1 year and 3 (14%) for 5 years. The postoperative mortality rate was 20%; the mean survival time after surgery was 11.7 months.

Radical radiotherapy should be among the treatment options for patients having resectable squamous cell carcinoma of the esophagus. A prospective randomized trial, comparing radical radiotherapy with surgery is needed.

▶ As pointed out by Professor Hennessy in the Discussion, there is no controlled, prospective, randomized trial of radiotherapy vs. surgery for squamous carcinoma of the esophagus. The problem in evaluating the results in the present paper is the uncertainty of staging assessment. If the operable group undergoing radiotherapy was staged correctly, the results are not comparable to surgery. If all patients had lymph node involvement, the results of radiotherapy are much more comparable to surgery. Because the general figure for lymph node involvement is about 50%, it is difficult to ascribe an equivalent therapeutic result to radiotherapy.— S.I. Schwartz, M.D.

Chemotherapy and Radiation Therapy Before Transhiatal Esophagectomy for Esophageal Carcinoma
Orringer MB, Forastiere AA, Perez-Tamayo C, Urba S, Takasugi BJ, Bromberg J
(Univ of Michigan)
Ann Thorac Surg 49:348–355, 1990   19–7

Patients with esophageal cancer have had an extremely poor prognosis. Because most of the patients have local tumor invasion or distant metastases at the time of diagnosis, therapy has concentrated on palliation of dysphagia. In an attempt to improve long-term survival, preoperative chemotherapy and radiation have been added to transhiatal esophagectomy (THE). The results of multimodal therapy in 43 patients with esophageal carcinoma were evaluated.

The series included 32 men and 11 women whose average age was 62 years. None had undergone previous treatment, and all had tumors judged to be totally resectable. There were 22 squamous cell carcinomas and 21 adenocarcinomas. Treatment consisted of cisplatin, vinblastine, and 5-fluorouracil chemotherapy concurrent with 4,500 cGy radiation therapy for 21 days. Three weeks later, THE without thoracotomy was performed, with alimentary continuity established at the same operation.

Two patients died of sepsis before the planned surgery. Two patients who were operated on had incurable disease at exploration and did not undergo esophagectomy. In all but 1 of the 39 patients who had THE, gross total removal of all visible or palpable tumor was believed to have been obtained. Resected specimens showed no residual cancer in 11 (43%) of the 43 patients entered into the study. Thirteen patients (32%) were surgically staged as T_0. At a median follow-up of 27 months, 20 (46%) patients were alive and clinically disease free.

Survival was superior in those with no residual disease at surgery; the median length of survival for the group as a whole was 29 months. Intensive combined modality therapy appears to be able to achieve long-term survival, not just palliation, in many patients with esophageal cancer.

▶ The improved 2-year survival, compared with that of earlier patients, is of interest, but it is far too early to extrapolate from historical controls. Parker et al. (1) demonstrated that the addition of preoperative chemotherapy as an adjunct did not result in a statistically significant increase in either the 2-year or 5-year survival of patients with operative squamous carcinoma. Of 129 patients in their series, only 3 were able to complete preoperative chemotherapy and radiation therapy and then undergo resection. Perhaps most pertinent was the fact that the absence of tumor in the surgical specimen did not appear to confer any better chance for long-term survival.—S.I. Schwartz, M.D.

Reference

1. Parker GA, et al: *J Thorac Cardiovasc Surg* 95:1037, 1988.

20 The Stomach and the Duodenum

Lymph Node Metastases of Gastric Cancer: General Pattern in 1,931 Patients
Maruyama K, Gunvén P, Okabayashi K, Sasako M, Kinoshita T (Natl Cancer Ctr Hosp, Tokyo)
Ann Surg 210:596–602, 1989

20–1

The survival rates for gastric cancer, no matter what the stage of tumor node metastasis, have improved at this Japanese hospital in every 5-year period since 1962. To determine the importance of consistent, systematic dissection of various lymph nodes in this experience, lymph node metastases and survival rates were analyzed for 1,931 patients.

As tumors invaded deeper into the stomach wall, the incidence of metastasis rose. A clear relationship was seen between the position of the tumor and distribution of the perigastric deposits. Although the most common deposits were in some perigastric node stations, other stations such as those along the left gastric artery and common hepatic artery, around the celiac artery, and at the splenic hilus often had metastases. From 2% to 4% of patients with negative perigastric nodes had skip metastases to distant nodes.

Survival rates were better in those with deposits in perigastric nodes, but from 6% to 19% of patients with deposits along the left gastric artery and common hepatic artery, splenic artery, and celiac artery survived 5 years if nodes were dissected.

In patients undergoing resection aimed at cure, node dissection may be based on previous patterns of spread and survival in matched patients. Less extensive resection may suffice for the most superficial early tumors, but for advanced cancer more extensive dissection is recommended.

▶ The Japanese have for decades paid meticulous attention to lymphadenectomy in operations for proximal gut cancer. Akiyama has raised this to an art form in his tour-de-force procedures for esophageal cancer in which he does a combined radical neck dissection, complete thoracic node dissection, and celiac lymphadenectomy (1,2). In this current paper from the National Cancer Hospital in Tokyo, the authors state that they achieve, in 78% of all resections, an R2 resection, which removes perigastric nodes, nodes about the common hepatic artery, the left gastric artery, and celiac artery, and, for proximal cancers, the nodes in the splenic hilum, along the splenic artery, and the left cardiac nodes. I doubt if there is any series in the world that could match that achievement in more than 1,900 patients. Their achievement of survival in patients with nodes along the left gastric, common hepatic, and splenic and celiac arteries is a testimony to their care. There were no 5-year survivors among patients who had positive nodes around the middle colic artery.

Gastric cancer, fortunately, is much less common in America, and no group of American surgeons could in a lifetime develop this experience. Nonetheless, the excellent results of careful node dissection deserve emulation.—J.C. Thompson, M.D.

References

1. Akiyama H: *Curr Probl Surg* 17:65, 1980.
2. Akiyama H: *Am J Surg* 147:9, 1984.

Failure of Nutritional Recovery After Total Gastrectomy
Curran FT, Hill GL (Auckland Hosp, New Zealand)
Br J Surg 77:1015–1017, 1990   20–2

It is often claimed that malnutrition is inevitable after total gastrectomy, but its cause is not clear. Energy intake, fecal fat and nitrogen, and body protein and fat stores were measured in 6 patients having total gastrectomy for adenocarcinoma or, in 1 patient, lymphoma. Five patients had a Roux-en-Y jejunal loop made and 1 received a Hunt-Lawrence pouch. Follow-up studies were performed a median of 45 months after surgery.

Daily energy intake from frequent small meals was close to the required intake of 2,284 kcal. The same was true for protein intake. Fecal fat excretion was consistently increased, markedly in 2 patients. Serum albumin levels were normal. In 2 patients, serum iron levels were slightly low, but the patients were not anemic. No significant weight change followed gastrectomy. Total body protein remained lower than predicted after operation. More than 75% of predicted total body fat was lost in 2 patients; the mean group values remained significantly lower than those predicted.

The malnutrition consequent to total gastrectomy appears to result from marked depletion of body reserves. The disease itself is more responsible than the operation. Curative total gastrectomy prevents further decline, but protein and fat stores do not recover despite a normal energy intake. Steatorrhea may be a contributing factor.

▶ This small, carefully studied group of patients demonstrates, somewhat contrary to the title of the paper, that those having total gastrectomy are able to maintain their preoperative weight. We have performed total gastrectomy for the Zollinger-Ellison syndrome on patients who were obese and they lost 10% to 15% of their body weight. One patient maintained her weight above 200 lbs for more than 3 years after total gastrectomy.

The majority of poor results after total gastrectomy for malignancy result from progression of the disease. Most poor outcomes in the so-called Roux-en-Y syndrome occur, in fact, in patients who had a Roux-en-Y reconstruction of a Billroth II subtotal gastrectomy as a putative cure for alkaline reflux gastritis. We have found total gastrectomy to be a remarkably effective operation with relatively few nutritional sequelae. We have found it unnecessary to construct any kind of reservoir pouch. We have reoperated on several of our patients for various reasons years after total gastrectomy and have found the Roux-en-Y limb to be greatly dilated, resembling a vertical, spindle-shaped stomach. It is usual for our patients to be able to eat 3 regular meals a day within 6 months of operation and to do so with surprisingly few problems with the dumping syndrome. Of more than 35 patients, only 2 have required temporary dietary supplementation with guar gel to slow gastric emptying. Within 1 year, both had resumed normal dietary habits.— J.C. Thompson, M.D.

Nutritional Consequences of Total Gastrectomy: The Relationship Between Mode of Reconstruction, Postprandial Symptoms, and Body Composition
Miholic J, Meyer HJ, Müller MJ, Weimann A, Pichlmayr R (Hannover School of Medicine)
Surgery 108:488–494, 1990   20–3

Many patients experience nutritional consequences after total gastrectomy, but the impact of the method of reconstruction and that of postprandial symptoms has not been clearly elucidated. Body composition, postprandial symptoms, and social performance were evaluated in 15 patients who underwent total gastrectomy with Roux-en-Y esophagojejunostomy and 26 who had jejunal interposition. Patients were similar in age, sex, initial tumor stage, interval since surgery, and premorbid body mass index (BMI). They were studied by history, anthropometric measurements, and bioelectrical impedance analysis.

In patients with Roux-en-Y reconstructions, the lowest postoperative BMI was 72% of the premorbid BMI, whereas in those with jejunal interposition, it was 79%. At the time of study, the relative BMI was 81% in patients who underwent Roux-en-Y procedures and 88% in those who underwent jejunal interposition (Fig 20–1). Muscle mass and lean body mass correlated independently with sex and with mode of reconstruction. These correlations were confirmed by multiple linear regression. Postprandial symptoms had no significant association with changes in body composition except that there was an inverse relationship between the Sigstad dumping score and the extracellular mass/body cell mass ratio.

Of patients younger than 60 years, 10 of 15 with jejunal interposition and 2 of 8 with Roux-en-Y reconstruction were able to return to work. Those who resumed working had significantly higher relative BMIs, lean body mass, and muscle mass than those who no longer worked.

It appears that preserving the duodenal transit should be the main consideration in gastric replacement after total gastrectomy. Patients with jejunal interposition lose significantly less weight and regain a higher per-

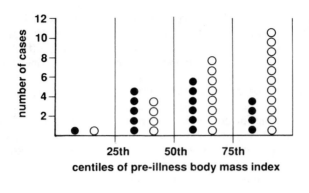

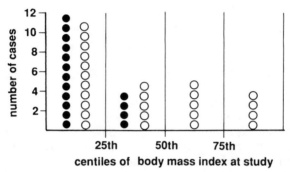

Fig 20-1.—Premorbid body mass index (BMI) (**top**) and BMI at study (**bottom**) expressed as quartiles of a reference population (corrected for sex and age). Patients who underwent later Roux-en-Y *(filled circles)* esophagojejunostomy and jejunal interposition *(open circles)* yielded no significantly different distributions of their pre-illness BMI, whereas at study a significantly (chi-square test; $P = .051$) larger proportion of the patients with Roux-en-Y reconstruction (75%) was below the 25th percentile than patients with jejunal interposition (44%). (Courtesy of Miholic J, Meyer HJ, Müller MJ, et al: *Surgery* 108:488-494, 1990.)

centage of preoperative BMI than do patients with Roux-en-Y esophago-jejunostomy.

▶ This study compares nutrition after total gastrectomy in patients with a classic Roux-en-Y esophagojejunostomy and those in whom a 50-cm limb of jejunum is interposed between the esophagus and the first part of the duodenum to preserve normal duodenal passage of ingested food. The study confirms the generally good nutritional status after total gastrectomy in those patients who survived for a median of 3 years after total gastrectomy for malignancy. As the authors note, in this retrospective study, it is not possible to determine why one operation was assigned to a patient over another. The differences between the 2 anastomoses are small but significant and confirm widespread impressions that activation of pancreatic and biliary mechanisms by food transit in the duodenum is important in maintenance of absorption of food. We have not used this procedure, but it appears worthy of trial.—J.C. Thompson, M.D.

Surgical Treatment of Gastric Carcinoma: A Retrospective Analysis With Special Regard to the Value of Total Gastrectomy as the Operation of Choice

Meyer H-J, Jaehne J, Pichlmayr R (Medizinische Hochschule Hannover, Germany)

J R Coll Surg Edinb 34:258–262, 1989 20–4

Although the incidence of gastric carcinoma is decreasing, it remains a leading cause of death from cancer. Early diagnosis and appropriate surgical excision are the most important requirements for a successful outcome. No consensus yet exists on the extent of resection and the place of total gastrectomy as the operation of choice. The outcome in 1,510 cases of early and advanced gastric carcinoma was reviewed.

The patients had a mean age of 61.6 years; there were 959 men and 551 women. In about half (760) the tumor involved more than one third of the stomach. Follow-up was available for 98.3% of the patients. The overall rate of resectability was 75%, representing 714 total, 313 distal subtotal, and 108 proximal gastrectomies. During the study period, 1968–1987, the frequency of total gastrectomy rose from 25.2% to 81.1%.

Operative mortality was 12.4% for all resections and did not differ significantly between distal subtotal and total gastrectomies. Over time, morbidity and mortality rates associated with total gastrectomy declined as surgical techniques improved. In the study institution, postoperative mortality with total gastrectomy has decreased to approximately 2%.

The lack of a significant difference in 5-year survival rates between total and subtotal gastrectomy may result from a selection bias of patients. Nevertheless, total gastrectomy now appears to be a safe, accepted procedure. Other studies have shown that stage-dependent gastrectomies result in a poorer outcome than routine total gastrectomy.

▶ This paper is a retrospective analysis of the efficacy of total gastrectomy in treatment of gastric cancer in more than 1,500 patients operated on during a 19-year period at Hannover. The previous paper from the same clinic apparently selected a few of these patients to study nutritional sequelae. The increased frequency of total gastrectomy during the study period is a manifestation of the acceptance by the authors of total gastrectomy as the treatment of choice for most patients with gastric cancer. Certainly, there is no need to do total gastrectomy in a patient with a pyloric carcinoma when the line of resection in the mid-stomach can be shown by frozen-section biopsy to be free of tumor. There is a well-recognized extensive proximal submucosal migration of tumor cells in patients with distal cancer of the stomach.

Total gastrectomy, in our hands, is actually a simpler and more rapid procedure than is distal 85% gastrectomy. The problem, of course, is that patients must always be cautioned to take vitamin B_{12} to offset loss of parietal cell intrinsic factor. This sounds simple, but several of our patients have gotten into trouble by forgetting to take their B_{12} shots. Everyone in the family must know about it, and the patient must be lectured repeatedly on the necessity of regular B_{12} injections.—J.C. Thompson, M.D.

Quantitative Analysis of Nodal Involvement With Respect to Survival Rate After Curative Gastrectomy for Carcinoma

Okusa T, Nakane Y, Boku T, Takada H, Yamamura M, Hioki K, Yamamoto M
(Kansai Med Univ, Osaka, Japan)

Surg Gynecol Obstet 170:488–494, 1990   20–5

In Japan, the survival rate after curative gastrectomy for carcinoma of the stomach has steadily improved. Previous authors have reported on the relationship between the survival rate and level of lymph node involvement, but few have examined in depth the relationship between lymph node metastases and survival. Whether the survival rate after curative gastrectomy is related to the total number of lymph nodal metastases and/or the frequency of metastases was investigated in 433 patients with carcinoma of the stomach. Regional lymph nodes of the stomach were numbered according to anatomical location, and patients were classified into 3 groups according to the site of the stomach tumor. Investigators also classified the grade of gastric resection according to extent of lymph nodal dissection.

Forty-five percent of 433 patients who underwent curative gastrectomy for carcinoma had lymph nodal metastases. The mean number of lymph nodes dissected per patient was 23.4. Of a total of 10,130 dissected lymph nodes, 13% contained metastases. The number and frequency of metastases increased with the degree of invasion into the gastric wall. Positive nodes were found more frequently in carcinoma of the diffuse type than in carcinoma of the intestinal type. There was also a marked increase in the frequency of positive nodes with more advanced stages of carcinoma and with greater vascular invasion.

The 5-year survival rate for patients with no metastases—group A—was 81%; for those with up to 25% frequency of metastases—group B, it was 66%; for those with up to 50% frequency of metastases—group C, it was 30%; and for those with more than 50% metastases—group D, it was only 23%. Based on the number of lymph node metastases, the 5-year survival rates were 81% for group A, 63% for group B, 47% for group C, and 29% for group D.

The frequency and number of involved nodes increased as carcinoma progressed, and they were closely related to other prognostic factors. There were correlations between the 5-year survival rate and the number and frequency of involved nodes. Both parameters had prognostic significance.

▶ In 1981 the Japanese Research Society for Stomach Cancer published a *vade mecum* for the study and therapy of gastric cancer (1). The article was entitled "The General Rules for Gastric Cancer Study," and these rules have been strictly applied throughout Japan for the past decade. This stringent application has resulted in comparability among centers all over Japan and has led to huge series of patients available for study. The authors here have looked into whether the number and frequency of node metastases influence survival and have found that both do. No surprises here. What is a surprise is that group D patients who had a more than 50% incidence of metastases (and the largest number of lymph node metastases) had a 5-year survival rate of more than 20%. We are told that all of these patients had "curative" gastrectomy, but this high rate of survival in patients with high rates of metastases is vastly different from experience in the United States. No one in America has comparable data, so we should learn from these series.—J.C. Thompson, M.D.

Reference

1. Japanese Research Society for Stomach Cancer: *Japanese J Surg* 16:121, 1981.

CT Diagnosis of Perforated Duodenal Diverticulum

Goodman P, Raval B, Zimmerman G (Univ of Texas, Houston)
Clin Imaging 13:321–322, 1989   20–6

Perforated duodenal diverticulum is a rare but potentially fatal condition that may be difficult to diagnose clinically or with conventional radiography. In 1 instance the diagnosis was made preoperatively by CT.

Woman, 52, had a 2-day history of infraumbilical and left lower quadrant pain, a temperature of 102° F, and leukocytosis. Her white blood cell count was 16,000. She had a history of a single gallstone that caused infrequent pain in the right upper quadrant, but she described this pain as being entirely different. There was no clinical evidence of pancreatitis; abdominal radiography showed nonspecific bowel gas. Computed tomography showed a midabdominal 3-cm cavity containing air, fluid, and some orally administered contrast material. The cavity was adjacent to an opacified loop of proximal small bowel, and it was associated with increased density of adjacent mesenteric fat. The adjacent inferior pancreatic head and proximal right ureter seemed normal. These findings were suggestive of inflammation of a small bowel diverticulum or an abscess secondary to perforation. At surgery the only visible anomaly was induration of the base of the mesentery at the junction of the third and fourth portions of the duodenum, but further exploration revealed an abscess cavity that contained a small amount of turbid fluid. When this cavity was palpated, a tract was revealed that extended from the abscess to a perforated diverticulum in the retroperitoneal aspect adjacent to the fourth portion of the duodenum. The surgeon performed a Kocher maneuver to mobilize the duodenum, but the tract could not be visualized. The diverticular sac was excised and a double-layer primary closure of the duodenal wall was performed. Histologic examination of the excised material revealed inflammation and fibrinopurulent and necrotic debris. The patient recovered uneventfully.

Upper gastrointestinal radiography is superior to CT in demonstrating the actual site of perforation or the course of a tract, but CT permits demonstration of small amounts of retroperitoneal gas and fluid. This information is important to evaluate the extent of abnormality and its relationship to adjacent vital structures. Computed tomography provides early diagnosis of a perforated duodenal diverticulum and permits prompt surgical treatment of this potentially life-threatening condition.

▶ This paper is included for interest—it is the only preoperatively diagnosed case of duodenal diverticulitis that I am aware of. The picture appears classic and demonstrates for the zillionth time the unique value of abdominal CT.— J.C. Thompson, M.D.

Upper GI Bleeding in an Urban Hospital: Etiology, Recurrence, and Prognosis
Sugawa C, Steffes CP, Nakamura R, Sferra JJ, Sferra CS, Sugimura Y, Fromm D (Wayne State Univ, Detroit)
Ann Surg 212:521–527, 1990   20–7

Acute upper gastrointestinal bleeding (UGIB) continues to be a common cause of hospital admission and morbidity and mortality. Data were reviewed on 469 patients admitted to a surgical ward of an urban hospital. The number of admissions totaled 562, because 53 patients had to be readmitted 93 times; this indicates a recurrence rate of 20%.

Bleeding, diagnosed endoscopically in all cases, was most commonly caused by an acute gastric mucosal lesion (135 patients, 24%), esophageal varices (121 patients, 22%), gastric ulcer (108 patients, 19%), duodenal ulcer (78 patients, 14%), Mallory-Weiss tear (61 patients, 11%), and esophagitis (15 patients, 3%). For the majority of patients (504), nonoperative therapy was sufficient. Endoscopic treatment was used in 144 cases. In 58 cases (10.5%), operations were performed; this group included 29% of the ulcers. Emergency operations to control hemorrhage were required in only 2.5% of all cases.

The rate of major surgical complications was 11%; the mortality rate was 5.2%. Of the 58 deaths (12.6%), 36 were attributable directly to UGIB. Factors associated with death included shock at admission (systolic blood pressure of less than 80), transfusion of more than 5 units, and the presence of esophageal varices.

Usually, UGIB can be treated nonoperatively, including endoscopic treatment, when diagnostic endoscopy establishes the source of bleeding. Operations can be done subsequently in selected patients, with low rates of morbidity and mortality resulting.

▶ This article was selected because it reflects current shifts in the etiology of major UGIB, and because the authors support my own deep conviction that early endoscopy is vital in such patients, especially in selecting those who can be managed nonoperatively. Sequestration of that group of patients allows the surgeon to concentrate on those who require operation. As recently as a decade ago, almost all gastrointestinal surgeons would have agreed that a bleeding duodenal ulcer was the major cause of massive UGIB. If you were now to study a group of patients outside the inner city, especially patients in whom alcholism was not rampant, results might differ slightly. In our patients, varices, gastritis, and duodenal ulcer are still the major causes of massive UGIB. Early endoscopy allows the identification of patients with varices who will be treated differently, patients with bleeding gastritis (in whom we try everything in the world before operating), and patients with Mallory-Weiss hemorrhage who almost never need operation.

The operative and overall mortality rates reported here indicate, I believe, the excellent care that this desperately ill group of patients received. If you must operate on somebody with diffuse bleeding gastritis, total gastrectomy may be life-saving; many of these patients cannot tolerate an unsuccessful lesser operation.—J.C. Thompson, M.D.

Enhanced Hyperplasia of Gastric Enterochromaffin-like Cells in Response to Omeprazole-Evoked Hypergastrinemia in Rats With Portacaval Shunts: An Immunocytochemical and Chemical Study
Axelson J, Ekelund M, Sundler F, Håkanson R (Univ of Lund, Sweden)
Gastroenterology 99:635–640, 1990   20–8

Long-term hypergastrinemia leads to proliferation of the histamine-storing enterochromaffin-like cells present in the oxyntic mucosa of the rat stomach. A similar effect is associated with portacaval shunting, which does not increase the serum level of gastrin. The effect of the potent antisecretory agent omeprazole was examined in rats with portacaval shunts. Omeprazole, μmol/kg, was given orally for 8–10 weeks before the animals were killed.

Portacaval shunt surgery reduced serum gastrin levels. Omeprazole increased gastrin levels comparably in these rats and in those that were sham operated. Omeprazole treatment countered the effect of portacaval shunting in reducing oxyntic mucosal weight and thickness. Shunt surgery led to diffuse hyperplasia of enterochromaffin-like cells, and omeprazole had an even more marked effect on these cells. Parallel changes occurred in the histamine concentration and histidine decarboxylase activity.

Portacaval shunting may increase the ability of enterochromaffin-like cells to respond to gastrin. Alternatively, it may increase plasma levels of intestinal agents that no longer are degraded by the liver, 1 of which has a trophic effect on the enterochromaffin-like cells.

▶ The finding that in some rats given long-term omeprazole therapy carcinoid-like tumors of the stomach developed sent a shock wave through the ivory towers in which investigators study control of gut function. To a much greater degree, those waves battered the boardrooms of multinational pharmaceutical corporations. The fight to see who could suppress acid secretion most effectively had been wrested from the manufacturers of H_2-receptor antagonists (with progressively longer half-lives) by the manufacturer of a drug (omeprazole) that interferes with the proton pump in the parietal cell to halt acid production in its tracks. Since then, countless studies have attempted to delineate the true effects of ablation of acid output. The well-established increased incidence of gastric cancer in patients who had previously undergone subtotal gastrectomy for peptic ulcer disease was in the minds of everyone, and if the causal agent for postgastrectomy cancer was diminished acid secretion, were not all patients given agents that greatly diminished acid output potentially at risk? If so, was not the agent that actually halted acid secretion not the most risky?

The current study is one of a number of Håkanson and colleagues in Lund who have attempted to delineate responsible mechanisms and to understand the severity of the threat. They confirm that hypergastrinemia does cause hyperplasia, but that some other factor, presumably something normally extracted by the liver, may also contribute.—J.C. Thompson, M.D.

Long-Term Clinical Results After Proximal Gastric Vagotomy
Soper NJ, Kelly KA, van Heerden JA, Ilstrup DM (Mayo Clinic and Found, Rochester, Minn)
Surg Gynecol Obstet 169:488–494, 1989   20–9

Proximal gastric vagotomy for peptic ulcer has been accepted by many Europeans as the surgical procedure of choice for peptic ulcer. However, this approach is not well accepted in the United States, partly because of concern over reported high recurrence rates and partly because of the greater technical difficulty of the procedure as compared with truncal vagotomy. The incidence of recurrent peptic ulcers and the eventual clinical outcome after proximal gastric vagotomy were documented in a large group of patients with long-term follow-up.

Between 1973 and 1981, 396 patients underwent proximal gastric vagotomy for peptic ulcer. The original site of peptic ulcer was duodenal in 293 patients (74%), midgastric in 14 (4%), pyloric or prepyloric in 46 (12%), and combined gastric, pyloric, prepyloric, and duodenal in 43 (11%). Of the 396 patients, 274 (69%) underwent PGV because of intractability, 68 (17%) for obstruction, 46 (12%) for active or recent bleeding, and 8 (2%) because of perforation. Follow-up was by questionnaire, telephone inquiry, or direct interview. Routine postoperative endoscopy or acid studies were not used. The postoperative follow-up ranged from 5 to 13 years. Complete follow-up data were available for 382 (96%) patients.

None of the patients died in the early postoperative period. Fifty patients (13%) died during follow-up of unrelated diseases. Only 8 patients (2%) required reoperation for nonulceratve complications. Fifty-five patients (14%) had documented recurrent ulcers. An additional 10 patients complained of recurrent ulcer-like pain but refused to undergo further testing. Twenty-four patients had a recurrent ulcer in the duodenum and 6 had a recurrent gastric, pyloric, or prepyloric ulcer. Of the 16 patients who required operation for the recurrences, 4 were treated on an emer-

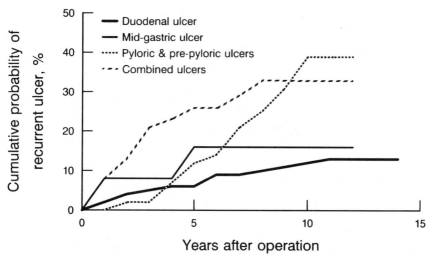

Fig 20–2.—Cumulative expected probabilities of recurrent ulceration (Kaplan-Meier) after proximal gastric vagotomy for peptic ulcer disease. (Courtesy of Soper NJ, Kelly KA, van Heerden JA, et al: *Surg Gynecol Obstet* 169:488–494, 1989.)

gency basis. Kaplan-Meier estimates of the probabilities of peptic ulcer recurrence after proximal gastric vagotomy were 6% at 5 years and 12% at 10 years for duodenal ulcer, 16% at 5 years and 16% at 10 years for gastric ulcer, 12% at 5 years and 39% at 10 years for pyloric or prepyloric ulcer, and 26% at 5 years and 33% at 10 years for combined ulcers (Fig 20–2).

Proximal gastric vagotomy has an acceptable long-term recurrence rate when used to treat duodenal, and perhaps midgastric, ulcers. Alternative operations should be performed for pyloric or prepyloric ulcers and for combined ulcers.

▶ This is another in a series of papers that have concluded that selective proximal vagotomy (or proximal gastric vagotomy) is a good (perhaps the best) operation for patients with duodenal ulcer disease, even though the recurrence rate is high. The authors' findings that prepyloric ulcers have a higher recurrence rate corroborates the experience of Amdrups' group (1), who found a significantly higher 5-year recurrence rate with prepyloric ulcer (16.5%) than with duodenal ulcer (9.2%). Adami et al. (2) agreed, and I think that we can now say with conviction that selective proximal vagotomy is not a good operation for pyloric or prepyloric ulcers. The question of whether it is a good procedure for mid-gastric ulcer, as suggested by Jordan [3] and others, is still not clear to me. Clinical results after subtotal gastrectomy and Billroth's I anastomosis for gastric ulcer have not been equaled, and I believe it to be the procedure of choice.

I would agree with these authors and with Paul Jordan (4) that selective proximal vagotomy is the operation of choice for duodenal ulcer disease. Jordan has even extended indications for selective proximal vagotomy to patients who are bleeding and patients who have perforation. Nearly everyone now agrees, I believe, that selective proximal vagotomy is not a good operation for patients with duodenal ulcer disease who are operated on because of gastric outlet obstruction.—J.C. Thompson, M.D.

References

1. Anderson D, et al: *World J Surg* 6:86, 1982.
2. Adami, H-O, et al: *Ann Surg* 199:393, 1984.
3. Jordan PH: *Arch Surg* 116:1320, 1981.
4. Jordan PH: *Ann Surg* 205:572, 1987.

Effects of Aging on Duodenal Bicarbonate Secretion
Kim SW, Parekh D, Townsend CM Jr, Thompson JC (Univ of Texas, Galveston)
Ann Surg 212:332–338, 1990   20–10

Bicarbonate secretion by the gut mucosa maintains the pH within the mucus gel at neutrality, even when the intraduodenal pH is very low. Because aging can affect secretory function in the gastrointestinal tract, basal and acid-stimulated bicarbonate secretion by the proximal duodenal mucosa was measured in rats of differing age.

Basal bicarbonate secretion was comparable in the various groups of rats, but secretion in response to luminal acid was reduced in animals aged 1 year and 2 years compared with those aged 3 months (Fig 20–3). Infusion of vasoactive intestinal polypeptide and intraluminal administration of prostaglandin E_2 induced bicarbonate secretion in a dose-dependent manner in all age groups.

This study demonstrated an age-related reduction in acid-stimulated duodenal bicarbonate secretion in the rat. The increased occurrence of duodenal ulcer with advancing age may be the result in part of a progres-

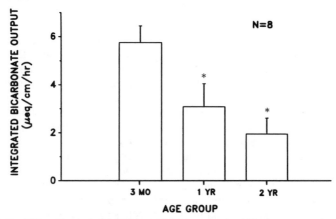

Fig 20–3.—Effect of luminal acid (100 mmol/L HCl) on duodenal bicarbonate secretion in rats of 3 age groups. Results in this figure are 1-hour integrated values and expressed as mean ± SEM. * = $P <$ .05 vs. 3-month-old rats. (Courtesy of Kim SW, Parekh D, Townsend CM Jr, et al: *Ann Surg* 212:332–338, 1990.)

sive breakdown of mucosal defense against acid in the proximal duodenum.

▶ The problem is that incidence of duodenal ulcer in man seems to increase linearly with age, although gastric acid secretion appears to decline with aging. After Isenberg et al. (1) showed impairment of secretion of duodenal mucosal bicarbonate in duodenal ulcer patients, the authors studied duodenal bicarbonate production and found that it decreases dramatically with age. This does not necessarily prove anything, but it does provide a possible explanation for the surprisingly increased incidence of duodenal ulcer in old people.—J.C. Thompson, M.D.

Reference

1. Isenberg JI, et al: *N Engl J Med* 316:374, 1987.

Time Trends in Peptic Ulcer Surgery, 1956 to 1986: A Nation-Wide Survey in Sweden
Gustavsson S, Nyrén O (Univ Hosp, Uppsala, Sweden)
Ann Surg 210:704–709, 1989   20–11

The epidemiology of peptic ulcer disease has changed considerably during the past century. Although duodenal ulcer was rarely encountered in the 1800s, it became several times more common than gastric ulcer between 1900 and 1950. In recent decades, however, mortality statistics and hospital admission rates have shown a decline in peptic ulcer. Trends in peptic ulcer surgery throughout Sweden for the past 30 years were examined.

All surgical departments were asked to provide information on the number and sex distribution of patients with elective and emergency operations for gastric and duodenal ulcers performed in 1956, 1966, 1976, and 1986. The number of reoperations and the exact catchment areas of the hospitals were also requested. Complete information was obtained from 39 of 81 responding hospitals.

In a population of 7 million people, a total of 860 elective operations for peptic ulcer were performed in 1986, for a rate of elective operations of 12.2/100,000 inhabitants. The rate of operations performed for perforation was 6.4/100,000 inhabitants in 1986. During the 4 selected study years the rate of elective procedures declined steadily, from 72.1 to 10.7/100,000 persons. The decline was equally pronounced for both ulcer sites, but male predominance became less marked. In 1956, 80% of elective operations were performed in men, whereas in 1986, operations in men were only 50% more common than in women. During the 30-year period the number of operations for perforation decreased by 50%.

In the past 30 years, elective ulcer surgery rate fell by 85% in Sweden. The reasons for this decline are not clear, because the trend started long before the advent of fiberoptic endoscopy, highly selective vagotomy, or

H_2-receptor antagonists. A similar trend has been reported in the United States.

▶ The vast epidemiologic decrease in peptic ulcer is fascinating; I addressed the problem in an editorial (1) nearly a decade ago. Since then, the decreased incidence has continued. This study from Uppsala, for example, reports a sevenfold diminution in the number of elective operative procedures for peptic ulcer in the 30-year period ending in 1986. In common with other reports, the authors noted a great decline in the male/female ratio (4.5 to 1.5:1); this study differs from previous ones in that surgery for gastric ulcer diminished just as much as for duodenal ulcer.

There does not seem to be agreement among the many studies I have reviewed as to the diminution in operations for bleeding and perforation. Anyone can see that the total rate of ulcer surgery has decreased (indeed, hospitalizations for all peptic ulcer disease have fallen dramatically in the past 3 decades). It is fascinating to note that these changes occurred long before introduction of H_2-receptor antagonist therapy.

Because the disease is greatly diminishing in frequency, how is it that the dollar value of sales of drugs to treat ulcer disease leads all others? And continues to climb? We continue to see complicated manifestations of long-standing ulcer disease, both primary and recurrent, but the trend is clear.—J.C. Thompson, M.D.

Reference

1. Thompson JC: *N Engl J Med* 307:550, 1982.

Laparoscopic Treatment of Perforated Peptic Ulcer
Mouret P, François Y, Vignal J, Barth X, Lombard-Platet R (Hôp Claude Bernard; Hôp Edouard Herriot, Lyon, France)
Br J Surg 77:1006, 1990   20–12

The results of laparoscopic treatment in 5 patients with perforated peptic ulcer were reviewed. Two patients had a history of ulcer disease. In all 5, pneumoperitoneum was observed. The interval from perforation to laparoscopy was 10–24 hours.

General anesthesia was used. The entire peritoneal cavity was cleaned using a cannula placed through a second incision. Four perforations were identified at laparoscopy. Fibrin sealant and an omental patch were used to seal 3 perforations. A large antral perforation was converted to a gastrostomy. Abdominal drainage was instituted in 3 patients, and all patients had a nasogastric tube in place. Antibiotics were given intravenously along with ranitidine or cimetidine, and the patients were given parenteral nutrition.

The postoperative was uneventful in 4 patients. Repeated endoscopy in 3 patients showed a sealed ulcer. Septic shock developed in the patient who underwent conversion to a gastrostomy; this patient was also being treated for laryngeal cancer and died later of progressive disease. Laparoscopic treatment of perforated ulcer avoids wound complications and may allow more thorough cleaning of the entire peritoneal cavity. Definitive surgery, if necessary, may be easier if there are no adhesions.

▶ Just because something can be done, there is no reason to conclude that it should be done. As a result of the explosive popularity of laparoscopic cholecystectomy, I am sure we will see attempts to perform nearly every intra-abdominal procedure by laparoscopy (or, as our circulating nurse calls them, operations by remote control). The method might well be successful in relatively simple ulcer perforations in patients who do not require or are not candidates for acid-reducing operations. The technique may ultimately have application when ulcers perforate acutely in patients without an antecedent history. It is certainly possible for surgeons to develop great skill at doing these procedures as it were, by remote control, but the great variety of pathology caused by perforated ulcer, and the high incidence of unexpected operative findings, cause me to opt strongly for open operative closure at present.—J.C. Thompson, M.D.

Gastrocolic Fistula as a Complication of Benign Gastric Ulcer: Report of Four Cases and Update of the Literature
Soybel DI, Kestenberg A, Brunt EM, Becker JM (Washington Univ; Univ of Utah)
Br J Surg 76:1298–1300, 1989   20–13

Four patients were seen with gastrocolic fistulas complicating benign gastric ulcers. This brings to 108 the total number of cases reported in the English language literature. In a review of 30 cases described in the past decade, the data indicated an unusually high percentage of young female patients (younger than 50 years). Overall, 75% of the patients took steroids or nonsteroidal anti-inflammatory agents.

Gastrocolic fistulas should be suspected in patients complaining of weight loss, diarrhea, and fecal vomiting. Small fistulas may not be suspected when other complications of ulcer disease (e.g., bleeding or a perforated viscus) also are present. In some instances, medical management may suffice. Surgery involves en bloc resection, including the fistula, and surrounding colon and gastric segments.

▶ This report was chosen to remind us that gastrocolic fistulas do not necessarily indicate malignancy of the stomach or colon. We have seen them with benign gastric ulcer as reported here and with colonic diverticulitis. Clues to their presence are weight loss, diarrhea, foul eructations, and feculent gastric aspirates. If a fistula is suspected, the best diagnostic study is barium enema. The next best study is another barium enema. Upper or lower endoscopy with biopsy should settle the question of malignancy. The diarrhea results from the profound enteritis caused by coliform organisms in the proximal gut. Diarrhea can be halted by bowel sterilization. If the patient is in desperate condition, a transverse colostomy proximal to the fistula will allow diarrhea to subside. Because we can now sterilize the bowel with moderate effectiveness, colostomy is rarely required.

One last question is why do all these young women have gastrocolic fistulas? The Australian experience with gastric ulcer in young women eventually traced all of the episodes to major intakes of aspirin or related compounds.— J.C. Thompson, M.D.

Long-Term Follow-Up of 2529 Patients Reveals Gastric Ulcers Rarely Become Malignant

Lee S, Iida M, Yao T, Shindo S, Okabe H, Fujishima M (Kyushu Univ, Fukuoka; Karatsu Gastric Inst; Kitasato Univ, Kanagawa, Japan)
Dig Dis Sci 35:763–768, 1990   20–14

There is controversy over the relationship between gastric ulcer and gastric cancer. Previous epidemiologic studies have estimated the rate of malignant transformation in gastric ulcer at .5% to 12.3%, but only patients with an open ulcer in the acute phase were considered. The relationship between peptic ulcer and gastric cancer was assessed by verifying the original ulcer and subsequent cancer sites, reevaluating the diagnostic accuracy of the initial data, and comparing the mortality from gastric cancer in patients with ulcer with the expected mortality from gastric cancer in the population without ulcers.

Between 1963 and 1975, 2,529 patients aged 11–87 years (average age, 47 years) had diagnoses of gastric or duodenal ulcer, or both. Of the patients, 1,482 had gastric ulcer, 715 had duodenal ulcer, and 330 had both gastric and duodenal ulcers. Two patients had a stomal ulcer. Between 1985 and 1986, follow-up data were obtained by interview. The follow-up period ranged from 9 to 23 years. The clinical and pathologic data from patients in whom gastric cancer developed during the follow-up were reviewed retrospectively. Death certificates were obtained for all patients who died during the follow-up period.

Of the 2,529 patients, 486 (19.2%) died and the outcome was unknown for 18 (.7%). There were 38 patients in whom gastric cancer developed or who died of gastric cancer. In 9 patients, gastric cancer was detected at the same site as the initially diagnosed gastric ulcer, and in 22 patients it was detected at a different site. (The site of gastric cancer was not given on the death certificate of the remaining 7 patients.) Gastric cancer was suspected or could not be completely ruled out in 7 of the 9 patients in whom gastric cancer was detected at the same site. A diagnosis of benign ulcer was made in the remaining 2 patients. However, the possibility that the initially diagnosed gastric ulcer represented a phase of the malignant cycle could not be excluded.

Statistical analysis revealed that the number of deaths from gastric cancer in patients with gastric ulcer was significantly low compared with that expected and computed for the age- and sex-matched general population. These findings indicate that malignant transformation of a benign gastric ulcer is rare.

▶ First of all, the title is misleading. Overall, 715 patients had duodenal ulcers and 2 had stomal ulcers. The second caveat is that this is a retrospective study carried out by chart review and questionnaire. A third footnote should be directed to the concept of ulcer scar as compared to open ulcer. It might be possible in a prospective study to be sure that everything called a scar was at one time an ulcer, but looking through more than 1,400 old charts of patients with gastric ulcer and concluding that whenever a scar is mentioned it is the same as an open gastric ulcer, leaves me skeptical. Nonetheless, the point the authors make—namely, that many patients have benign gastric ulcers and few of these become malignant—seems valid.

This is an interesting paper, but it suffers from all of the problems of a late chart review.—J.C. Thompson, M.D.

Recurrence in Early Gastric Cancer
Ichiyoshi Y, Toda T, Minamisono Y, Nagasaki S, Yakeishi Y, Sugimachi K (Inst of Gastroenterology of Hofu, Yamaguchi; Kyushu Univ, Fukuoka, Japan)
Surgery 107:489–495, 1990   20–15

Early gastric cancer is potentially curable surgically, but there may be recurrence after curative resection. The records of 503 patients who had curative resection for early gastric cancer over a 24-year period were reviewed to determine the incidence and patterns of recurrence, characteristic findings related to clinicopathologic features or surgical procedures, and the possibility of improving the prognosis.

In the period reviewed, 97 patients died. Seventeen died of recurrence of gastric cancer, 72 of unrelated causes, and 8 of unknown causes. Cumulative recurrence mortality rates were 2.2% at 9 years for mucosal cancer and 8.4% at 8 years for submucosal cancer. There were no deaths as a result of recurrence after 9 years (Fig 20–4). Submucosal cancer had a significantly higher recurrence rate. Recurrence of hematogenic metastasis in liver, lung, or bone occurred in 9 cases, recurrence in the residual stomach in 5, and recurrence in lymph nodes in 3. Of 12 patients with recurrence of hematogenic or lymph node metastasis, 83% died within 5 years after surgery. All 5 patients with recurrence in the residual stomach survived for more than 5 years.

Submucosal cancers with a macroscopically elevated appearance, lymph node metastasis, and evidence of vessel invasion were at high risk for hematogenic recurrence. These patients require adjuvant chemotherapy. Metastasis to group 2 lymph nodes was found in 1.5% of cases, but because macroscopic diagnosis of nodal status was often inaccurate, complete dissection should be performed whether or not metastasis is identified. The 5 recurrences in the residual stomach were thought to be overlooked lesions of multiple carcinoma. These were detected at an ad-

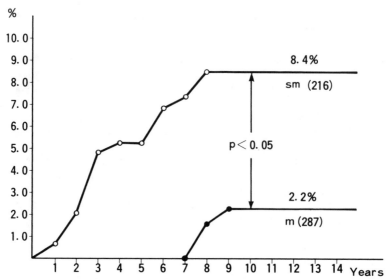

Fig 20–4.—Cumulative recurrence mortality rate in early gastric cancer. *Figures in parentheses,* number of cases; *sm*, submucosal cancer; *m*, mucosal cancer. (Courtesy of Ichiyoshi Y, Toda T, Minamisono Y, et al: *Surgery* 107:489–495, 1990.)

vanced stage. Meticulous and regular postoperative follow-up should detect these recurrences at an early stage.

▶ This is another retrospective chart review from Kyushu University—the record room there must be a beehive. One problem is that "early" is not defined in the term "early gastric cancer." Presumably, it refers to tumors limited to the mucosa and submucosa. Anyhow, a cumulative 3% mortality rate from *recurrent* gastric cancer is a great testimony to the vigilance of postoperative endoscopic survey. As shown in Figure 20–4, if you made it to 9 years in this postoperative study, you appear to have achieved immortality (or at least freedom from death caused by recurrent cancer).—J.C. Thompson, M.D.

21 The Small Intestine

Duodenojejunostomy as an Alternative to Anastomosis of the Small Intestine at the Ligament of Treitz
Nauta RJ (Georgetown Univ Hosp)
Surg Gynecol Obstet 170:172–174, 1990   21–1

Anastomosis is technically difficult near the first jejunal branches during repairs to the duodenum or resection of the small intestine near the origin of the superior mesenteric vessels. Although duodenojejunostomy is not often used for reconstruction of the upper part of the gastrointestinal tract, the procedure can restore continuity without the technical problems of an end-to-end duodenojejunostomy or the complications of gastrojejunostomy (Fig 21–1).

Man, 75, had a preoperative diagnosis of sentinel bleeding from an aortoduodenal fistula, which was confirmed at operation. Because of a large hole in the duodenum, primary repair might have resulted in critical narrowing of the duodenum. Using the GIA stapling device, the fourth portion of the duodenum was

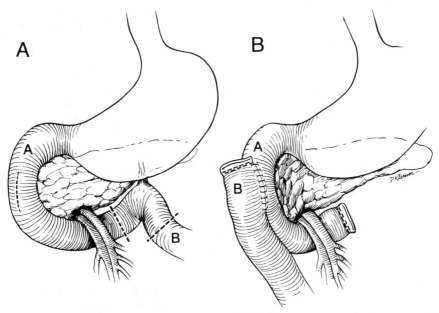

Fig 21–1.—Technique for reconstruction. Longitudinal duodenostomy, **A,** is made after resection of distal portion of duodenal or proximal portion of jejunal section. Proximal end of jejunum, **B,** is mobilized through a transverse mesocolonic rent, and side-to-side duodenjejunostomy is performed. (Courtesy of Nauta RJ: *Surg Gynecol Obstet* 170:172–174, 1990.)

resected. A retrocolic side-to-side duodenojejunostomy was created between the mobilized small intestine and the duodenum after a Kocher maneuver, reestablishing the integrity of the gastrointestinal tract.

When resection of the small intestine is necessary at the ligament of Treitz or in close proximity to the origin of the mesenteric vasculature, this technique offers a convenient means of reconstructing the upper portion of the gastrointestinal tract. This alternative method obviates the need to visualize or mobilize the transected duodenal stump to construct an anastomosis.

▶ Any time you have to resect a segment of proximal jejunum (because of trauma, because of involvement in adjacent pathology, e.g., colon cancer or colon diverticulitis, or in revision of previous Roux-en-Y procedures) repair by jejunojejunostomy immediately adjacent to the ligament of Treitz is always difficult. The proximal jejunum is tethered by short direct vessels, and attempts to mobilize it are hazardous. This is an excellent solution to the problem and, like most excellent solutions, is simple, easy, and safe. I wish I had thought of it.— J.C. Thompson, M.D.

Long-Term Outcome of Reversal of Small Intestinal Bypass Operations
Dean P, Joshi S, Kaminski DL (St Louis Univ)
Am J Surg 159:118–124, 1990   21–2

It is estimated that approximately 25,000 persons in the United States underwent jejunoileal bypass operations for morbid obesity between 1969 when the procedure was first described and 1980 when a moratorium was declared on its performance. Data were reviewed on experience with reversal operations performed in patients who had complex metabolic complications associated with the jejunoileal bypass procedure.

Between 1971 and 1978, approximately 800 patients underwent jejunoileal bypass operations at the present institution. Between 1979 and 1987, 43 patients underwent reversal operations of those procedures because of metabolic complications. Primary indications for reconstruction included electrolyte imbalance, malnutrition, and diarrhea in 16 patients, as well as cirrhosis in 9, nephrolithiasis in 9, arthritis in 7, and pathologic bone fractures in 1. Many patients had multiple metabolic complications. Twenty-nine patients had simultaneous gastroplasty and 14 did not. Hospitalization required for reconstruction ranged from 6 to 32 days and averaged 8.2 days. All patients were followed continuously for at least 18 months after reconstruction.

Two of the 9 patients with cirrhosis died of liver failure after reconstruction; both had preoperative ascites. Postoperative needle aspiration liver biopsies performed between 18 and 37 months after reconstruction in the 7 surviving patients with cirrhosis but without ascites indicated improvement in histologic appearance in 4 and no change in 3. Symptoms in all 16 patients operated on for electrolyte imbalance, malnutrition, and diarrhea improved after reconstruction. Five of the 7 patients with arthritis and all 9 with nephrolithiasis were improved after reconstruction.

Gastroplasty performed simultaneously with reconstruction produced no benefit in alleviation of metabolic complications but significantly decreased body weight when compared with results in patients who had reconstruction without gastroplasty. Although the survival rate at last follow-up was 95%, 12 patients (mean age, 47 years) were physically disabled to some degree because of their obesity and obesity operations.

Asymptomatic patients who do not require any medications to treat complications of jejunoileal bypass operation and who have no histologic evidence of hepatic fibrosis should be observed for late serious metabolic consequences. Prophylactic reversal is not recommended.

▶ What is remarkable is that only about 5% of jejunoileal bypass patients underwent reconstruction. Of course, some may have gone elsewhere and some may have died quietly at home. Nonetheless, as we and many other institutions have noted, only a fraction of patients have required reestablishment of full gut continuity. One major factor is the patients' fear that a rehook-up will lead to resumption of morbid obesity. There is, of course, as in nearly every other "disease," a full spectrum of reactions; if you expose a room full of people to a standard dose of influenza virus, only a portion of them will contract the disease. In jejunoileal bypass, the spectrum is totally diverse. Of the small number of patients we have treated, 3 have thrived for more than 2 decades and have ascribed their successful life to the operation. About 4 times as many have required reanastomosis, however, and the remaining 50% have varying degrees of disability. I fully agree that reversal of the operation should be undertaken only for cause.—J.C. Thompson, M.D.

Incidence and Frequency of Complications and Management of Meckel's Diverticulum
Lüdtke F-E, Mende V, Köhler H, Lepsien G (Univ of Göttingen, Germany)
Surg Gynecol Obstet 169:537–542, 1989   21–3

Data on 84 patients with Meckel's diverticula treated at 1 institution in a 27-year period were reviewed retrospectively. In the 50 patients in group 1, the diverticulum was an incidental result of a laparotomy indicated for other reasons. The 34 patients in group 2 underwent surgery because of complications of Meckel's diverticula. The diverticula occurred mainly in children and young adults and most frequently in males; 75% of patients were younger than 25 years. Patients with complications were younger (mean age, 10 years) than patients with bland diverticula (mean age, 23 years). Children younger than 2 years were most endangered from complications.

Obstruction and diverticulitis were the most frequent complications of the diverticula (Fig 21–2); 15 patients had an obstruction. Diverticulitis was found in 15 patients, indicating the important role that inflammatory changes play in the appearance of complications. Peptic ulcers were

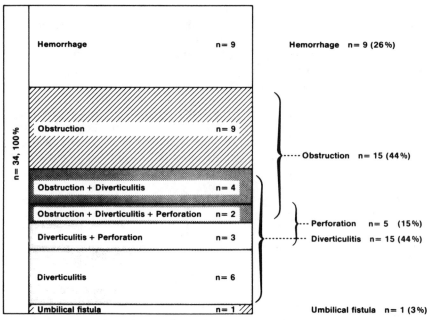

Fig 21–2.—Observed complication of Meckel's diverticulum; diverticulitis, obstruction, and perforation were often found simultaneously. (Courtesy of Lüdtke F-E, Mende V, Köhler H, et al: *Surg Gynecol Obstet* 169:537–542, 1989.)

found in 7 patients and transrectal hemorrhages caused by Meckel's diverticula were found in 9. All 5 instances of perforation were combined with diverticulitis.

Meckel's diverticulum is seldom diagnosed preoperatively. Diagnostic procedures were useful only in patients with hemorrhage. Prophylactic resection is indicated when Meckel's diverticula are discovered. The base of the diverticulum should be checked carefully for heterotopic tissue, especially in patients with hemorrhage.

▶ The general consensus in America for the past decade or so has been that Meckel's diverticula found incidentally at operation should be left alone. Now comes this group from Göttingen saying that they should be removed. The problem is, we never know the true risk of complications in a rare condition; we know how many patients have pathologic Meckel's diverticula, but we do not know the denominator, or how many people during a similar time span in the same locale went through life with innocent Meckel's diverticula. Because complications of Meckel's diverticula are so rare, it seems difficult to me to justify their incidental removal. Although the authors state that they have removed 3.1 diverticula yearly for the past 27 years (a total of 84), only 34 patients had complications; therefore, an average of slightly more than 1 pathologic diverticulum was removed per year. This seems to me unlikely to justify an argument for removal of all normal Meckel's diverticula.—J.C. Thompson, M.D.

Childhood Intussusception

Skipper RP, Boeckman CR, Klein RL (Children's Hosp Med Ctr, Akron, Ohio)
Surg Gynecol Obstet 171:151–153, 1990   21–4

Intussusception remains the most frequent cause of intestinal obstruction and acute abdomen in children. Data on 157 patients in whom a diagnosis of intussusception was confirmed in 1977–1988 were reviewed. Of the children, 107 (68%) were boys and 145 (92%) were 3 years and younger.

Symptoms were present for longer than 72 hours in only 19% of the group. Emesis, pain, and hematochezia were the most common presenting features. Only 28% of patients had diarrhea, and 16% had an abdominal mass. Barium enema reduction succeeded in 66% of attempts. Laparotomy was necessary in 64 children, and 30 required bowel resection. Barium enema reduction most often succeeded when attempted within 24 hours of the onset of symptoms. A total of 21 children had 27 episodes of intussusception, 2 after laparotomy. There were 2 deaths; 1 of sepsis before treatment and 1 nonabdominal illness.

Attempted reduction by barium enema is the logical initial approach to intussusception of the bowel in childhood. Laparotomy is reserved for patients in whom this fails and those who are extremely ill. Recurrences also are treated with barium enema reduction.

▶ Surgeons will be paying off their debts to Mark Ravitch well into the next century. Time and again when studying successful approaches to difficult problems, we find that the answer was provided by Dr. Ravitch. Hydrostatic reduction of childhood intussusception is used all over the world. Reports from China document the successful use of water enemas in thousands of cases. If all of the safety criteria established by Dr. Ravitch are stringently adhered to, barium enema reduction is safe and efficient and should work in two thirds to three quarters of all patients. As the authors here note, the chief limiting factor is duration of symptoms. The longer the child has the intussusception, the less likely that hydrostatic reduction will be successful. If it is not successful, the surgeon should resort swiftly to operation.—J.C. Thompson, M.D.

Clinical Relapse of Crohn's Disease Under Standardized Conservative Treatment and After Excisional Surgery

Dirks E, Goebell H, Schaarschmidt K, Förster S, Quebe-Fehling E, Eigler FW (Univ of Essen, Germany)
Dig Dis Sci 34:1832–1840, 1989   21–5

Strict criteria governed the definition of clinical relapse and the indications for resection in 205 patients with Crohn's disease. Parameters examined included symptoms, clinical and laboratory findings, Crohn's disease activity index, and the clinical relapse rate in relation to localization of the disease.

The 131 women and 74 men had a mean age of 29.7 years; the mean total duration of disease 96 months. Disease was localized to the small bowel in 25% and to the large bowel in 25% of patients; 50% had ileocolitis. Excisional surgery was performed in 93 patients. The indications for surgery were a life-threatening situation, absolute nonresponse to drug treatment, and severe intervisceral fistulas. A standardized drug regimen consisted of salazosulfapyridine and prednisone.

The mean follow-up was 43 months. The relapse rate was lower (20%) in surgical patients than in patients treated conservatively (51%) (Fig 21–3). Differences between the 2 regimens were significant in patients with colitis (18% vs. 67%) and those with ileocolitis (20% vs. 49%), but no differences were observed between the treatment groups in ileitis (25% to 30% relapses in both after 4 years). Symptoms, clinical and laboratory findings, and Crohn's disease activity index were also more favorable in patients undergoing resection. Further research is needed to determine the value of earlier surgery in patients with less severe disease.

▶ The message to take home from this paper is this: Recognizing that there is no cure for Crohn's disease, patients who are operated on for colitis or for ileocolitis seem to fare much better, over a short period at least, than do patients who are not operated on. The authors, gastroenterologists and surgeons, suggest that a trial of earlier operation might be warranted. If this is attempted, the

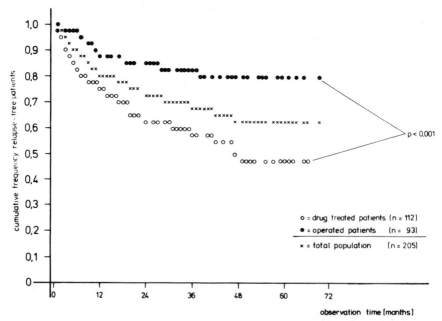

Fig 21–3.—Cumulative frequency of relapse-free patients for the total 205 patients *(Xs),* for 112 drug-treated patients *(open circles),* and 93 operated-on patients *(filled circles);* the latter differ significantly (*P* < .001). (Courtesy of Dirks E, Goebell H, Schaarschmidt K, et al: *Dig Dis Sci* 34:1832–1840, 1989.)

surgeons in this trial should closely adhere to conservatism and take out only that segment of bowel causing the symptoms. They should not launch a jihad against all areas of bowel involved with Crohn's disease.

An important goal in medical therapy is to attempt to keep the dose of prednisone as low as possible. The cumulative ill effects of even moderately high doses of prednisone over long periods are often devastating.—J.C. Thompson, M.D.

Non-Hodgkin's Lymphomas of the Gastrointestinal Tract: An Evaluation of Paraffin Section Immunostaining
Wolf BC, Martin AW, Ree HJ, Banks PM, Smith S, Neiman RS (Boston Univ; Mt Sinai School of Medicine, New York; Mayo Clinic and Found, Rochester, Minn)
Am J Clin Pathol 93:233–239, 1990   21–6

The gastrointestinal tract is the most common site of primary extranodal lymphoma. Immunophenotyping of these tumors often is difficult because of the presence of admixed reactive and inflammatory cells. Paraffin-reactive antibodies detecting markers of B, T, histiocytic, and epithelial cells were used to analyze 34 non-Hodgkin's lymphomas of the gastrointestinal tract. For each patient, definite frozen-section immunophenotyping was available as a control.

Although a wide range of histologic subtypes was represented, most lymphomas were of the large cell type, particularly diffuse large cell and large cell immunoblastic lesions. Frozen-section studies yielded 31 tumors of B cell origin and 3 of T cell origin. Paraffin-reactive antibody studies confirmed a B cell lineage in 28 of 31 patients. Only 1 T cell lesion was identified in paraffin studies.

Immunohistologic staining for lymphoid and monocyte-histiocyte markers in paraffin-embedded tissues allows study of a large number of patients from various archival sources. Good cytologic detail is achieved. The lack of lineage-specific antibodies against T cell and monocyte-histiocyte antigens is a disadvantage. In addition, reliable studies require optimal fixation and processing of the tissues.

▶ First of all, why does anyone care whether a non-Hodgkin's lymphoma is primarily of B cell, T cell, histiocytic, or epithelial cell origin? The main reason is that they have different prognoses, and they are treated by different chemotherapeutic regimens. In the past, immunostaining of frozen sections was necessary because the process of fixation leeched out all of the antigens that could be studied. Newer antibodies can react with some of the antigens that remain post fixation. The present authors tell us that process works well if the tumor is of B cell origin but is not particularly good with T cell antigens. Even when immunostaining works in paraffin sections, the effectiveness depends on optimal fixation and processing of tissue. Immunostaining of frozen sections remains the gold standard.—J.C. Thompson, M.D.

Lethal Short-Bowel Syndrome

Hancock BJ, Wiseman NE (Univ of Manitoba, Winnipeg)
J Pediatr Surg 25:1131–1134, 1990
21–7

Improved nutritional methods have enhanced the formerly dismal outlook for infants with extreme short-bowel syndrome, but many still die of either the short bowel itself or complications of aggressive management. Data on 7 infants who died of short-bowel syndrome were reviewed.

Causes included volvulus in 3 infants, and multiple atresias and total intestinal aganglionosis in 2 each. Survival times ranged from 2 weeks to 8 months. All infants had 1–3 operations and received total parenteral nutrition. Of the 7 infants, 4 had no functional small bowel beyond the ligament of Treitz. Liver failure secondary to parenteral nutrition was the cause of death in 1 infant; the others died after withdrawal of treatment, most of them remaining hospitalized until death. Enteral feeding was attempted in 2 infants but was not tolerated.

In these infants, laparotomy is appropriate to make a diagnosis. Infants with volvulus may undergo second-look laparotomy to reassess the state of the bowel; otherwise, aggressive management is not indicated for infants with such extensive bowel loss. Excessive morbidity and unnecessary surgery should be avoided when death is inevitable.

▶ Every time a surgeon operates on a newborn baby with bile vomiting and finds midgut volvulus, or multiple atretic segments, he or she is faced with the problem of what to do—whether to excise the involved bowel and hope for ultimate nutritional rehabilitation, or simply close the abdomen and take the bad news to the parents that the child will not live. These authors from Winnipeg suggest that infants with less than 6 cm of viable jejunoileum will inevitably die. They conclude that a decision to withhold further treatment in such children would be reasonable at the time the diagnosis is established. The only hope is development of small bowel transplantation (see Abstract 21–8).—J.C. Thompson, M.D.

Successful Segmental Intestinal Transplantation in Enterectomized Pigs

Kimura K, LaRosa CA, Blank MA, Jaffe BM (State Univ of New York, Brooklyn)
Ann Surg 211:158–164, 1990
21–8

Both rejection and graft-vs.-host disease are potential barriers to successful small bowel allotransplantation. A study was conducted to determine whether segmental intestinal allografts can, in conjunction with low-dose cyclosporine, maintain outbred pigs with surgically created short bowel syndrome. Control animals had the entire small bowel removed; recipient animals had 3–4 m of jejunum transplanted orthotopically.

Control animals died of malabsorption after a mean of about 2 months. Animals given jejunal allografts but not cyclosporine died of rejection within 9 days on average, but allograft recipients who received cyclosporine, 10 mg/kg, daily starting on the day of surgery, survived for a mean of 81 days and gained body weight. Of 11 animals, 3 lived longer than 6 months before being killed. The transplanted bowel retained its mucosal integrity and lacked significant lymphocytic infiltration. Short-segment jejunal allografts, combined with cyclosporine immunosuppression, significantly improve the outlook for pigs with surgical short bowel syndrome.

▶ The bottom line, it should be noted, is that no one has successfully achieved small bowel allografting. The problem, apparently, is that the bowel is an immunologic bomb stuffed with highly reactive cells designed to protect the organism from foreign invaders, and when these cells are put into another organism, they excite a vast reaction. When the host does not reject them, the immune cells in the graft may take on the host itself, i.e., they may incite a graft-vs.-host reaction.

Jaffe and colleagues at SUNY Downstate have been grappling with this problem for years, and this is a report of small initial progress. They got a segment of bowel to live for a mean of 81 days. They killed the remaining 3 of the 11 pigs at 6 months; you can surmise that the pigs were not doing too well. This is a step.—J.C. Thompson, M.D.

22 The Colon and the Rectum

The Epidemiology of Appendicitis and Appendectomy in the United States
Addiss DG, Shaffer N, Fowler BS, Tauxe RV (Centers for Disease Control, Atlanta)
Am J Epidemiol 132:910–925, 1990   22–1

There have been few population-based epidemiologic studies of appendicitis despite the fact that appendectomy for acute appendicitis is one of the most frequently performed procedures in the United States. Data from the National Hospital Discharge Survey for the years 1979 to 1984 were analyzed.

During the study period, approximately 561,000 appendectomies were performed annually, of which 53% were primary. Appendectomy accounted for an estimated 1 million hospital days per year. The discharge diagnosis was acute appendicitis in 85% of these cases. The crude incidence of acute appendectomy was 11/10,000 population, and that of incidental appendectomy, 12/10,000 population. The highest incidence of appendicitis occurred in persons aged 10–19 years; this age group had an incidence of 23.3/10,000 population.

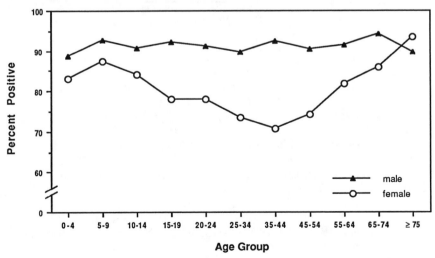

Fig 22–1.—Diagnostic accuracy of primary appendectomies performed in the United States, by age group and sex, from 1979 to 1984. Diagnostic accuracy was defined as the proportion of all primary appendectomies with a discharge diagnosis of appendicitis. (Courtesy of Addiss DG, Shaffer N, Fowler BS, et al: *Am J Epidemiol* 132:910–925, 1990.)

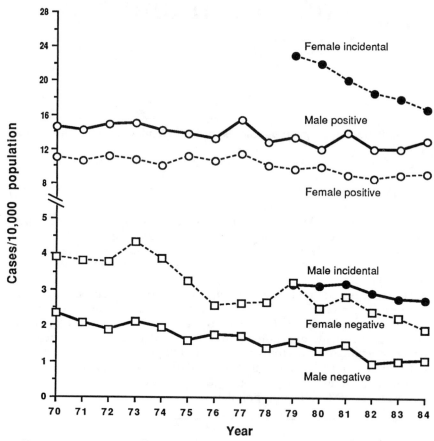

Fig 22–2.—Appendicitis and appendectomy trends (per 10,000 population) in the United States from 1970 to 1984, by year, sex, and type of appendectomy (primary positive, primary negative, and incidental.) (Courtesy of Addiss DG, Shaffer N, Fowler BS, et al: *Am J Epidemiol* 132:910–925, 1990.)

In all age groups, males had higher rates of appendicitis than females. Appendicitis rates in whites were 1.5 times higher than in nonwhites, and rates were highest in the west north central region. Appendicitis rates were 11.3% higher in the summer than in the winter. Women aged 35–44 years had the highest rate of incidental appendectomy. Their rate of 43.8/10,000 population per year was 12.1 times higher than that in men of the same age. Overall diagnostic accuracy was lower in females than in males—78.6% vs. 91.2%. In females, diagnostic accuracy fell sharply during childbearing years, whereas it did not vary appreciably with age in males (Fig 22–1). The incidence of appendicitis decreased by 14.6% between 1970 and 1984 (Fig 22–2), but the reasons for this decline are unknown.

A life-table model indicates that the lifetime risk of appendicitis is 8.6% for males and 6.7% for females. The lifetime risk of appendectomy is 12% for males and 23.1% for females. Overall, surgeons perform an estimated 36 incidental procedures to prevent 1 case of appendicitis. The preventive value of incidental procedures is considerably lower in the elderly.

▶ This epidemiologic survey of appendectomy is filled with information you have always wondered about; the only problem is that sometimes the line between appendectomy for appendicitis and incidental appendectomy, is faintly drawn. Nonetheless, where else would you find that whites are 1.5 times more likely to have appendicitis than nonwhites, and that the summertime risk is 11% greater than in winter? I suspect that the overall diagnostic accuracy is 79% for women and 91% for men. The fall of nearly 15% in the incidence of appendicitis between 1970 and 1984 coincides, I believe, with conventional wisdom (whatever that is). At the next conversational lull, you can brightly remark that 8.6% of men and 6.7% of women in the United States will have appendicitis, and that it is necessary to do 36 incidental appendectomies to prevent a single attack of appendicitis.—J.C. Thompson, M.D.

Primary Adenocarcinoma of the Appendix
Evans DA, Hamid BNA, Hoare EM (Trafford Gen Hosp, Manchester, England)
J R Coll Surg Edinb 35:33–35, 1990   22–2

Data were reviewed on 13 patients (mean age, 70 years) with primary adenocarcinoma of the appendix treated in 1972–1984. Acute appendicitis was the most common preoperative diagnosis. No patient was suspected of having primary appendiceal carcinoma before surgery. Appendectomy alone was the primary procedure in 10 patients, 4 of whom later had a successful right hemicolectomy. The tumor was a chance finding at postmortem examination in 1 patient. Histologically, 7 tumors were of the colonic type and 6 were cystadenocarcinomas.

The mean follow-up of survivors was for 70 months. Of 7 patients who underwent appendectomy alone, 4 were alive with a mean survival of 59 months; the 3 who died had a mean survival of 16 months. Appendectomy was followed by early elective right hemicolectomy in 3 patients, 2 of whom died after a mean of 41 months.

Past studies suggest that hemicolectomy increases survival in patients with primary adenocarcinoma of the appendix. Although there are sound anatomical reasons for advising this course, these data indicate that appendectomy alone may be associated with long survival, and that the addition of right hemicolectomy is not necessarily curative.

▶ These problems seem to appear more on board questions than in real life. The astute student knows that right colectomy is indicated for carcinoid tumors of the appendix larger than 2 cm in diameter and for all primary adenocarcinomas. Because the proper diagnosis is usually not made initially, reoperation is indicated. This paper from Manchester suggests that survival is increased by right colectomy, but the procedure is certainly not necessarily curative.—J.C. Thompson, M.D.

Cecal Diverticulitis Presented as a Cecal Tumor

Kaufman Z, Shpitz B, Reina A, (Meir Gen Hosp, Kfar Saba; Tel Aviv Univ Sackler Faculty of Medicine, Israel)
Am Surg 56:675–677, 1990   22–3

Cecal diverticula are the most common causes of massive lower gastrointestinal tract bleeding, but the most frequent complication is diverticulitis. A cecal mass is usually found at laparotomy. Data were reviewed on 7 patients in whom cecal diverticulitis presented as a cecal mass; they were treated during an 8-year period.

Patients most often had right lower quadrant pain and moderate fever, which had been present for 1–3 days. All patients had tenderness in the right lower abdomen, as well as signs of local peritoneal irritation, but no mass. All were thought preoperatively to have acute appendicitis. The masses found at surgery were 4–7 cm in size and were located in the antimesenteric border of the cecum; 2 patients had a pericecal abscess. Right hemicolectomy was necessary in 2 patients. Two other patients had wedge resection of the cecal wall with primary closure of the cecum; 3 patients had diverticulectomy. The postoperative course was uneventful. True cecal diverticulae with acute inflammation and edema were found in 5 patients; 2 had false diverticula with acute inflammation.

Cecal diverticulitis is part of the differential diagnosis of cecal wall tumor. Usually, it is possible to separate the cecal mass and perform a diverticulectomy.

▶ The situation is familiar. The middle-aged to elderly patient is operated on with a preoperative diagnosis of acute appendicitis and, lo and behold, a large inflammatory mass involving the cecum is found in the right lower quadrant. What is the etiology, and what to do? The etiology may of course be an appendiceal abscess or a perforated cecal diverticulitis or a perforated cecal carcinoma, or even, I guess, a cecal perforation caused by a chicken bone. They all look the same from the outside, and they should probably all be handled the same, i.e., they should be treated by resection and ileoascending or ileotransverse colostomy. If you find that you are dealing with a perforated cecal carcinoma you should, if possible, increase the scope of your operation to remove all cancer tissue. Differentiation between perforated cecal cancer and perforated cecal diverticulitis can be very difficult. If the mass has perforated and if there is great spillage of pus, we do an ileostomy and transverse colostomy mucus fistula. It took me a long time to learn that.—J.C. Thompson, M.D.

Rates of Morbidity and Mortality After Closure of Loop and End Colostomy

Mileski WJ, Rege RV, Joehl RJ, Nahrwold DL (Northwestern Univ; VA Lakeside Med Ctr, Chicago)
Surg Gynecol Obstet 171:17–20, 1990   22–4

It often is claimed that closing a loop colostomy is associated with less risk of morbidity and mortality than taking down an end colostomy and performing an anastomosis, but this has not been confirmed. The outcome of loop colostomy closure and end colostomy closure were compared in 93 consecutive patients operated on in 1978–1986; 62 loop colostomies and 31 end colostomies were closed.

The preoperative hemoglobin was lower in patients with loop colostomy and the time to closure was significantly longer. Most colostomies were performed for complications of diverticular disease and colon cancer. Closure of end colostomies took longer and was associated with greater blood loss, although not increased transfusion needs. The overall mortality was 4.3%. Complications were comparably frequent in the 2 surgical groups. Wound infection occurred in 9% of patients having primary closure and in 5% of those having delayed closure.

Morbidity was comparable after closure of loop and end colostomies in this series. Closure must be approached cautiously in patients with lower serum albumin levels and those dependent on steroids. Primary closure of the skin at the stomal site is safe and shortens the hospital stay.

▶ The only advantage that I know for a loop colostomy is that it can be constructed quickly, which can be an advantage in desperately ill patients with obstructing left colon carcinoma. Otherwise, it is not as efficient as an end colostomy in providing for diversion of enteric flow, and this study shows that loop colostomy cannot be closed with less risk. Indeed, we should all take head of the mortality rate of nearly 5% in closure of a loop colostomy. Whenever you think of doing a 3-stage operation for obstructed colon, you should think of the cumulative risk of morbidity and mortality attendant on each stage. The cumulation provides strong impetus to adoption of 1- or 2-stage procedures whenever possible.—J.C. Thompson, M.D.

Endometriosis of the Colon: Its Diagnosis and Management
Collin GR, Russell JC (New Britain Gen Hosp, New Britain, Conn)
Am Surg 56:275–279, 1990   22–5

Endometriosis can occasionally result in colonic symptoms. The most common areas of involvement are the rectosigmoid and sigmoid colon, the appendix, and the ileum. Data were reviewed on 9 patients (mean age, 41 years) who had endometriosis of the colon to develop some recommendations concerning the diagnosis and management of this condition.

The most common symptom was crampy abdominal pain; diarrhea, constipation, abdominal distention, and blood per rectum were also noted. Seven patients had a history of dysmenorrhea and 4 of endometriosis. Plain abdominal films showed signs of obstruction in all patients. Of 6 patients undergoing a barium enema, 6 had an extramucosal defect in the rectosigmoid or sigmoid colon (Fig 22–3); the other patient had total obstruction of the colon. An extramucosal mass compressing the lumen was found by endoscopy in all 5 patients who underwent the procedure. Resection with primary anastomosis was performed in 6 patients. The re-

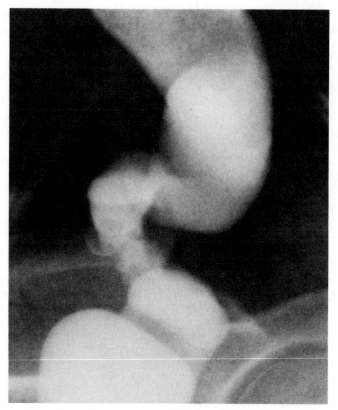

Fig 22–3.—Barium enema shows extramucosal defect causing compression of the sigmoid colon resulting from endometriosis. (Courtesy of Collin GR, Russell JC: *Am Surg* 56:275–279, 1990.)

maining 3 had resection with sigmoid end-colostomy and Hartmann's pouch; all 3 had successful reversal of the colostomies within 1 year. An adenocarcinoma of the colon was found in 1 patient, although the tumor was not thought to be the cause of her symptoms.

Endometriosis of the colon should be considered in evaluating women with colonic symptoms, particularly in those with a history of dysmenorrhea or cyclic changes in bowel habits. Surgical resection is the preferred treatment for relief of symptoms.

▶ Endometriosis is one of those conditions that is apt to catch the surgeon unaware. We are asked to see a patient with bowel dysfunction, and we ponder the list of likely causes and often operate without a firm diagnosis, only to find, to our surprise, dense adhesions and clumps of strange-looking tissue. On frozen section this turns out to be endometrium. The preoperative diagnosis is rare but can be suspected in women with strong histories of gynecologic complaints. Therapy should be conservative, more or less along the lines of treatment for Crohn's disease. Involved segments should be resected conservatively, and no attempt should be made to completely eradicate all endometriosis.—J.C. Thompson, M.D.

The National Polyp Study: Patient and Polyp Characteristics Associated With High-Grade Dysplasia in Colorectal Adenomas
O'Brien MJ, Winawer SJ, Zauber AG, Gottlieb LS, Sternberg SS, Diaz B, Dickersin GR, Ewing S, Geller S, Kasimian D, Komorowski R, Szporn A, and the Natl Polyp Study Workgroup (Mem Sloan-Kettering Cancer Ctr, New York; Boston City Hosp)
Gastroenterology 98:371–379, 1990   22–6

Most colorectal carcinomas are thought to develop within preexisting adenomas. Because adenomas are common in persons older than age 40, it is important to discover what patient and polyp characteristics are associated with high-grade dysplasia. Data were reviewed on patients included in the National Polyp Study, a multicenter trial initiated to evaluate effective surveillance of adenoma patients.

The 2,363 patients had a total of 5,066 polyps. Of these, 66.5% were adenomas, 11.2% were hyperplastic, and 22.3% were classified as "other." Of 3,371 adenomas removed from 1,867 patients, 86.1% showed mild dysplasia, 7.7% moderate dysplasia, and 6.2% high-grade dysplasia. Histologic types included tubular (70.4%), villous A (16.7%), villous B (8.2%), villous C (3.9%), and villous D (.8%).

The percentage of adenomas with high-grade dysplasia increased significantly with increasing adenoma size (Fig 22–4). and with increasing

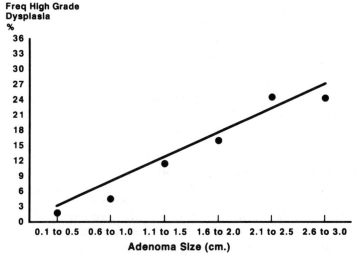

Fig 22–4.—National Polyp Study. Frequency of high-grade dysplasia in adenomas by size *(filled circles,* observed; *line,* expected regression line). Test for association: $\chi^2_{3} = 251.8$, $P < .0001$; test for linear trend: $\chi^2_{1} = 243.5$, $P < .0001$. (Courtesy of O'Brien MJ, Winawer SJ, Zauber AG, et al: *Gastroenterology* 98:371–379, 1990.)

villous component. Relative to tubular adenomas, the odds ratio increased to 20.2 for villous C and D. Similarly, the mean adenoma size increased significantly as the proportion of villous component increased in the adenoma. The mean size of adenomas was significantly larger in the left colon than in the proximal colon.

High-grade dysplasia was more common in patients with multiple adenomas (13.8%) than in those with single adenomas (7.3%), and in patients with large adenomas (20.6%) than in those with small adenomas (4.6%). Whether the adenomas were single or multiple, villous adenomas were more likely than tubular adenomas to exhibit high-grade dysplasia. Increasing age, but not gender, was associated with high-grade dysplasia.

High-grade dysplasia represents an intermediate stage in the evolution of invasive carcinoma and is a valid marker of the potential for malignant transformation. The detailed model described here integrates multiple patient and adenoma factors associated with high-grade dysplasia in colorectal adenomas.

▶ Currently, conventional wisdom is that most colorectal cancers arise from adenomas, and that dysplastic adenomas are the most dangerous kind. The incidence of adenomas in patients older than 40 years in the United States is 30% or more (1,2). The authors of this huge multicenter project attempted, by multivariant analysis, to determine those risk factors for high-grade dysplasia (6.2% had high-grade dysplasia). The 4 major risk factors were multiplicity of adenomas, high histologic villous component, and size and age of patient. These data were very difficult to come by, and the study was expensive and time-consuming; we should all learn from it in order to make it worthwhile.— J.C. Thompson, M.D.

References

1. Arminski TC, McLean DW: *Dis Colon Rectum* 7:249, 1964.
2. Rickert RR, et al: *Cancer* 43:1847, 1979.

Hazard Rates for Dysplasia and Cancer in Ulcerative Colitis: Results from a Surveillance Program
Lashner BA, Silverstein MD, Hanauer SB (Univ of Chicago)
Dig Dis Sci 34:1536–1541, 1989   22–7

Patients with chronic ulcerative colitis are at considerably increased risk for cancer of the colon. The risk of colon cancer is related to the duration and extent of disease, and perhaps to younger age at symptom onset. The relationship between ulcerative colitis, dysplasia, and cancer was investigated in patients in a surveillance program. Patients were eligible if disease duration was longer than 8 years and its extent was proximal to the splenic flexure.

Annual colonoscopy was performed, with biopsy specimens taken every 10 cm from the cecum and from suspicious masses or polyps. Patients

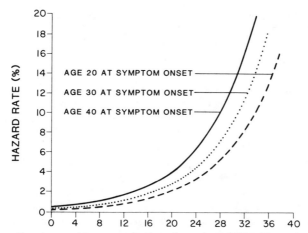

Fig 22–5.—Effect of age at symptom onset on hazard rates for HGD/Ca). These curves are examples illustrating hazard rates for HGD/Ca as a function of age of symptom onset for symptom onset at ages 20, 30, and 40 years. Hazard rates increase 38% for each decade increase in age at symptom onset as calculated from a Cox proportional hazards model. (Courtesy of Lashner BA, Silverstein MD, Hanauer SB: *Dig Dis Sci* 34:1536–1541, 1989.)

were classified as having no dysplasia, indefinite for dysplasia, low-grade dysplasia, high-grade dysplasia, and invasive carcinoma. The latter 2 categories were treated as a single lesion in the analysis (HGD/Ca).

The patients included 61 men and 38 women. The average age at symptom onset was 23 years, and the average duration of disease before entry into the study was 17 years; followup averaged 9 years after entry. The hazard rate for high-grade dysplasia or cancer in patients with pancolitis determined from symptom onset was 2.5% at 20 years, 4% at 25 years, 7% at 30 years, 13% at 35 years, and 20% at 40 years.

The risk for HGD/Ca increases with both the duration of disease and with age at symptom onset (Fig 22–5). Sex was not a significant predictor of HGD/Ca. The hazard rate for HGD/Ca increases 38% for each 10-year increase in age at symptom onset. The absolute risk of cancer in patients with ulcerative colitis is actually lower when disease onset occurs in childhood.

▶ Epidemiologic studies provide invaluable information on the natural history of disease, but when manifestations of the disease are highly variable, huge numbers of patients may be necessary in order to show accurate trends. Although a collection of 99 patients represents a major effort, it probably is nowhere nearly large enough a group to allow firm conclusions.

What is impressive here is that no support was found for the widely held conviction that early age of onset of ulcerative colitis is associated with high risk of cancer. The figures that I have always used are a risk of 5% per year, beginning at 10 years. This study shows half that risk at 20 years. Nonetheless, after 40 years the risk was 20%.—J.C. Thompson, M.D.

Ulcerative Colitis and Colorectal Cancer: A Population-Based Study

Ekbom A, Helmick C, Zack M, Adami H-O (Univ Hosp, Uppsala, Sweden; Ctrs for Disease Control, Atlanta)
N Engl J Med 323:1228–1233, 1990   22–8

Whereas ulcerative colitis is associated with colorectal cancer, the exact risk of colorectal cancer is unknown. In an attempt to provide an accurate assessment of this risk, a retrospective analysis was made of data on 3,117 patients with ulcerative colitis seen from 1922 through 1983 in a 6-county area in Sweden. Follow-up extended through 1984.

Colorectal cancer was diagnosed in 91 patients between 1958 and 1984. This was 5.7 times the expected number of cases. Forty-five patients died of colorectal cancer, 4.4 times the expected number. No difference in risk of colorectal cancer was seen between men and women, but the risk did increase with increasing extent of disease at diagnosis: patients with pancolitis had 14.8 times the expected risk of colorectal cancer, whereas those with ulcerative proctitis had a standardized incidence ratio of 1.7. Independently, the relative risk decreased with increasing age at diagnosis. When patients were divided into age groups of under 15 years, 15–29 years, 30–39 years, 40–49 years, 50–59 years, and 60 years or older, the relative risk of colorectal cancer decreased by about half for each increase in age group.

These findings suggest that patients in whom ulcerative colitis is diagnosed before age 15 years, or those with pancolitis, have extremely high relative risks of colorectal cancer. Such patients might best be treated with prophylactic proctocolectomy in lieu of close surveillance.

▶ As predicted in the first sentence of my discussion of Abstract 21–7, the study of larger groups may give different information. This study firmly supports the great hazard of cancer in those individuals who have chronic idiopathic ulcerative colitis before the age of 15. Similarly, patients with pancolitis were 15 times more apt to have cancer of the colon than the unaffected population. This is the strongest recommendation for prophylactic proctocolectomy (in a closely circumscribed group of patients with pancolitis, especially those who have the disease before age 15) that I have seen.—J.C. Thompson, M.D.

Carcinoma of the Colon and Rectum in Patients Less Than 20 Years of Age

Lewis CTP, Riley WE, Georgeson K, Warren JH (Univ of Alabama, Birmingham)
South Med J 83:383–385, 1990   22–9

In 1962–1987, 8 children and adolescents were treated for colonic adenocarcinoma at 3 large referral hospitals. The average age was 15 years. Symptoms had been present for an average of 7½ months; rectal bleeding was most prevalent. Only 1 patient had a palpable mass at the time of diagnosis. Six patients had stage C or D disease, and 6 lesions were poorly differentiated. Six tumors were removed, only 3 with curative intent. Only 3 patients lived longer than 6 months; 2 of them were well at 28 months and 40 months, respectively, and 1 was unavailable for follow-up 12 years after operation.

Children and adolescents who have gastrointestinal tract bleeding or unexplained abdominal complaints should be carefully evaluated and the possibility of colorectal cancer kept in mind. The aggressive nature of disease in this age group and the frequent presence of advanced disease at diagnosis contribute to a poor survival rate.

▶ Anyone who passes blood per rectum should be suspected of having colon cancer, even children. The youngest in this series was a 9-year-old boy! Although Abstract 22–8 gave evidence of the dangers of cancer development in children with ulcerative colitis, the great majority of children in whom colon cancer develops have no preexisting illness. Although women with colon cancer outnumber men, among children, boys are affected twice as commonly. All series agree that the disease is deadly.—J.C. Thompson, M.D.

Anterior Versus Abdominoperineal Resections in the Management of Mid-Rectal Tumours
Graf W, Påhlman L, Enblad P, Glimelius B (Uppsala Univ, Sweden)
Acta Chir Scand 156:231–235, 1990   22–10

Since the circular stapler was introduced into clinical practice, a larger proportion of patients with midrectal tumors have been treated with anterior resection rather than abdominoperineal resection. The effects of this new technique on the local recurrence rate and survival were evaluated in 2 consecutive series of patients treated for cancer in the mid-rectum.

In the first series, 81 patients underwent curative operations before the stapling instrument was in general use; 65 patients had abdominoperineal resection and 16 had anterior resection. Only 2 anastomoses were stapled; the other 14 were handsewn. The median follow-up was 132 months. In the second series, 156 patients underwent curative operations for tumors in the mid-rectum. Of these, 105 had an abdominoperineal resection and 51 had anterior resection. The circular stapling device was used in all but 2 patients treated with anterior resection. Patients in the second series were randomized to receive pre- or postoperative radiotherapy. The median follow-up was 60 months.

Local recurrence rates did not differ significantly with either procedure, neither in the first or second series nor among the radiotherapy groups in the second series. In the first series, 39% of patients having anterior resection and 41% having abdominoperineal resection had recurrence; in the second series, 16% of patients who had anterior resection and 17% who had abdominoperineal resection had local recurrence. Cancer-specific survival did not differ between operations in any of the series.

The outcomes of patients with mid-rectal cancer were not adversely affected by use of the stapling technique. Neither local occurrence nor cancer-specific deaths increased with the increase in number of sphincter-saving operations.

▶ Introduction of the EEA stapling device has facilitated low anterior resections for midrectal cancers, and several series have addressed the question of whether this advantage has been purchased by a higher rate of cancer recurrence. Different studies report different results. This paper from Uppsala seems clearly to show no increase (in fact, a decrease) in local recurrence. Again, large numbers of patients will be required to finally answer this question.—J.C. Thompson, M.D.

Levamisole and Fluorouracil for Adjuvant Therapy of Resected Colon Carcinoma

Moertel CG, Fleming TR, Macdonald JS, Haller DG, Laurie JA, Goodman PJ, Ungerleider JS, Emerson WA, Tormey DG, Glick JH, Veeder MH, Mailliard JA (Mayo Clinic and Found, Rochester, Minn; Fred Hutchinson Cancer Research Ctr, Seattle; Temple Univ; Univ of Pennsylvania; Grand Forks Clinic, Grand Forks, ND; et al)

N Engl J Med 322:352–358, 1990   22–11

A series of 1,296 patients with resected colon cancer, either locally invasive (stage B_2) or involving regional nodes (stage C), were randomly assigned to observation or to treatment for 1 year with levamisole plus fluorouracil. Patients with stage C disease could also be randomly assigned to treatment with levamisole alone. The median follow-up was 3 years (range, 2 to 5½ years).

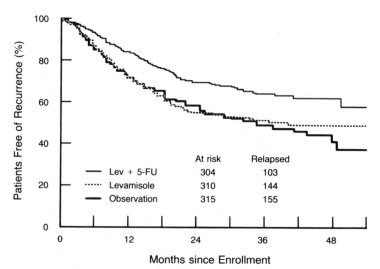

Fig 22–6.—Recurrence-free interval. Lev + 5-FU denotes combination therapy with levamisole and fluorouracil. (Courtesy of Moertel CG, Fleming TR, Macdonald JS, et al: *N Engl J Med* 322:352–358, 1990.)

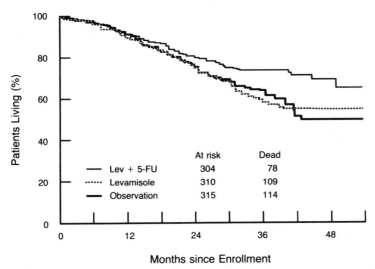

Fig 22–7.—Survival among all eligible patients in study. Lev + 5-FU denotes combination therapy with levamisole and fluorouracil. (Courtesy of Moertel CG, Fleming TR, Macdonald JS, et al: *N Engl J Med* 322:352–358, 1990.)

The results of using levamisole plus fluorouracil in patients with stage B_2 disease were equivocal. For those with stage C disease, however, treatment with combination therapy lowered the risk of recurrence by 41% and reduced overall mortality by 33%. Levamisole alone had no apparent effect on patients with stage C disease. Recurrence-free intervals are plotted in Figure 22–6 and are carried out to 52 months, at which point fewer than 10% of patients could be followed. Survival among all eligible patients in the study is plotted in Figure 22–7. Toxicity from levamisole alone was infrequent and usually consisted of mild nausea, occasional dermatitis, or leukopenia. Combined treatment produced similar effects and diarrhea as well, but the effects usually were not severe and did not interfere significantly with patient compliance. Second primary cancers occurred in 3.2% of patients.

Adjuvant treatment with levamisole and fluorouracil should be offered to all patients with stage C colon cancer after putatively curative resection. Patients should have a white blood cell count of at least 4,000/µL and a platelet count of at least 130,000/µL for treatment, which may be started 3 weeks after surgery when the patient is ambulatory and in good nutritional condition.

▶ As a cause of cancer death, the colon is second only to the lungs. Despite huge efforts, no reliable screening method has evolved. For years we have read one discouraging report after another from the National Bowel Cancer Study regarding failure of radiation or chemotherapy to avert death. This report is highly encouraging. It involved studies of nearly 1,300 patients with locally invasive or regional node involvement, and it was carried out by an outstanding group of leading chemotherapists. Their finding that stage C patients had a

41% reduction in the chance of recurrence, and that the death rate was cut by one third overall in patients given the combination of levamisole and 5-FU, is the best news in years. An added gift is the apparent low toxicity of the regimen.—J.C. Thompson, M.D.

The Double Stapling Technique for Low Anterior Resection: Results, Modifications, and Observations
Griffen FD, Knight CD Sr, Whitaker JM, Knight CD Jr (Louisiana State Univ)
Ann Surg 211:745–752, 1990   22–12

An earlier report described a modification of low rectal anastomosis with end-to-end anastomosis using a double-stapling technique with a linear stapler. A review was made of experience with stapled colorectal anastomoses in 75 patients. The series included 33 men and 42 women

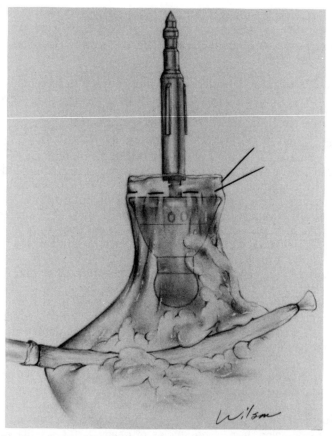

Fig 22–8.—After selection of the proper cartridge, the anvil shaft assembly is detached from the central rod, placed in the proximal bowel through the pursestring, and the suture is tied into the groove on the shaft. (Courtesy of Griffen FD, Knight CD Sr, Whitaker JM, et al: *Ann Surg* 211:745–752, 1990.)

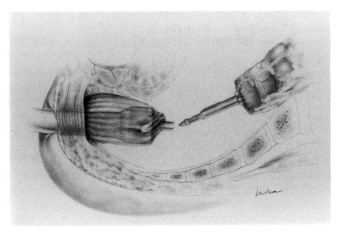

Fig 22–9.—The premium CEEA staple is introduced into the rectal segment with the anvil shaft assembly removed and the center rod with the trocar attachment retracted within the cartridge. The instrument is advanced, placing the cartridge against the linear staple row. The center rod is extended, passing the trocar into the abdominal cavity adjacent to the staple line, following which the trocar is removed. (Courtesy of Griffen FD, Knight CD Sr, Whitaker JM, et al: *Ann Surg* 211:745–752, 1990.)

(mean age, 65 years); two thirds patients were at least 70 years old. Fifty patients had carcinoma of the rectosigmoid colon, 20 had diverticulitis, 3 had carcinoma of the ovary; and 1 each had volvulus and rectal prolapse.

Technique. During the procedure the surgeon mobilizes the rectosigmoid colon, applies a TA-55 stapler at the lower limit of the resection, and places a double row of staples. After the proper cartridge is selected, the anvil shaft assembly is detached from the central rod and placed in the proximal bowel through the pursestring; the suture is tied into the groove on the shaft (Fig 22–8). The circular stapler is introduced into the rectal segment with the anvil shaft assembly removed and the center rod containing the trocar attachment retracted into the cartridge. The instrument is advanced until the cartridge reaches the row of linear staples. Then the center rod is extended and the trocar is passed into the abdominal cavity adjacent to the staple line. The trocar is removed (Fig 22–9), and the anvil shaft is inserted into the rod. The circular stapler is closed and activated to form a circular end-to-end inverting anastomosis. Mattress sutures are placed across the anastomosis if it is technically feasible. The circular stapler is opened and removed. Any leaks are repaired with silk sutures. After drainage is placed, the abdomen is closed in the usual manner. The pelvic peritoneum is not sutured.

Among 75 patients, 2 had anastomotic leaks and 2 had stenoses that required treatment. There were no deaths. This modification of the end-to-end anastomosis technique allows a lower anastomosis in some patients. The procedure is safe and easily performed.

▶ The bête noire of low anterior resections for colon cancer is anastomotic leakage. This method of stapled anastomosis using a unique trocar attachment reduces the leakage to less than 3%. The technique appears worthwhile.—J.C. Thompson, M.D.

Anorectal Melanoma: Clinical Characteristics and Results of Surgical Management in Twenty-Four Patients

Slingluff CL Jr, Vollmer RT, Seigler HF (Duke Univ; Durham VA Hosp, NC)
Surgery 107:1–9, 1990   22–13

Although primary malignant melanoma of the anorectum accounts for only about 1% of all primary melanomas, it is usually discovered late and metastasis is common. Data on 24 patients who underwent abdominoperineal resection in a 15-year period were reviewed retrospectively. The patients had a mean age of 64 years, and there was a predominance of women to men (2.4:1).

Most patients had rectal bleeding, often misdiagnosed as hemorrhoids; 3 patients also had asymptomatic anorectal masses. All of the lesions arose in the mucosa of the anorectum at or near the anorectal junction, and most were 2 cm or larger. On histologic evaluation, 19 lesions had a junctional pattern and 3 a nodular pattern; 2 were unclassified.

Within 45 days of diagnosis, 13 patients underwent resection. Because of local recurrence, 3 patients underwent resection later in their clinical course. Those surgically free of disease received specific active immunotherapy. Patients with unresectable metastatic disease were treated with chemotherapy. The most common metastatic sites during follow-up were the lung, liver, and pelvis.

During a mean follow-up of 2.2 years, 20 of 24 patients died of progressive melanoma. Of the remaining 4 patients, 1 died of a seizure disorder and 3 had a recent diagnosis (1–18 months). In patients with stage I disease, abdominoperineal resection did not significantly alter the length of survival. The median survival was significantly longer with stage I (29 months) than with stage II (11 months) or stage III (9 months) disease (Fig 22–10).

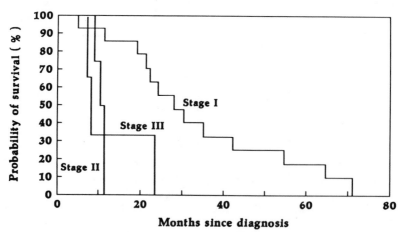

Fig 22–10.—Kaplan-Meier survival curves for patients with anorectal melanoma in stage I, II, or III. Nodal metastases defined stage II disease, and distant metastases defined stage III disease. Survival of patients with stage I disease was prolonged relative to survival of patients with stage II disease ($P = .0003$) and patients with stage III disease ($P = .022$). (Courtesy of Slingluff CL Jr, Vollmer RT, Seigler HF: *Surgery* 107:1–9, 1990.)

Melanoma of the anorectal canal has increased biologic aggressiveness and a high risk for metastasis. Earlier diagnosis, combined modality therapy, and treatment of the regions of highest risk for metastasis may improve the prognosis in these patients.

▶ The disease is deadly regardless of operation; no one survived for more than 6 years. One of the authors' conclusions appears strange to me. In the Discussion they note that abdominoperineal resection has not been effective, so that it may be reasonable to attempt even more aggressive surgery in selected patients. What is the rationale? It seems to me that they have shown that this is a systemic disease, a disease unlikely to respond to any local measure. The authors quote series that record a less than 10% 5-year survival, but no one survived for more than 6 years in this carefully studied series.—J.C. Thompson, M.D.

The Recalcitrant Perineal Wound After Rectal Extirpation: Applications of Muscle Flap Closure
Anthony JP, Mathes SJ (Univ of California, San Francisco)
Arch Surg 125:1371–1377, 1990   22–14

Once a perineal wound becomes chronic, local wound care seldom succeeds and further surgery usually is necessary. Data on 13 consecutive patients who had muscle flap closure of chronic postproctectomy perineal wounds in 1979–1988 were reviewed. The wounds had persisted for longer than 1 month despite local care. Their average duration was 42 months, and the average wound size after débridement was 44 cm². Nine patients had undergone 18 unsuccessful operations before muscle flap surgery, most often débridement and curettage.

After wide débridement, the wound was covered with a gracilis, gluteus maximus, inferior gluteal thigh, or rectus abdominis flap. An abdominoperineal approach was used for immediate reconstruction in 2 patients. The other patients had muscle flap closure after a chronic perineal wound developed.

The average time to healing after muscle flap closure was 3 weeks. Minor complications occurred in 4 patients; there were no major complications requiring reoperation, and no flap losses. During an average follow-up of 3.5 years, 12 patients remained well. One patient had wound recurrence after 6 months and has done well since closure with a rectus abdominus flap.

Débridement and muscle flap coverage are effective measures for patients with chronic perineal wounds after proctectomy. Immediate flap closure should be considered for those with severe skin damage from radiation exposure or active suppuration, as they are especially likely to have chronic wounds.

▶ Obviously, the best management is prevention, and the incidence of chronic open perineal wounds has greatly diminished since surgeons have learned assiduously to achieve hemostasis and to close the pelvic floor. These authors have extensive experience in closure of chronic ischemic suppurating wounds, and they apply the principle that the best way to get tissue with poor blood supply to heal is to bring in new tissue carrying its own blood supply. The authors remind us that the major risk factors for nonhealing perineal wounds are perioperative radiation, reoperations for recurrent cancer, and inflammatory bowel disease. Composite graft repair seems to be the ideal answer to this vexing problem.—J.C. Thompson, M.D.

23 The Liver and the Spleen

Focal Nodular Hyperplasia of the Liver
Brady MS, Coit DG (Mem Sloan-Kettering Cancer Ctr, New York)
Surg Gynecol Obstet 171:377–381, 1990   23–1

Focal nodular hyperplasia (FNH), a benign liver tumor, usually is found in women of reproductive age. Most patients are asymptomatic and have normal physical examinations. The tumor is often discovered incidentally at laparotomy or during investigation for another problem. A retrospective study was made of 24 patients (22 women) undergoing intraoperative biopsy or resection of FNH of the liver at Memorial Sloan-Kettering Cancer Center between 1978 and 1988. The mean age was 35 years. Eighteen had a history of oral contraceptive or conjugated estrogen use. Neither of the men had a history of hormone use.

Twenty-two tumors were solitary; 17 were in the left lobe of the liver. Fifteen patients had a previous or simultaneous malignant lesion. Six had other benign tumors. Thirteen tumors were resected with a wedge or subsegment of liver. Four patients had segmentectomy, and 5 had lobectomy for removal of the tumors. Two patients only underwent intraoperative biopsy. Computed tomography and arteriography were routinely done in patients in whom the tumor was diagnosed preoperatively. Scintigraphy of the liver with sulfur colloid, which has a distinct potential for the nonoperative diagnosis of FNH, was done in only 3 cases.

The data confirm that FNH occurs primarily in relatively young women and has an innocuous, often incidental, mode of presentation. Oral estrogen may be related to the development of these tumors. Other tumors were found with an unexpectedly high frequency in this series. Hepatic scintigraphy with sulfur-colloid-labeled tracer is essential in patients with a primary hepatic tumor that appears benign on CT and arteriography. Increased uptake of tracer by the tumor is characteristic of FNH and may permit nonsurgical management in certain patients.

► In the past we have not regarded focal nodular hyperplasia per se as an indication for major hepatic resection. The issue of malignant degeneration has not been defined. There have been no reported incidences of spontaneous rupture or hemorrhage into the necrotic center. These lesions are usually asymptomatic, but if it is thought that symptoms can be ascribed to a lesion, resection is indicated. Iwatsuki et al. (1) reported 8 patients with moderate to severe pain who experienced complete relief after resection. Resection was carried out in 11 patients who had vague but annoying symptoms and 78% had complete relief.—S.I. Schwartz, M.D.

Reference

1. Iwatsuki S, et al: *Surg Gynecol Obstet* 171:240, 1990.

Mesenchymal Hamartoma of the Liver: A 35-Year Review

DeMaioribus CA, Lally KP, Sim K, Isaacs H, Mahour GH (Wilford Hall US Air Force Med Ctr, Lackland AFB, Texas; Children's Hosp of Los Angeles; Univ of California, Los Angeles)
Arch Surg 125:598–600, 1990   23–2

Mesenchymal hamartoma of the liver occurs almost exclusively in infants and children; approximately 140 such patients have been described. Data on 18 patients with mesenchymal hamartoma seen at a children's hospital in 1952–1986 were reviewed. The 9 boys and 9 girls had a mean age at diagnosis of 16 months. Progressive abdominal distention was present in 13 patients. In 2 patients the liver mass was detected incidentally at autopsy after death from other causes. A right upper quadrant mass was found in 9 patients; 1 had a left upper quadrant mass, and the remaining 8 had hepatomegaly alone.

Ultrasonography and CT were the most useful diagnostic tests. Laboratory evaluation, plain films of the abdomen, and contrast studies were not helpful. Hepatic lobectomy was performed on 9 patients, and excision of the tumor only on 5. One child had associated congenital heart disease and underwent needle biopsy of the lesion only; another had a biopsy and marsupialization of the lesion. At a mean of 5 years after surgery, all 13 patients available for follow-up were well and symptom free.

The lesions were large, rounded, or irregular masses weighing as much as 1,898 g. Although the exact pathogenesis of mesenchymal hamartoma is not certain, it may represent aberrant development of primitive mesenchyme in the portal tracts, most likely from bile ducts. Because the lesion is benign, an overly aggressive surgical approach is not usually justified. Nevertheless, excision or marsupialization of the lesion is recommended in all patients once the diagnosis is established.

▶ This is a complete review of the literature on an unusual hepatic tumor. The only issue that can be added suggests that radiotherapy may effect some reduction of the size of the lesion as a result of hyalinization of the mesenchymal components. Surgical excision remains the treatment of choice. As the article points out, this must be regarded as a lesion distinctly different from the cystadenoma without mesenchymal stroma. Any potential malignant change of a cystadenoma without mesenchymal stroma has not been defined. On 3 occasions we have locally resected benign cystadenoma from the bile duct, and on 2 occasions from the ampulla of Vater, with long-term follow-up showing no evidence of recurrence.—S.I. Schwartz, M.D.

Treatment of Highly Symptomatic Polycystic Liver Disease: Preliminary Experience With a Combined Hepatic Resection-Fenestration Procedure

Newman KD, Torress VE, Rakela J, Nagorney DM (Mayo Clinic and Found, Rochester, Minn)
Ann Surg 212:30–37, 1990   23–3

In symptomatic patients with polycystic liver disease sometimes all conservative treatment options are exhausted. Surgery is the next alternative. The value and consequences of combined hepatic resection and cyst fenestration were assessed in 9 highly symptomatic patients with polycystic liver disease. All 9 underwent resection of 2 or more liver segments and extensive fenestration of residual cysts in the remnant liver (Fig 23–1).

Symptomatic relief and reduction in abdominal girth were obtained in 8 surviving patients, who were followed for an average of 17 months. There was no progression of cystic disease clinically or on CT, and hepatic function was preserved. Complications, which developed in 5 patients, included transient right pleural effusion and thrombosis of an arteriovenous fistula. One patient who had hepatic cyst fenestration and had received a cadaveric renal transplantation previously died after surgery of intracerebral hemorrhage after having coagulopathy, hyperbilirubinemia, and sepsis.

Certain highly symptomatic patients with massive polycystic liver disease may benefit from combined hepatic resection and fenestration. The risk from the procedure appears to be acceptable. Previous liver surgery

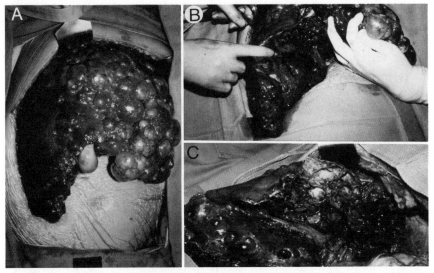

Fig 23–1.—A, intraoperative photographs of massively enlarged polycystic liver, showing polycystic liver *(right)* and spared parenchyma *(left)*. **B,** anticipated transection plane between spared and polycystic liver. **C,** remnant liver after left hepatectomy. Resection of cystic segments 7 and 8 was subsequently completed. (Courtesy of Newman KD, Torress VE, Rakela J, et al: *Ann Surg* 212:30–37, 1990.)

and immunosuppressive therapy may increase the risk. The duration of benefit from this combined procedure has yet to be determined.

▶ I certainly agree with the authors that there is a small but definite group of patients with polycystic liver disease for whom hepatic resection and fenestration are indicated. I have operated on 3 such patients, however, in whom the liver mass interfered with gastric filling and resulted in marked early satiety and, in 1 case, gastric outlet obstruction. All patients were women who had been taking oral contraceptives for variable periods of time. The anatomical planes are difficult to define, but resection can usually be carried out along nonanatomical planes with minimal bleeding.—S.I. Schwartz, M.D.

Repeat Hepatectomy for Recurrent Malignant Tumors of the Liver
Lange JF, Leese T, Castaing D, Bismuth H (Hôp Paul Brousse, Université Paris-Sud, Villejuif, France)
Surg Gynecol Obstet 169:119–126, 1989   23–4

Between 1972 and 1987, 34 repeat hepatectomies were performed for recurrent malignant tumors of the liver in 28 patients. There was no operative mortality. The morbidity rate was 15%, and none of the patients experienced postoperative hepatic insufficiency. Only 5 of the repeat hepatectomies involved 3 or more hepatic segments. Thirteen repeat hepatectomies were performed on 11 patients with hepatocellular carcinoma. The interval between primary and repeat hepatectomy was less than 1 year in 7 patients. Serial measurements of serum α-fetoprotein levels and ultrasound were valuable adjuncts to management. Four patients were alive during a mean follow-up of 33 months (range, 11–48 months); only 1 had tumor recurrence.

Ten repeat hepatectomies were performed in 9 patients with colorectal metastases. All but 1 of the recurrent tumors was discovered during the first 2 years after the primary hepatectomy. Five patients were still alive, 1 with recurrent disease, during a mean follow-up of 13 months (range, 6–41 months). Three of 4 patients who died had multiple hepatic metastases at initial hepatectomy.

Eleven resections were performed on 8 patients with recurrent miscellaneous malignant tumors. Four were alive at a mean follow-up of 28 months (range, 20–36 months), including 3 with recurrent disease. Two patients who underwent repeat hepatectomy for endocrine hepatic metastases were both alive.

Repeat hepatectomies for recurrent malignant tumors of the liver are technically highly feasible. Segmentectomy is the operation of choice. The results are beneficial in a minority of patients, particularly in those with hepatocellular carcinoma, colorectal metastases, and endocrine tumor metastases.

▶ The demonstration that some, although admittedly few, of the patients are alive and tumor free for more than 2 years provides evidence that the procedure is reasonable. Griffith et al. (1) reported 9 patients who underwent repeat liver resection for isolated hepatic recurrence. The median follow-up was 21 months. Five of the patients were free of recurrent disease in 9, 19, 31, 50, and 67 months after their second hepatic resection.— S.I. Schwartz, M.D.

Reference

1. Griffith KD, et al: *Surgery* 107:101, 1990.

Surgical Therapy for Recurrent Liver Metastases From Colorectal Cancer
Stone MD, Cady B, Jenkins RL, McDermott WV, Steele GD Jr (New England Deaconess Hosp, Boston)
Arch Surg 125:718–722, 1990   23–5

Forty percent of the patients with recurrent disease after hepatic resection for liver metastases from colorectal cancer will initially have only liver metastases. Data were reviewed on experience with repeated surgical treatment for liver-only recurrence after previous hepatic resection for colorectal metastases.

Six women and 4 men aged 45–67 years underwent repeated hepatic procedures. The primary colon cancer stage was A in 2 patients, C1 in 2, C4 in 4, and D in 1; the stage was not known in 1 patient. Intraoperative ultrasound enabled identification of 3 unsuspected metastases and determination of unresectability of 2 metastases during 11 procedures. The initial hepatic surgeries included 5 anatomical lobectomies, 1 extended left-sided lobectomy, 2 wedge resections, a left lateral segmentectomy, and a right trisegmentectomy. The second hepatic procedures included 1 lobectomy and 8 wedge resections of 1 or 2 lesions.

Three patients were disease free at 31, 41, and 48 months, respectively, after the first procedure and at 15, 31, and 43 months after the second. Five patients were still free of hepatic disease at last follow-up. Patients whose initial metastases were less than 6 cm in diameter and had single liver recurrences after hepatic resection were apparently the best candidates for additional surgery.

These findings and a review of the literature suggest that surgical treatment of recurrent liver metastases from colorectal cancer is feasible and safe. This treatment approach is associated with long-term disease-free survival in up to 38% of carefully selected patients.

▶ Results of a multi-institutional study describe indications for resection of colorectal carcinoma metastatic to the liver (1). The finding of a 33% 5-year survival provides substantial evidence that the procedure is indicated. Huguet et al. (2) reported on repeated hepatic resection for primary metastatic carcinoma of the liver; the 3-year actuarial survival was 64%, and the mortality rate was 5%. I have personally removed recurrent hepatic metastases in 3 patients after major hepatic resection. All 3 patients remain alive 6 months, 1 year, and 3 years subsequent to the re-resection. In view of the low mortality associated with hepatic resection, it is reasonable to adopt an aggressive attitude in selected cases.—S.I. Schwartz, M.D.

References

1. Hughes KS, et al: *Surgery* 103:278, 1988.
2. Huguet C, et al: *Surg Gynecol Obstet* 171:398, 1990.

Central Bisegmentectomy of the Liver: Experience in 16 Patients
Hasegawa H, Makuuchi M, Yamazaki S, Gunvén P (Natl Cancer Ctr Hosp, Tokyo)
World J Surg 13:786–790, 1989   23–6

Central bisegmentectomy of the liver, or "central hepatectomy," involves en bloc removal of the left medial and right anterior segments of the organ. The procedure was performed in 14 patients with hepatocellular carcinoma (HCC) and mild to moderate liver dysfunction. Two other patients had metachronous liver metastases of rectal cancer.

In later cases a hemihepatic vascular occlusion technique was used to reduce bleeding and conserve partial perfusion of the lifer. Operating times ranged from 5 to 11 hours and blood loss from .6 to 7.5 liters.

One patient who previously had undergone hepatic artery embolization died postoperatively with multiple bleeding ulcers. Complications included 2 bile leaks and a low-grade wound infection. Four patients were alive 5–11 years after hepatectomy without evidence of disease. The overall median survival presently is 34 months. Two patients are alive with recurrent tumor.

Central bisegmentectomy remains indicated for HCC and metastatic disease involving the central segments of the liver where it is necessary to preserve hepatic function. The operation may be suitable when there are contraindications to extended right or left bisegmentectomy or trisegmentectomy.

▶ This is truly a technical feat for which the authors should be complimented. The survival data are most encouraging. The effects of preoperative chemotherapy or embolization are certainly not defined by the data. One of the issues related to the management of malignant hepatic tumors is the preoperative assessment. I agree with the findings of Sitzmann et al. (1) that our best predictive yield for the choice of operative procedure is also achieved with arteriographically enhanced CT. The other issue related to technique is concerned with the effect of hemodilution on transfusion requirements of the liver resection. Sejourne and associates (2) have demonstrated that intraoperative hemodilution in patients undergoing liver resection reduces the requirements for all blood products without increasing the complication rate.—S.I. Schwartz, M.D.

References

1. Sitzmann JV, et al: *Am J Surg* 159:137, 1990.
2. Sejourne P, et al: *Lancet* 2:1380–1382, 1989.

Long-Term Injection Sclerotherapy Treatment for Esophageal Varices: A 10-Year Prospective Evaluation
Terblanche J, Kahn D, Bornman PC (Univ of Cape Town; Groote Schuur Hosp, Cape Town, South Africa)
Ann Surg 210:725–731, 1989   23–7

The role of injection sclerotherapy in the long-term management of patients with acute variceal bleeding remains controversial. The results of long-term injection sclerotherapy were assessed in 245 patients treated between 1975 and 1985.

The study included 169 men and 76 women whose mean age was 46 years. Alcoholic (57%) and cryptogenic (16%) cirrhosis were the main causes of portal hypertension. Within 3 months of entering the study, 105 patients died; outcome was thus assessed in the 140 remaining patients.

Esophageal varices were eradicated in 123 (88%) of the final study group. A median of 5 injections during a mean of 9.25 months were necessary for eradication. In 37 patients varices recurred after a mean of

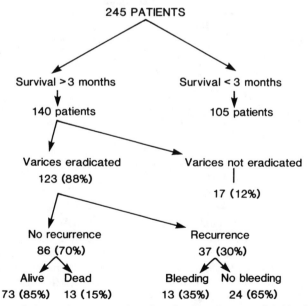

Fig 23–2.—Eradication and recurrence of esophageal varices. (Courtesy of Terblanche J, Kahn D, Bornman PC: *Ann Surg* 210:725–731, 1989.)

15.7 months. Further variceal bleeding was common in these patients (35%). At the end of the study, 73 patients were alive with a clear esophagus at a mean of 21.6 months after eradication (Fig 23–2). Complications were common; 1 in 4 sclerotherapy treatments was followed by a complication. Follow-up endoscopy revealed mucosal slough or local ulceration at the injection site in 114 patients, but this condition rarely led to serious problems. An injection site leak occurred in 17 patients. Rupture of the esophagus, the most serious complication, occurred in 4 patients who were injected electively, 2 of whom died.

Survival rates were 54% at 1 year and 29% at 5 years. Liver failure was the most common cause of death. The Pugh-Child's risk grade and number of variceal bleeds before entering the study influenced prognosis; patients with first bleeds had a lower rate of survival. Patients whose varices are difficult to eradicate should undergo either a portosystemic shunt or a devascularization and transection procedure.

▶ The rate of eradication of esophageal varices with sclerotherapy is extremely impressive. Santangelo et al. (1) demonstrated that prophylactic sclerotherapy of large varices in patients with chronic alcoholic cirrhosis would not provide any clinical benefit. Garrett et al. (2) indicate that, although sclerotherapy may successfully control hemorrhage, the influence of this therapy on long-term survival is limited. Spina and associates (3) reported a prospective controlled trial comparing endoscopic sclerotherapy with the distal splenorenal shunt in the elective treatment of variceal hemorrhage in cirrhotic patients. Preliminary data seem to indicate that a distal splenorenal shunt in patients with good liver function prevents variceal bleeding more effectively than endoscopic sclerotherapy, but there is no difference in survival between the 2 groups.—S.I. Schwartz, M.D.

References

1. Santangelo WG, et al: *J Med* 318:814, 1988.
2. Garrett, KO, et al: *Surgery* 104:813, 1988.
3. Spinar GP, et al: *Am Surg* 211:178, 1989.

Current Status of the Distal Splenorenal Shunt in China
Jin G (Zhejiang Med Univ, Hangzhou, Zhejiang, China)
Am J Surg 160:93–97, 1990   23–8

Bleeding from esophageal varices is the second major cause of upper gastrointestinal tract hemorrhage in China. Animal studies have shown that high-pressure gastroesophageal venous blood can be shunted by way of the short gastric and splenic veins. The first distal splenorenal shunt (DSRS) was performed in China in 1979. The preliminary results and current status of DSRS in China were reviewed.

In 1979–1989, the DSRS was performed in 302 patients with esophagogastric varices. Of 249 patients classified, 112 were in Child's class A,

97 in class B, and 40 in class C. Portal hypertension was caused by post-hepatic cirrhosis in 217 patients, schistosomiasis in 28, alcoholic cirrhosis in 3, and biliary cirrhosis in 1. Therapeutic selective shunts were performed in 200 patients with variceal bleeding; 102 received prophylactic shunts. Emergency surgery was performed in 10 patients. The original Warren shunt was performed in 264 patients, with various modifications applied in another 38; 202 patients had simultaneous ligation of the splenic artery. Overall, the operative death rate was 6%. After 3 months to 10 years of follow-up, there was an 8% recurrent bleeding rate, a 1% incidence of encephalopathy, and a survival rate of 72.3% to 100%.

The DSRS is safe and effective in the treatment of esophagogastric variceal bleeding. It can also be performed prophylactically in patients with Child's class A or B disease.

▶ This encouraging report is highlighted by an extremely low incidence of encephalopathy. This is doubtless related to the extent of the hepatocellular dysfunction and also to the fact that only 3 of the patients had alcoholic cirrhosis. Experience throughout the world suggests that the DSRS is particularly appropriate in nonalcoholic patients with lower degrees of dysfunction. In patients with advanced hepatocele dysfunction, in our experience, the incidence of encephalopathy varied little regardless of the shunt employed.—S.I. Schwartz, M.D.

Peritoneovenous Shunting as Compared With Medical Treatment in Patients With Alcoholic Cirrhosis and Massive Ascites
Stanley MM, Ochi S, Lee KK, Nemchausky BA, Greenlee HB, Allen JI, Allen MJ, Baum RA, Gadacz TR, Camara DS, Caruana JA, Schiff ER, Livingstone AS, Samanta AK, Najem AZ, Glick ME, Juler GL, Adham N, Baker JD, Cain GD, Jordan PH, Wolf DC, Fulenwider JT, James KE, and the VA Cooperative Study on Treatment of Alcoholic Cirrhosis With Ascites (VA Med Ctr, Hines, Ill)
N Engl J Med 321:1632–1638, 1989   23–9

The best management for patients with alcoholic cirrhosis who have marked ascites remains uncertain. A total of 299 men seen in a 5.5-year period with alcoholic cirrhosis and persistent or recurrent severe ascites were randomized to receive either intensive medical treatment or the LeVeen peritoneovenous shunt. Patients with normal or only mildly abnormal liver function were placed in risk group 1; those with more marked dysfunction or previous complications made up group 2, and those with severe prerenal azotemia without kidney disease were placed in group 3. Survival curves for the 3 risk groups are shown in Figure 23–3.

Twenty-five patients assigned to medical management eventually received shunts. The median time to resolution of ascites was 5.5 weeks in patients treated medically and 3 weeks in patients who had surgery. Time to recurrence of ascites was much prolonged in the surgical group. Hospital times were longer for medically treated patients. The incidence of

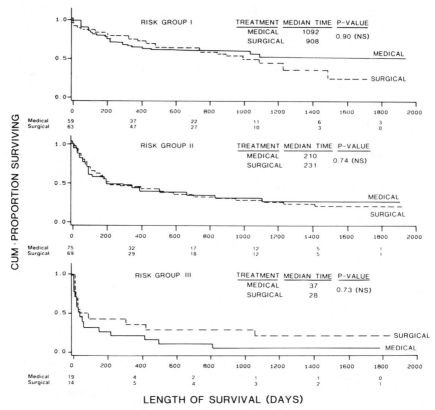

LENGTH OF SURVIVAL (DAYS)

Fig 23–3.—Survival curves for patients treated medically and surgically in 3 risk groups. Survival was not changed by treatment. However, median length of survival differed significantly between risk groups. *Abbreviation: NS,* not significant. (Courtesy of Stanley MM, Ochi S, Lee KK, et al: *N Engl J Med* 321:1632–1638, 1989.)

infection, gastrointestinal bleeding, and encephalopathy was comparable in the medical and surgical groups.

The LeVeen shunt provides greater relief of ascites in a shorter time than does intensive medical care, and ascites recurs more rapidly in the latter patients. Overall mortality is similar with both approaches. Peritoneovenous shunting is indicated when ascites is not adequately managed medically.

▶ The conclusions of this article suggest that peritoneal venous shunting does provide a cost-effective method of managing these patients. Once the intractability of ascites has been defined, it seems appropriate to provide for peritoneal venous shunting. Although it was not demonstrated that postoperative coagulopathy is eliminated by removal of ascitic fluid during the operation, it is of interest that there is little disadvantage in removing that fluid and replacing it with saline.—S.I. Schwartz, M.D.

Technique and Preliminary Results of Extracorporeal Liver Surgery (Bench Procedure) and of Surgery on the In Situ Perfused Liver
Pichlmayr R, Grosse H, Hauss J, Gubernatis G, Lamesch P, Bretschneider HJ
(Medizinischen Hochschule Hannover; Univ of Göttingen, Germany)
Br J Surg 77:21–26, 1990   23–10

Advances in the field of hepatic transplantation have made possible new surgical methods of treating liver disease. Data were reviewed on 9 patients who underwent ex situ operation of the liver and 3 who underwent surgery on an in situ hypothermic perfused liver after vascular isolation (table).

For the ex situ approach, the principles used were those of liver grafting, with a number of variations. Bypass is mandatory because there is always an anhepatic period of several hours. All patients had venovenous bypass from the portal vein and inferior vena cava to the axillary vein. Hypothermic liver perfusion was performed in situ after clamping of the suprahepatic and subhepatic vena cava and dissection above the subhepatic clamp.

In ex situ surgical procedures on the liver, small arterial branches or essential liver veins must be preserved. Vascular interruption must be avoided in those areas of the organ to be preserved. Such an error led to death in 1 patient. When the essential structures to be preserved are freed, liver resection can then be performed in the conventional manner. In patients undergoing vascular isolation and in situ hypothermic perfusion, complete dissection of the posterior wall of the retrohepatic vein is performed. The suprahepatic vena cava need not be dissected from the diaphragm. Hypothermic perfusion with HTK-Bretschneider solution always followed incision or transection of the portal vein, and the arterial system was clamped, not perfused. Individual findings governed the method of resection.

Initial experience with the ex situ technique suggests its value in patients with hepatocellular tumors or metastases who do not have severe impairment of liver function or bile secretion. In situ hypothermic infusion may be applicable to resections in regions where preservation of an essential hepatic vein is critical, or in atypical resections in the depth of the liver.

▶ This is a description of an elegant surgical technique, but one that has rare applicability. It is hard to imagine that any of the malignant tumors would have been cured by this approach. One would wonder whether the huge focal nodular hyperplasia could not have been enucleated with inflow occlusion if necessary, even leaving part of the tumor. I realize it is a philosophical issue, but there does come a time when a good operation should be limited because it does not provide appropriately good results.— S.I. Schwartz, M.D.

Operations and Follow-up Data After ex Situ Operation on the Liver in 9 Patients

Patient no.	Age (years)	Diagnosis	Indication group*	Operation	Operation time† (h)	Intraoperative complications	Maximum ischaemic damage		Postoperative follow-up
							SGOT (units/litre)	GLDH (units/litre)	
1a	40	Metastasis from leiomyosarcoma Extrahepatic metastasis	III	Segmental resection (II, III, V, VI, VII, VIII) (4·5 kg) Reimplantation of segments I and IV	16 (6)	Bleeding	740	560	Uneventful Good palliation Discharged after 8 weeks
2a	46	Multiple metastases (colonic carcinoma)	III	Segmental resection (V, VI, wedge VII)	15 (5)	None	450	40	Uneventful ?Palliation Discharged after 2 weeks
3a	52	Klatskin tumour Recurrent cholangitis	III	Right extended hemihepatectomy (trisegmentectomy) Partial resection and reconstruction of inferior vena cava	12 (4)	None	19	180	Reduced liver function during 2 weeks Discharged after 4 weeks
4a	58	Metastasis of colonic carcinoma Infiltration of vena cava Cholestasis Post non-A, non-B hepatitis	III	Right extended hemihepatectomy (trisegmentectomy) Reconstruction of inferior vena cava	11 (7)	Delayed reperfusion	27	250	Hepatic insufficiency Sepsis Died after 44 days
5a	30	Huge focal nodular hyperplasia in segment IV Compression of inferior vena cava	II	Segmental resection (I, IV)	11 (4)	None	80	60	Uneventful Discharged after 2 weeks

6a	57	Sigmoid carcinoma Infiltration of right hepatic vein	III	Left extended hemihepatectomy (2 kg)	11 (6)	None	678	1150	Delayed recovery Discharged after 8 weeks
7a	48	Klatskin tumour with extrahepatic metastasis Cholestasis	III	Left extended hemihepatectomy Gastrectomy Pancreatectomy, splenectomy Reconstruction of hepatic artery (saphenous vein interposition)	16 (6)	Delayed reperfusion of segment V	792	1243	Hepatic insufficiency, transplantation, sepsis, multiple organ failure Died after 50 days
8a	62	Klatskin tumour with infiltration of left and right portal vein Cholestasis	II	Hilar resection Reconstruction of portal vein	18 (9)	Bad reperfusion oedema	984	362	Hepatic insufficiency, transplantation after 22 h Remains in critical condition
9a	54	Klatskin tumour with moderate cholestasis	II	Right extended hemihepatectomy (trisegmentectomy) Reconstruction of hepatic artery and portal vein	13 (4)	Delayed reperfusion	770	1000	Deterioration of liver function on 3rd day, requiring liver transplantation on the 17th postoperative day Retransplantation 2 days later (initial non-functioning organ) Sepsis, multiple organ failure Died on 23rd day

Abbreviations: SGOT, serum glutamic oxaloacetic transaminase; *GLDH*, glutamic lactate dehydrogenase.
*See Table 3 of original article.
†Values in parentheses show the length of the anhepatic phase of the operation.
(Courtesy of Pichlmayr R, Grosse H, Hauss J, et al: *Br J Surg* 77:21–26, 1990.)

Current Management of the Budd-Chiari Syndrome

Klein AS, Sitzmann JV, Coleman J, Herlong FH, Cameron JL (Johns Hopkins Med Insts)

Ann Surg 212:144–149, 1990   23–11

The Budd-Chiari syndrome, which results from hepatic venous outflow occlusion, is rare but often fatal. Numerous surgical procedures have been proposed for decompression of the congested liver by converting the portal vein into an outflow tract.

In a 15-year period, 26 patients were treated. The median age at diagnosis was 37 years; 21 were female. Nine had polycythemia vera; 6 were taking estrogen therapy; 5 had previous hepatitis A or B infection; and 4 had cirrhosis. The most common presenting feature was ascites. Hepatic function at diagnosis was only slightly abnormal. Hepatic vein catheterization confirmed the diagnosis of the Budd-Chiari syndrome in all cases. Inferior vena cavography revealed caval occlusion in 4 patients, significant caval obstruction in 13, and a normal vena cava in 9. The diagnosis and treatment are outlined in the chart.

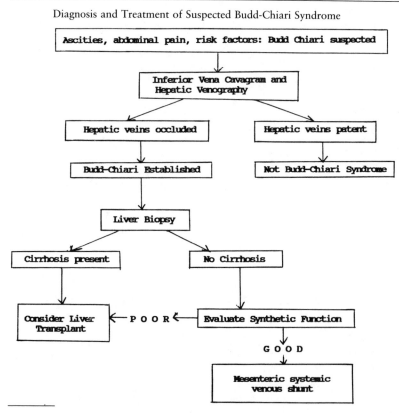

Diagnosis and Treatment of Suspected Budd-Chiari Syndrome

(Courtesy of Klein AS, Sitzmann JV, Coleman J, et al: *Ann Surg* 212:144–149, 1990.)

Interpretation of the vena cavogram was useful for selecting appropriate surgical procedures. Twenty-three patients had percutaneous liver biopsy before surgery with no morbidity or mortality; well-established cirrhosis was noted on biopsy in 4 cases. Thirty mesenteric-systemic venous shunts were done on all patients. In 11, a mesocaval shunt was performed. In 1 case, conversion to a mesoatrial shunt was required as a second procedure. A mesoatrial shunt was done as the initial procedure in 15 patients. Graft thrombosis in 2 of these patients prompted 1 and 2 revisions, respectively.

Hospital mortality was 31%. The other 18 patients were discharged well with patent shunts. Follow-up ranged from 9 months to 13 years (median, 43 months). Five patients died between 5 months and 84 months after surgery. The 3- and 5-year actuarial survival rates were 65% and 59%, respectively.

Untreated hepatic venous thrombosis leads to progressive liver failure and death. Most patients with the Budd-Chiari syndrome can be safely, successfully treated with appropriate selection of mesocaval shunt, mesoatrial shunt, or orthotopic liver transplantation.

▶ Recently Orloff and Girard (1) reported on the long-term results with side-to-side portal caval shunt. Of thirteen patients subjected to the operation, eleven were alive and well 3-16 years after the operation. All were free of acites without diuretic therapy. Hepatic function returned to normal in all but two. No patient had portalsystemic encephalopathy.—S.I. Schwartz, M.D.

Reference

1. Orloff MJ, Girard B: *Surg Gynecol Obstet* 168:33, 1989.

Liver Transplantation for the Budd-Chiari Syndrome

Halff G, Todo S, Tzakis AG, Gordon RD, Starzl TE (Univ of Pittsburgh; VA Med Ctr, Pittsburgh)
Ann Surg 211:43–49, 1990   23–12

The Budd-Chiari syndrome encompasses a spectrum of diseases ranging from a veno occlusive disorder with small vessel occlusion to thrombosis of the major hepatic and/or inferior vena cava. Treatments range from anticoagulation to liver transplantation. Data on 23 patients who underwent orthotopic liver transplantation for Budd-Chiari syndrome with end-stage liver disease were reviewed retrospectively. Patients were followed for up to 14 years.

There were no serious complications or postoperative anticoagulation. Budd-Chiari syndrome recurred in 3 patients, all of whom died. No other patient had evidence of recurrent Budd-Chiari syndrome in postoperative liver biopsy specimens. The actuarial survival rates were 68.8% at 1 year, 44.7% at 3 years, and 44.7% at 5 years. These rates were not statistically different from those of previously reported studies.

Orthotopic liver transplantation for Budd-Chiari syndrome can be performed with acceptable rates of morbidity and mortality. It is the treatment of choice for patients with end-stage liver disease and Budd-Chiari syndrome. The best treatment for patients with Budd-Chiari syndrome and intermediate degrees of liver failure has not yet been established.

▶ The finding of recurrent disease is an interesting one that warrants investigation. Jennings et al. (1) reported a (2)-stage approach to the surgical management of the acute Budd-Chiari syndrome complicated by inferior vena caval obstruction. This entailed initial hepatic decompression by a subhepatic meso-atrial shunt with subsequent takedown of that shunt combined with conversion to an intrahepatic portacaval shunt. Klein and Cameron (2) indicated that most cases are amenable to mesocaval and mesoatrial shunting, and only those patients with documented cirrhosis or fulminant hepatic failure should be managed by orthotopic liver transplantation.— S.I. Schwartz, M.D.

References

1. Jennings RH, et al: *Surg Gynecol Obstet* 169:501, 1989.
2. Klein AS, Cameron JL: *Am J Surg* 160:128, 1990.

The Management of Splenic Trauma in a Trauma System
Molin MR, Shackford SR (Univ of California, San Diego; Univ of Vermont, Burlington)
Arch Surg 125:840–843, 1990   23–13

The splenic salvage rates in adults after splenic trauma treated at large teaching hospitals ranges from 40% to 50%. To determine whether similar rates could be achieved in community trauma centers that see a lower volume of splenic injuries, have a greater number of surgeons managing trauma victims, and treat a higher percentage of blunt injuries 117, patients with splenic injury treated at a level I center and 311 patients treated at 4 level II centers in 1984–1988 were studied. Splenectomy was performed in 252 (59%) patients and splenorrhaphy in 160 (37%); 16 (4%) patients were observed. Splenic injury was diagnosed by peritoneal lavage in 69%, CT in 20%, physical examination in 9%, and other methods in 2%. Treated patients included 24 with grade I injury, 70 with grade II, 74 with grade III, 8 with grade IV, and 252 with grade V.

The splenic salvage rate at the level I center was 50%, compared with only 38% at the level II centers. However, selective splenorrhaphy was successful at the level II centers in which the volume of splenic injury was lower.

Selective splenorrhaphy can be safely applied at community trauma centers even if the patient volume is relatively low. It is associated with fewer septic complications than splenectomy and requires less transfusion. The rate of splenic salvage improves with experience.

▶ This is another in a series of articles demonstrating that many patients can be managed without splenectomy and thus without increasing the risk of postsplenectomy sepsis. Villalba et al. (1) recently reported 51 consecutive adult patients with ruptured spleens sustained from blunt trauma. Two thirds of them were hemodynamically stabilized at the time of admission and placed on a regimen of bed rest. Nonoperative treatment was successful in 97% of those patients. There have been no long-term sequelae.—S.I. Schwartz, M.D.

Reference

1. Villalba M, et al: *Arch Surg* 125:836, 1990.

Nonoperative Management of Blunt Splenic Trauma: A Multicenter Experience
Cogbill TH, Moore EE, Jurkovich GJ, Morris JA, Mucha P Jr, Shackford SR and co-investigators Stolee RT, Moore FA, Pilcher S, LoCicero R, Farnell MB, Molin M (Gundersen/Lutheran Med Ctr, La Crosse, Wis; Denver Gen Hosp; Univ of Colorado; Harborview Med Ctr; Univ of Washington; et al)
J Trauma 29:1312–1317, 1989   23–14

Many splenic injuries once treated by splenectomy are now managed with nonoperative techniques because of the lifelong risk of overwhelming infection after splenectomy. Although salvage techniques have been accepted for selected pediatric splenic injuries, some reports have discouraged the use of such methods in adults. A multicenter study evaluated outcome in 112 patients treated during a 5-year period with splenic salvage techniques.

The patient group represented 14% of the blunt splenic injuries treated at 6 institutions during the study period. Nonoperative management was defined as the intentional observation of a proven splenic injury. The patients ranged in age from 1 to 83 years; 40 (36%) were younger than age 16 years. On the splenic organ injury scale (table), 28 (25%) were class I, 51 (45%) class II, 31 (28%) class III, and 2 (2%) class IV. No splenic injury was class V. Only 25% of the patients were free of associated injuries.

Ninety-nine patients (88%) were successfully treated without surgery. Twelve of the 13 failures were caused by ongoing hemorrhage, sudden hematocrit decrease, or localized abdominal pain and tenderness. The failure rate was higher in adults (17%) than in children (2%). The overall mortality was 3%, and none of the 4 deaths resulted from the splenic or other intra-abdominal injury. Nonoperative management had a higher success rate in patients with class I–class II injuries than in patients with class III–class IV injuries.

Splenic salvage techniques are appropriate and successful when certain criteria are followed. Patients selected should have no hemodynamic instability after minimal initial fluid resuscitation. Class I–III splenic trauma must be confirmed by imaging techniques, and associated abdom-

Splenic Organ Injury Scale

Class I	Nonexpanding subcapsular hematoma <10% surface area.
	Nonbleeding capsular laceration with <1 cm deep parenchymal involvement.
Class II	Nonexpanding subcapsular hematoma 10–50% surface area.
	Nonexpanding intraparenchymal hematoma <2 cm in diameter.
	Bleeding capsular tear or parenchymal laceration 1–3 cm deep without trabecular vessel involvement.
Class III	Expanding subcapsular or intraparenchymal hematoma.
	Bleeding subcapsular hematoma or subcapsular hematoma >50% surface area.
	Intraparenchymal hematoma >2 cm in diameter.
	Parenchymal laceration >3 cm deep or involving trabecular vessels.
Class IV	Ruptured intraparenchymal hematoma with active bleeding.
	Laceration involving segmental or hilar vessels producing major (>25% splenic volume) devascularization.
Class V	Completely shattered or avulsed spleen.
	Hilar laceration which devascularizes entire spleen.

(Courtesy of Cogbill TH, Moore EE, Jurkovich GJ, et al: *J Trauma* 29:1312–1317, 1989.)

inal organ injury should be excluded by physical examination and CT with oral and intravenous contrast.

▶ This provides a database on which we can judge our own hospital performance. Pickhardt et al. (1) assessed a 10-year period in which 314 adults had splenic injury identified at emergency laparotomy. There were blunt injuries in 72% of the patients. In 1978 splenorrhaphy was accomplished in only 29% of patients; the operative splenic salvage rate rose to 63%. Grade 4 disrupture required splenectomy in 88% of cases; most patients with grades 1, 2, and 3 injuries could be managed with suturing techniques or application of hemostatic gauges.—S.I. Schwartz, M.D.

Reference

1. Pickhardt B, et al: *J Trauma* 29:1386, 1989.

HIV-1-Associated Thrombocytopenia: The Role of Splenectomy

Tyler DS, Shaunak S, Bartlett JA, Iglehart JD (Duke Univ)
Ann Surg 211:211–217, 1990   23–15

Thrombocytopenia often occurs in patients with HIV-1. The safety of splenectomy in 8 patients with HIV-1-associated thrombocytopenia (HAT) and its role in seropositive patients who become thrombocytopenic were investigated.

One patient responded completely, 5 responded partially, and 2 did not respond to treatment. None of the patients died during surgery, and perioperative morbidity was minimal. The HIV-1 infection did not progress to AIDS or AIDS-related complex after splenectomy in any of the asymptomatic patients. There was no increase in susceptibility to infections by encapsulated organisms as a result of splenectomy after a mean follow-up of 13.25 months. Data on 79 other patients reported in the literature were also reviewed. The response rate among these patients appeared to be greater than in the present series. An algorithm was developed to define the role of splenectomy in patients with HAT (Fig 23–4).

Although patients with HAT tolerated splenectomy well, the long-term follow-up data on these patients suggest that complete responses are not common. Therefore, splenectomy should be reserved for patients with medically refractory HAT.

▶ The algorithm presented by this group is an appropriate one. The criteria for splenectomy applied to patients with idiopathic thrombocytopenic purpura should be essentially the same as those applied to patients with HAT. As the authors point out, their finding that complete responses are uncommon in this group of patients is counter to other reports (1).—S.I. Schwartz, M.D.

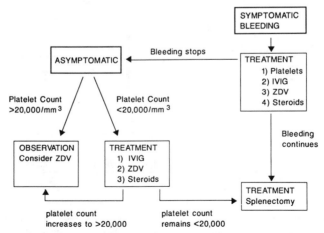

Fig 23–4.—Algorithm for the treatment of patients with HIV-1-associated thrombocytopenia. (Courtesy of Tyler DS, Shaunak S, Bartlett JA, et al: *Ann Surg* 211:211–217, 1990.)

Reference

1. Ferguson CM: *Surg Gynecol Obstet* 167:300, 1988.

Splenectomy for Hypersplenism in Chronic Lymphocytic Leukaemia and Malignant non-Hodgkin's Lymphoma
Delpero JR, Houvenaeghel G, Gastaut JA, Orsoni P, Blache JL, Guerinel G, Carcassonne Y (Inst of Cancer, Marseille, France)
Br J Surg 77:443–449, 1990   23–16

The value of splenectomy in the management of malignant lymphoma remains controversial. Sixty-two patients with splenomegaly and presumed hypersplenism complicating chronic lymphocytic leukemia (CLL) or malignant non-Hodgkin's lymphoma (NHL) were studied. Massive splenomegaly occurred in 34 patients. Forty-nine patients had a platelet

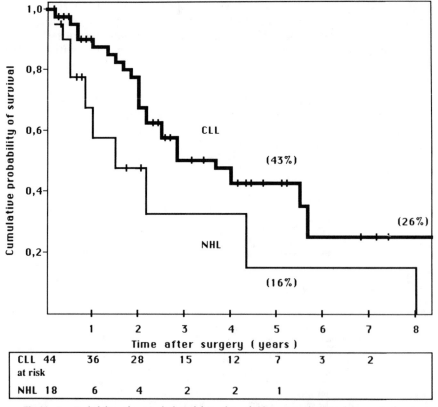

| CLL 44 at risk | 36 | 28 | 15 | 12 | 7 | 3 | 2 |
| NHL 18 | 6 | 4 | 2 | 2 | 1 | | |

Fig 23–5.—Probability of survival plotted from date of splenectomy for 44 splenectomized patients with chronic lymphocytic leukemia, 1 postoperative death, and 3 deaths unrelated to leukemia are included, and 18 splenectomized patients with non-Hodgkin's lymphoma. (Courtesy of Delpero JR, Houvenaeghel G, Gastaut JA, et al: *Br J Surg* 77:443–449, 1990.)

count of less than $100 \times 10^9/L$ and 16 were anemic. Splenectomy was done most often because of failure to respond to medical measures or inability to begin or tolerate adequate chemotherapy (Fig 23–5).

One patient died postoperatively, and 18 had complications. Eighty-nine percent of patients responded within a month of splenectomy, and 63% had an ongoing complete response after a median follow-up of 26 months. Seven patients failed to respond to splenectomy and 15 relapsed. These patients had lower platelet counts preoperatively. Marrow failure did not preclude a complete response to splenectomy. Actuarial 5-year survival rates after splenectomy were 43% in the group with CLL and 16% in patients with NHL.

Splenectomy may be a worthwhile palliative measure in lymphoproliferative disorders (e.g., CLL and NHL). It may allow patients to resume or begin full-dose chemotherapy, and may preclude the need for immediate treatment in some patients. Those who respond well may have a better chance of surviving.

▶ There is general agreement that splenectomy can offer effective palliation for these patients. Kehoe et al. (1) presented a review of 46 patients with non-Hodgkin's lymphoma having palliative splenectomy. The median survival was 18 months, with 2-year and 5-year survivals of 44% and 26%, respectively. Splenectomy generally provided satisfactory reversal of hematologic abnormalities. Friedman et al. (2) recently reported benefits related to reversal of thrombocytopenia and improved survival, and ability to tolerate chemotherapy, in patients with systemic mass cell disease.— S.I. Schwartz, M.D.

References

1. Kehoe JE, et al: *Cancer* 55:1256, 1985.
2. Friedman B, et al: *Surgery* 107:94, 1990.

Elective Subtotal Splenectomy: Indications and Results in 33 Patients
Guzzetta PC, Ruley EJ, Merrick HFW, Verderese C, Barton N (Children's Natl Med Ctr, Washington, DC; George Washington Univ; NIH, Bethesda, Md)
Ann Surg 211:34–42, 1990   23–17

The risk of postsplenectomy sepsis has made preservation of splenic function desirable whenever possible. The results of elective subtotal splenectomy were reviewed in 33 patients (30 children and 3 adults) operated on between 1981 and 1989. Twenty patients had the procedure to prevent azathioprine-induced neutropenia after renal transplantation, and 9 had the procedure because of type I Gaucher disease. Miscellaneous indications included cholesteryl ester storage disease, chronic myelogenous leukemia, thalassemia major, and splenic cyst.

There were no operative deaths, and no reoperation was necessary because of bleeding. Thirty patients (91%) had a functioning splenic remnant documented by radionuclide scanning. One patient became neutropenic but had no evidence of viral infection; the thalassemic patient improved only transiently. In all other cases the underlying disorder was controlled.

Subtotal splenectomy is an effective and safe procedure in patients with a variety of nontraumatic conditions. Careful surgery, especially if massive splenomegaly is present, can provide long-lasting control of hypersplenism.

▶ Rubin et al. (1) reported 11 children who underwent partial splenectomy for hypersplenism related to Gaucher's disease in an attempt to prevent postsplenectomy sepsis. Hematologic improvement followed partial splenectomy in 7 of 11 patients. No child acquired overwhelming postsplenectomy infection. It is more appropriate to perform partial splenectomy and leave a remnant attached to the splenic artery per se rather than to transpose splenic tissue into the omentum, because the latter does not provide for an appropriate circulation necessary to phagocytize encapsulated bacteria.—S.I. Schwartz, M.D.

Reference

1. Rubin M, et al: *J Pediatr Surg* 21:125, 1986.

24 The Biliary Tract

Ambulatory Cholecystectomy Without Disability
Ledet WP Jr (West Calcasiu Hosp, Sulphur, La)
Arch Surg 125:1434–1435, 1990   24–1

To examine the feasibility of ambulatory cholecystectomy, data were analyzed on 200 consecutive outpatient cholecystectomies done during 4 years at a small community hospital. The procedure involved minor modifications of the usual cholecystectomy procedure so that it could be done easily by general surgeons.

Technique.—The incision is a right-upper-quadrant transverse abdominal skin crease incision, varying in length from 5 to 10 cm. Each abdominal wound layer is closed with running sutures of blue monofilament polybutester. Each layer is injected with a solution of .25% bupivacaine hydrochloride with epinephrine bitartrate. The rectus abdominus muscle is injected with 30 mg of long-acting dexamethasone sodium phosphate diluted in 20 mL of normal saline and 10 mL of .25% bupivacaine and epinephrine. Prochlorperazine maleate was given as one 15-mg spansule every 6 hours for the first 48 hours. Patients were followed by telephone after discharge 2 times a day for the first 5 or 6 days.

All patients in this series were discharged within 3–10 hours after the procedure. About 20% complained of nausea after discharge, and about 5% of these had some vomiting. There were no cases of wound infection, hernia, thrombophlebitis, or pulmonary embolization.

Ambulatory cholecystectomy can greatly reduce the long- and short-term morbidity associated with this procedure and lead to savings of up to one fourth the cost of a routine inpatient cholecystectomy. It allows the general surgeon to treat patients with cholecystectomies in the manner in which the surgeon is accustomed and still greatly decrease the hospital stay. The morbidity associated with ambulatory cholecystectomy appears to be similar to that of laser laparoscopic cholecystectomy.

▶ This interesting series is relatively unique in its approach to the problem. Outpatient laparoscopic laser cholecystectomy easily represents the more popular approach. Reddick et al. (1) presented their first experience with the procedure, reporting on 83 patients. A patient laparoscopic cholecystectomy, usually performed without a laser, is being done with increasing frequency at all institutions and an increasing number of gallbladders are being removed. The technique has certainly been associated with a low morbidity rate and is well received by patients. There is little question that we are obliged to include the training of laparoscopic cholecystectomy in our residency programs. Whether the procedure is applicable to patients with truly asymptomatic gallstones is not yet defined.—S.I. Schwartz, M.D.

Reference

1. Reddick EJ, et al: *Am J Surg* 160:485, 1990.

Choledochoscopy: A Cost-Minimization Analysis

Nagorney DM, Lohmuller JL (Mayo Clinic and Found, Rochester, Minn)
Ann Surg 211:354–359, 1990   24–2

Although it has been claimed that choledochoscopy for the prevention of retained bile duct stones would be cost effective, no economic evaluations have been performed to confirm this. In a cost-minimization analysis of choledochoscopy as a routine adjunct to common duct exploration, data on 287 patients who had choledochoscopies during surgery for biliary tract calculi in 1981–1987 were reviewed.

Common duct exploration was positive for calculi in 75% of patients. Choledochoscopy detected residual stones after duct exploration in 10%. Residual stones were found after 12.5% of positive duct explorations and after 2.7% of negative duct explorations. Retained stones were noted in 4.5% of the patients postoperatively. Choledochoscopy had a sensitivity of 67%, a specificity of 100%, and a negative predictive value of 95%. The analysis demonstrated that the total cost of either selective or routine choledochoscopy significantly exceeded the total cost of obtaining a stone-free duct for patients with retained stones through extraction

Unsuspected and Retained Stone Rates With Choledochoscopy: Selective Literature Review

Author	Year	Scope Flexible/Rigid	Patients	Unsuspected Stones (%)	Retained Stones (%)
Nora et al.[1]	1977	R	208	25	1.9
Kappas et al.[2]	1979	R	121	18	6.6
Feliciano et al.[3]	1980	R	140	14	8.9
Yap et al.[4]	1980	F	149	14	1.3
Rattner/Warshaw[5]	1981	R	144	24	4
Kappas et al.[6]	1981	R	148	—	1.6
Chen et al.[7]	1983	F	339	24	4.4
Escat et al.[8]	1984	R	380	12	2
Dayton et al.[9]	1984	R	121	—	5.7
Escat et al.[10]	1985	R	441	10	2
Jakimowicz et al.[11]	1986	F	320	7.1	1.6
Markowitz et al.[12]	1987	F	102	—	0
Present series	1989	F & R	287	10.1	4.9

Note: Dash indicates rate undefined.
(Courtesy of Nagorney DM, Lohmuller JL: *Ann Surg* 211:354–359, 1990.)

using a T tube tract or endoscopic papillotomy (table). Choledochoscopy is effective in obtaining a stone-free duct. However, to make its routine or selective use competitive economically, a careful assessment of fee structures is necessary.

▶ There is little question that the modern scenario of medicine will be directed at minimizing the cost. An article such as this will assume greater importance. Choledochoscopy does represent an important addition to the surgery of the biliary tract and should be used selectively. The high success rate associated with extraction of retained stones through the T tube tract and via endoscopic retrograde cholangiopancreatography has appropriately changed the attitude related to cleaning the duct at the initial procedure.—S.I. Schwartz, M.D.

The Effect of Ursodiol on the Efficacy and Safety of Extracorporeal Shock-Wave Lithotripsy of Gallstones: The Dornier National Biliary Lithotripsy Study

Schoenfield LJ, Berci G, Carnovale RL, Casarella W, Caslowitz P, Chumley D, Davis RC, Gillenwater JY, Johnson AC, Jones RS, Jordan LG, et al. (Crawford-Long Hosp, Atlanta; Cedars-Sinai Med Ctr, Los Angeles; Univ of Iowa; Northwestern Mem Hosp, Chicago; Methodist Hosp of Indiana, Indianapolis; et al)
N Engl J Med 323:1239–1245, 1990   24–3

When treating gallstones with extracorporeal shock-wave lithotripsy, clinicians administer the bile acid ursodiol to dissolve the gallstone fragments. The value of this practice was assessed in a 10-center study in which 600 symptomatic patients with 3 or fewer radiolucent gallstones 5–30 mm in diameter were enrolled. Gallstones were visualized by oral cholecystography. The patients were randomly assigned to receive ursodiol or placebo for 6 months beginning 1 week before lithotripsy.

The stones were fragmented in 97% of the patients. The fragments were 5 mm in diameter or smaller in 46.8%. Overall, 21% of the patients receiving ursodiol and 9% receiving placebo had gallbladders free of stones after 6 months. Of those with completely radiolucent stones smaller than 20 mm, 35% receiving ursodiol and 18% receiving placebo were free of stones after 6 months. Biliary pain, usually mild, occurred in 73% of all patients, but this included only 13% of those free of stones after 3 months and 6 months. Few adverse effects were noted. The only side effect occurring with a significantly different frequency in the 2 groups was diarrhea: 32.6% in the ursodiol group were affected, compared with 24.7% in the placebo group.

Extracorporeal shock-wave lithotripsy with ursodiol is more effective than, and is as safe as, lithotripsy alone in the treatment of symptomatic gallstones. Treatment is more effective in patients with solitary compared with multiple stones, with radiolucent rather than slightly calcified stones, and with smaller rather than larger stones.

▶ With the advent of laparoscopic cholecystectomy, the lithotripsy of gallstones is becoming a disappearing modality of therapy. The percentage of patients who become stone free is extremely low, and the percentage of patients who remain stone free is even less. Lithotripsy also does not address the thesis expressed by Langenbush many years ago that the gallbladder is removed not because it contains stones but because it forms stones. Griffith et al. (1) reported an experience in 6 patients with symptomatic gallstones managed with cholecystolithotomy. All stones were cleared after 1 procedure. But there seems to be little advantage to this technique, compared to larparoscopic cholecystectomy. Cotton et al. (2), have reported on their experience with endoscopic laser lithotripsy of large bile duct stones.—S.I. Schwartz, M.D.

References

1. Griffith DP, et al: *Arch Surg* 125:1114, 1990.
2. Cotton PB, et al: *Gastroenterology* 99:1128, 1990.

Emergency Surgery for Severe Acute Cholangitis: The High-Risk Patients
Lai ECS, Tam P-C, Paterson IA, Ng MMT, Fan S-T, Choi T-K, Wong J (Univ of Hong Kong; Queen Mary Hosp, Hong Kong)
Ann Surg 211:55–59, 1990
24–4

Emergency biliary decompression in patients with severe acute cholangitis (SAC) is associated with formidable morbidity and mortality risks. A retrospective record review was conducted to identify the high-risk population among patients with fulminant calculous cholangitis who underwent emergency surgical decompression.

During a 4½-year period, 41 men and 45 women aged 28–97 years with SAC secondary to choledocholithiasis, in whom biliary sepsis was evident despite an adequate trial of conservative therapy, underwent emergency ductal exploration under general anesthesia. Additional procedures included cholecystectomy in 55 patients, cholecystostomy in 5, and transhepatic intubation in 2. Septicemic shock occurred in 55 patients before operation; 30 of these patients were hypotensive at the time of anesthesia induction despite active resuscitation. Hospital mortality was defined as death within the same hospitalization after emergency biliary tract operation, regardless of cause. Patients with primary or metastatic disease as the cause of biliary obstruction were excluded.

Seventeen patients (20%) died and 43 others (50%) had significant postoperative complications; 17 patients had more than 1 complication. Univariate analysis of 14 clinical and 11 biochemical parameters identified 10 variables that significantly correlated with postoperative hospital mortality rates (table). The postoperative outcomes of the 30 patients who remained in septicemic shock before operation was similar to outcomes in patients who were resuscitated successfully.

Multivariate analysis identified 5 variables with independent predictive value, including the presence of concomitant medical problems, pH less than 7.4, total bilirubin more than 90 μmol/L, a platelet count of less than 150×10^9/L, and serum albumin level of less than 30 g/L. Among patients in whom 3 or more risk factors were present, the postoperative

Factors Associated With Postoperative Mortality in Patients With
Severe Acute Cholangitis

Factors	Survival (n = 69)	Died (n = 17)	Probability
Age (yrs)	64 ± 14	73 ± 10	0.02
Platelet ($\times 10^9$/mL)	176 ± 108	98 ± 73	0.01
Urea (mmol/L)	9 ± 10	18 ± 9	0.002
Creatinine (mmol/L)	0.13 ± 0.08	0.23 ± 0.13	0.0001
Albumin (g/L)	36 ± 7.7	31 ± 8.9	0.015
Total bilirubin (μmol/L)	71 ± 2.3	115 ± 1.6	0.03
Duration of fever (hrs)*	6.8 ± 22	1.1 ± 31	0.04
Duration of hypotension (hrs)*	0.02 ± 22	1.24 ± 12	0.03
Percentage of patients with CMP†	26	71	0.002
Percentage of patients with pH <7.40†	17	53	0.006

Note: Values represented mean ± SD. Statistical analysis with 2-tailed Student's *t* test unless specified.
　*Logrithmic transformation.
　†Statistical analysis by χ^2 test with Yates' correction.
　(Courtesy of Lai ECS, Tam P-C, Paterson IA, et al: *Ann Surg* 211:55–59, 1990.)

mortality rate was 55% and the postoperative morbidity rate was 91%. Among patients in whom 2 or fewer risk factors were present, the postoperative mortality rate was 6% and the postoperative morbidity rate, 34%.

Because thrombocytopenia developed even with transient hypotension, timely ductal compression would improve the postoperative outcome in these patients. For the high-risk population, the use of nonoperative biliary drainage by percutaneous or endoscopic approaches as an initial intervention could potentially benefit these patients.

▶ The authors provide a series of risk factors that should suggest nonoperative biliary drainage in a given group of patients at severe risk. Kinoshita et al. (1) reviewed data on 125 patients treated for acute cholangitis. Seven of 11 patients with acute obstructive suppurative cholangitis recovered from shock after percutaneous transhepatic drainage and later successfully underwent surgery. Leese et al. (2) reported results suggesting acute cholangitis be treated by urgent endoscopic biliary decompression after resuscitative measures. Emergency surgery should be reserved for those in whom endoscopic decompression has failed or when they do not improve.—S.I. Schwartz, M.D.

Reference

1. Kinoshita H, et al: *World J Surg* 8:963, 1984.
2. Leese T, et al: *Br J Surg* 73:998, 1986.

Mirizzi Syndrome and Cholecystobiliary Fistula: A Unifying Classification

Csendes A, Díaz JC, Burdiles P, Maluenda F, Nava O (Univ of Chile, Santiago)
Br J Surg 76:1139–1143, 1989   24–5

The Mirizzi syndrome, first described in 1948, was said to consist of the combination of a stone impacted at the neck of the gallbladder or cystic duct and a functional disorder of a putative sphincter within the common hepatic duct. Both are considered to be stages in the evolution of a single pathologic condition. A new classification of patients with Mirizzi syndrome and cholecystobiliary fistula was developed.

Of 17,395 patients operated on for gallstones, 219 (1.3%) were considered to have Mirizzi syndrome and/or a cholecystobiliary fistula. Four evolving stages were defined, ranging from the type I lesion (the original Mirizzi syndrome) to the type IV lesion (presence of a cholecystobiliary fistula with complete destruction of the entire wall of the common bile duct) (Fig 24–1).

Overall, 10.5% of patients had type I lesions and 4.1% had type IV lesions; 41.1% had type II and 44.3% had type III lesions. In type II and III lesions, the fistula involves less than one third or up to two thirds, respectively, of the circumference of the common bile duct. Symptoms included biliary pain, jaundice, and fever. Patients with type III and type IV lesions tended to be older than those with type I and type II lesions (table).

Treatment varies according to type of lesion. Cholecystectomy plus choledochostomy was effective in type I lesions. Type II lesions can be treated by suture of the fistula or choledochoplasty with the remnant of the gallbladder. Choledochoplasty is recommended for type III lesions and bilioenteric anastomosis for type IV. Operative mortality and postoperative morbidity both increase according to the severity of the lesion.

▶ This excellent article provides a reasonable classification of the types of lesions, and the alternatives for surgical repair are most pertinent. Lubbers (1) reported a personal experience with 5 patients and published data from 19 addi-

Clinical Findings on Admission in 219 Patients With External Compression of the Common Bile Duct or Cholecystobiliary Fistula

	Classification			
Clinical findings	Type I (n = 23)	Type II (n = 90)	Type III (n = 97)	Type IV (n = 9)
Mean age (years)	44	42	53	62
Female (%)	65	77	77	100
Duration of symptoms >8 days (%)	43	43	39	55
Biliary pain (%)	100	94	97	100
Jaundice on admission (%)	83	84	92	67
Fever present for previous 5 days (%)	70	57	67	67
Rectal temperature >38°C (%)	35	33	53	34

(Courtesy of Csendes A, Díaz JC, Burdiles P, et al: *Br J Surg* 76:1139–1143, 1989.)

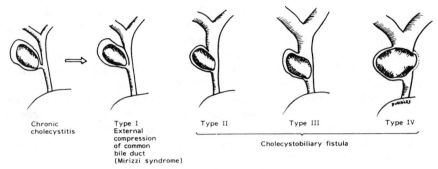

| Chronic cholecystitis | Type I External compression of common bile duct (Mirizzi syndrome) | Type II | Type III | Type IV |

Cholecystobiliary fistula

Fig 24–1.–Stages in the development of the Mirizzi syndrome and cholecystobiliary fistula. (Courtesy of Csendes A, Díaz JC, Burdiles P, et al: *Br J Surg* 76:1139–1143, 1989.)

tional cases. He concluded that involvement of the hepatic duct with gallstone disease may result in a wide variety of lesions of differing severity with no common pattern and suggested that the term "Mirizzi syndrome" has had no well-defined meaning and should be abandoned.—S.I. Schwartz, M.D.

Reference

1. Lubbers EJ: *World J Surg* 7:780, 1983.

Follow-Up 6 to 11 Years After Duodenoscopic Sphincterotomy for Stones in Patients With Prior Cholecystectomy

Hawes RH, Cotton PB, Vallon AG (Middlesex Hosp and Med School, London)
Gastroenterology 98:1008–1012, 1990   24–6

From 1975 to 1980, 163 patients who had retained or recurrent duct stones after previous cholecystectomy successfully underwent duodenoscopic sphincterotomy. Follow-up was possible in 148 patients in 1982 and in 115 of them in 1986 after a mean interval of 8 years. The mean age at the time of sphincterotomy was 62 years.

Clinical Findings at Follow-Up

	1982	1986
Patients contacted	148	115
Asymptomatic	98 } 73%	56 } 83%
Died (unrelated causes)	10	31
Dyspepsia	28 (19%)	15 (14%)
Biliary problems	12 (8%)	13 (11%)*

(Of the 13 patients, 10 had been identified as having symptoms in 1982; the other 3 were patients with new symptoms.

(Courtesy of Hawes RH, Cotton PB, Vallon AG: *Gastroenterology* 98:1008–1012, 1990.)

Biliary pathology was identified in 5 patients at the earlier follow-up (table). Three patients had sphincterotomy stenosis with stones, 1 had stones without stenosis, and 1 had stenosis only. Only 2 patients had continuing problems after further follow-up. Significant bacterial contamination of bile was present in 60% of the 44 patients undergoing check endoscopy, but this did not correlate with symptoms.

Comparable findings are reported from series with shorter follow-up intervals. The long-term outlook is comparable to that seen with surgery, and warrants the continued use of endoscopic treatment in patients with duct stones. The most serious short-term complications of this treatment result from the sphincterotomy.

▶ The results of this series are encouraging. The success rate achieved by this and other groups, coupled with the explosive interest in laparoscopic cholecystectomy, has changed the pattern of managing many of these patients. Ikeda et al. (1) reported a large series of patients who had undergone sphincterotomy and stone extraction; only 4% had further biliary problems.—S.I. Schwartz, M.D.

Reference

1. Ikeda S: et al: *Endoscopy* 20:13, 1988.

Surgical Aspects of Sclerosing Cholangitis: Results in 178 Patients
Martin FM, Rossi RL, Nugent FW, Scholz FJ, Jenkins RL, Lewis WD, Gagner M, Foley E, Braasch JW (Lahey Clinic Med Ctr, Burlington, Mass; New England Deaconess Hosp, Boston)
Ann Surg 212:551–558, 1990   24–7

Sclerosing cholangitis, an insidious, uncommon inflammatory disease, affects the biliary ductal system, resulting in obliteration and fibrosis of the ducts. Ultimately, biliary cirrhosis occurs. Several medical treatments have been suggested, but little success has been reported. Multiple surgical approaches for the relief of obstruction or cholangitis have also been described, with less than satisfactory results reported. Data were reviewed on 178 patients treated for sclerosing cholangitis at 1 center since 1950. Of these, 88 had associated inflammatory bowel disease; 72, no such history; and 18, iatrogenic injury or stone disease.

Of 233 biliary operations done, 75% produced temporary improvement after initial surgery. Subsequent operations resulted in lower success rates and higher mortalities. Radiologic findings included predominant extrahepatic disease in 29%, intrahepatic disease in 28%, and diffuse disease in 43%. No differences in survival were noted. Of 103 deaths, 73% were related to liver failure, bleeding, or sepsis. Of 14 patients undergoing portosystemic shunt, 13 died of related disease or surgical complications. Orthotopic liver transplantation, done in 16 cases, resulted in 8 deaths, mostly in patients who previously had extensive surgery. There

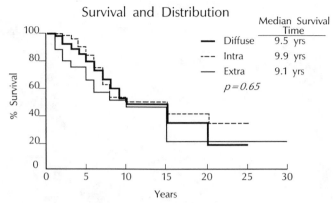

SCLEROSING CHOLANGITIS
Survival and Distribution

	Median Survival Time
— Diffuse	9.5 yrs
--- Intra	9.9 yrs
— Extra	9.1 yrs
	$p = 0.65$

Fig 24–2.—Patient survival and distribution of sclerosing cholangitis. Significance of differences of distribution was analyzed by the Mantel-Cox log-rank test. (Courtesy of Martin FM, Rossi RL, Nugent FW, et al: *Ann Surg* 212:551–558, 1990.)

were no differences in survival between the patients with inflammatory bowel disease, patients without that condition, and patients who had colectomy (Fig 24–2).

Surgical treatment in patients with sclerosing cholangitis should be kept to a minimum. For patients with portal hypertension, refractory cholangitis, advanced cirrhosis, or progressive liver failure, orthotopic liver transplantation should be offered as the treatment of choice.

▶ This is an excellent inclusive review of the subject. Wiesner et al. (1), who reported similar data, indicated that factors predicting survival were age, serum bilirubin, hemoglobin, and presence of inflammatory bowel disease with a degree of cirrhosis. Cameron et al. (2) recommend resection of the hepatic duct bifurcation and long-term transhepatic stenting for patients with sclerosing cholangitis with primary involvement of the extrahepatic bile ducts. Sclerosing cholangitis has emerged as one of the most important indications for liver transplantation when interhepatic involvement is pronounced. Eighty percent of patients given transplants because of sclerosing cholangitis have survived. As was pointed out in his discussion of this paper, Bismuth found cancer in 20% of specimens at the time of transplantation.—S.I. Schwartz, M.D.

References

1. Wiesner RH, et al: *Hepatology* 10:430, 1989.
2. Cameron JL, et al: *Ann Surg* 207:614, 1988.

Hepatobiliary Cystadenoma With Mesenchymal Stroma
Akwari OE, Tucker A, Seigler HF, Itani KMF (Duke Univ)
Ann Surg 211:18–27, 1990   24–8

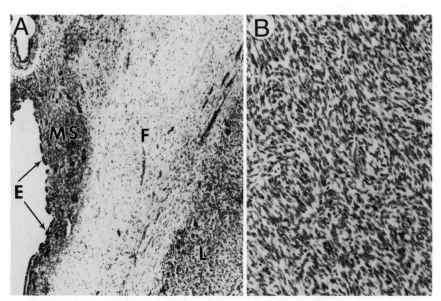

Fig 24–3.—**A**, a typical CMS tumor. A cyst is present, lined by cuboidal epithelial cells *(E)* with a subjacent layer of mesenchyma stroma cells *(MS)* and a layer of dense fibrous tissue *(F)*. Liver parenchyma *(L)* is also seen (original magnification, ×54). **B**, malignant transformation of the mesenchymal stroma in patient 3 resulted in this densely cellular sarcoma (original magnification, ×170). (Courtesy of Akwari OE, Tucker A, Seigler HF, et al: *Ann Surg* 211:18–27, 1990.)

Hepatobiliary cystadenoma with mesenchymal stroma (CMS tumor) is a distinct clinicopathologic entity. These tumors have been hypothesized to arise from ectopic rests of embryonic bile ducts. A subset of 53 patients in whom tumors were characterized by a mesenchymal cell layer interposed between an inner epithelial lining and an outer connective tissue layer was identified in a review of cystic hepatobiliary neoplasms.

Surgical Treatment of 53 Patients With CMS

Primary Operation	No. of Patients	No. of Patients Reoperated for Recurrence
Total excision of tumor	24 (3)	1
Left partial or total lobectomy	9 (1)	0
Partial right and left lobectomies	2	0
Partial excision or marsupialization	5 (4)	4, 1*, (1, 1*)
Tube drainage	1 (1)	1 (1*)
Roux-Y-limb drainage	2	0
Cholecystectomy	1	0
Total	44 (9)	6, 1*, (1, 2*)

Note: Numbers in parentheses represent patients with malignant CMS.
*Patients requiring more than 1 operation for recurrence.
(Courtesy of Akwari OE, Tucker A, Seigler HF, et al: *Ann Surg* 211:18–27, 1990.)

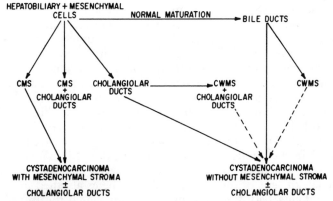

Fig 24–4.—The development of CMS necessitates a foci of primitive hepatobiliary and mesenchymal cells, which under normal maturation conditions give rise to the biliary duct system. Under suboptimal conditions, such as ischemia, these cells will develop into abnormal cholangiolar ducts. In young women, and under an unknown stimulus, these cells will become a CMS tumor that can also transform into a cystadenocarcinoma with mesenchymal stroma. If both this stimulus and ischemia are present, CMS will coexist with cholangiolar ducts. Cystadenoma without mesenchymal stroma *(CWMS)*, as well as cystadenocarcinoma without mesenchymal stroma, are neoplastic outgrowths of normal bile ducts or cholangiolar ducts subjected to carcinogens or ischemia. The transformation of CWMS into cystadenocarcinoma without mesenchymal stroma is, however, uncertain. (Courtesy of Akwari OE, Tucker A, Seigler HF, et al: *Ann Surg* 211:18–27, 1990.)

All of the patients were women. The tumors were benign on 44 patients (average age, 41 years) and were malignant in 9 patients (average age, 57 years). In 7 patients the malignancy arose from the epithelial layer, and in 2 patients, sarcomatous changes were found in the mesenchymal tissues.

Although all patients underwent surgery, 25% with benign hepatobiliary cystadenoma with mesenchymal stroma and 33% of those with malignant CMS had recurrence after primary resection. After a mean follow-up of 17 months, 44% of the women with malignant CMS were dead (Figs 24–3 and 24–4; table). Apparently, CMS occurs uniquely in young women, developing from nests of primitive embryonal cells. It has the potential for malignant transformation and, to prevent recurrence, should be completely resected during the primary operation.

▶ This is an excellent review of a rare lesion. The incidence of malignant transformation suggests that wide excision is indicated at the initial operation. We recently followed a patient with an unusual cystic lesion of the right lobe of the liver in whom we entertained this diagnosis. The ultimate diagnosis, however, was rhabdomyosarcoma of the diaphragm with invasion of the bare area of the liver. The cystic element of the disorder was a large hematoma within the right lobe of the liver.—S.I. Schwartz, M.D.

Gallstone Ileus
Clavien P-A, Richon J, Burgan S, Rohner A (Univ Hosp, Geneva)
Br J Surg 77:737–742, 1990

24–9

Gallstone ileus, which is often misdiagnosed and is associated with significant morbidity and mortality, is increasing in incidence. A series of 33 women and 4 men (median age, 78 years) had surgery for gallstone ileus during a 12-year period. The median length of follow-up was 6.2 years. Most of the patients had some serious concomitant illness.

In 17 patients the syndrome was diagnosed by plain abdominal radiographs on admission; in another 10 the diagnosis was made by ultrasonography, gastrointestinal contrast studies, or CT. Thus the diagnosis was made before operation in 73% of patients. Twenty-seven patients had obstructing stones in the terminal ileum, 5 in the proximal ileum or jejunum, 2 in the duodenum, and 3 in the colon. Six patients had more than 1 stone. The most commonly encountered fistula type was cholecystoduodenal; the site of the fistula could not be established in 8 cases.

Eight patients had a 1-stage procedure in which the impacted stone was removed, the fistula repaired, and cholecystectomy done; 2 of these patients died. Six patients had a 2-stage procedure in which enterolithotomy was followed by elective biliary surgery; none of these patients died. The remaining 23 patients had removal of the impacted stones only, and 5 of these patients died.

When feasible, a 1-stage procedure appears to be a valid option for treatment of gallstone ileus, and this may be the treatment of choice. A second procedure should be considered if additional stones are present and a 1-stage procedure is not feasible; for poor-risk patients, nonoperative treatment (e.g., shock-wave lithotripsy) should be considered.

▶ The data support the conclusions generally held. In a poor-risk patient, operated on for obstruction and with a significant inflammatory reaction in the right upper quadrant, enterotomy and removal of the obstructing gallstone are all that should be done. On the other hand, I would agree that a 1-stage procedure, including cholecystectomy, is appropriate if this can be carried out with little added risk to the patient.—S.I. Schwartz, M.D.

Carcinoma of the Gallbladder: Does Radical Resection Improve Outcome?
Donohue JH, Nagorney DM, Grant CS, Tsushima K, Ilstrup DM, Adson MA (Mayo Clinic and Found, Rochester, Minn)
Arch Surg 125:237–241, 1990   24–10

Resection of adjacent structures involved early in the course of gallbladder cancer has been advocated. Aggressive extirpation of the liver parenchyma and lymph nodes draining the gallbladder fossa seems to be critical in curing gallbladder carcinoma in patients with early invasion. Data on 111 patients with gallbladder cancer treated in 1972–1984 were reviewed to assess the effect of surgical resection on patient outcomes.

Distant metastases were present in 57% of patients, and 16% had nodal metastases without distant disease. The median survival was .5 years, and the 5-year survival rate was 13%. Patient outcome was predicted by clinical jaundice, tumor stage, and tumor grade. Although

DNA ploidy was measured in 70 patients, it was not a prognostic indicator. Cholecystectomy or radical cholecystectomy, including adjacent liver and regional lymph node resection, was performed in 36% of the patients and was potentially curative. Patients treated with radical procedures had a median survival of 3.6 years. Survival was .8 years after cholecystectomy. The 5-year survival rates were comparable (33% vs. 32%). Although radical cholecystectomy may benefit individual patients and is associated with low morbidity, there is no survival advantage compared with cholecystectomy.

▶ Primary gallbladder carcinoma remains a highly malignant disease. In Sweden there has been a marked increase in frequency during the past 15 years. Elvin et al. (1) and Nevin et al. (2) reported a dramatic fall in the survival rate with increasing tumorization of the gallbladder wall. The 5-year survival rate in patients with cancer localized to the mucosa-muscularis was approximately 80%, whereas it fell to less than 7% when all 3 layers of the gallbladder wall were involved. The use of subsegmental resection of the hepatic bed of the gallbladder from segments IV and V, accompanied by lymphadenectomy, is theoretically the appropriate approach. Haury et al. (3) reported 20 patients with gallbladder carcinoma treated with postoperative radiation; only 1 patient was alive for more than 5 years. The Japanese literature reports a disproportionately high incidence of high survival rate and length of survival. Nishino (4) described 44 patients, with a mean survival rate in the curative group of 49 months. It may well be that many of these patients had stage I carcinoma with no invasion of the muscle coat. It is also known that patients with papillary lesions represent a distinct subset having a better prognosis.—S.I. Schwartz, M.D.

References

1. Elvin A, et al: *Ann Radiol* 32:281, 1989.
2. Nevin JE, et al: *Cancer* 37:141, 1976.
3. Haury S, et al: *Br J Surg* 76:448, 1989.
4. Nishino H, et al: *Am Surg* 54:487, 1988.

Hepatic Segmentectomy With Caudate Lobe Resection for Bile Duct Carcinoma of the Hepatic Hilus
Nimura Y, Hayakawa N, Kamiya J, Kondo S, Shionoya S (Nagoya Univ, Japan)
World J Surg 14:535–544, 1990   24–11

Liver resection is used to treat bile duct carcinoma of the hepatic hilus, with varying degrees of success. However, the overall long-term survival rate after surgery is still low. In 1979–1989, surgical resection was performed in 55 of 66 patients with carcinoma of the hepatic hilus after improving jaundice by percutaneous transhepatic biliary drainage (PTBD). Selective cholangiography through PTBD was used to define the anatomical location and extent of the obstructing lesion in each segmental hepatic duct.

Percutaneous transhepatic cholangioscopy was performed after replac-

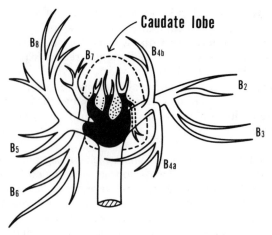

Fig 24–5.—The schema of the biliary tract and carcinoma of the hepatic hilus which involves caudate branches. B_2 indicates lateral posterior; B_3, lateral anterior; B_{4a}, medial inferior; B_{4b}, medial superior; B_5, anterior inferior; B_6, posterior inferior; B_7, posterior superior; B_8, anterior superior. (Courtesy of Nimura Y, Hayakawa N, Kamiya J, et al: *World J Surg* 14:535–544, 1990.)

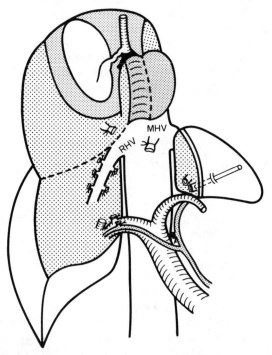

Fig 24–6.—The middle and anterior segment of the liver with entire caudate lobe in continuity with the extrahepatic bile duct are resected en bloc. (Courtesy of Nimura Y, Hayakawa N, Kamiya J, et al: *World J Surg* 14:535–544, 1990.)

Results of Aggressive Surgical Treatments

Author	No. of Resections		Morbidity	Mortality	Survival
	Resectability rate	Hepatectomy			
Longmire et al. [12]	6/34 (17.6%)	2	16/34 (47.1%)	5/34 (14.7%) Hx: 1/2 (50%)	8: >1 yr Longest: 15 yr
Fortner et al. [13]	9/25 (36.0%)	5		3/9 (33.3%) Hx: 3/5 (60.0%)	Bile duct resection: 7 mo Hepatectomy-liver transplantation: 8 mo
Launois et al. [28]	11/18 (61.1%)	Hx + LTX: 3 6		Hx + LTX: 2/3 (66.7%) 2/11 (18.2%) Hx: 1/6 (16.7%)	Liver transplantation (longest): 4 mo Mean: 521 days Hepatectomy (12–746 days)
Tsuzuki et al. [29]	16/31 (51.6%)	16	8/16 (50.0%)	Hx: 2/16 (12.5%)	Mean: 2 yr
Blumgart et al. [24]	18/94 (19.1%)	12		2/18 (11.1%) Hx: 2/12 (16.7%)	Mean: 17 mo
Gazzaniga et al. [30]	12/58 (20.7%)	5		3/12 (25.0%) Hx: 1/5 (20.0%)	Radical: 5-yr: 40%
Iwasaki et al. [31]	31/46 (67.4%)	9		0/31 (0%)	Mean: 2.2 yr Mean bile duct resection: 9.3 mo, mean hepatectomy 12.2 mo
Mizumoto et al. [32]	24/26 (92.3%)	13		1/26 (3.8%)	Mean: 3.6 yr (hepatectomy: 3.9 yr) 5-yr: 35% (hepatectomy: 44%)
Pinson and Rossi [33]	25/156 (16.0%)	9		1/25 (4.0%) Hx: 0/9 (0%)	Median: 7 mo Longest: 14.3 yr
Bengmark et al. [37]		22	9/16 (56.3%)	Hx: 6/22 (27.3%)	Median: 15 mo
Pichlmayr et al. [40]	52/108 (48.1%)	27 Hx + LTX: 16		9/52 (17.3%) Hx: 5/27 (18.5%)	Bile duct resection: 22 mo, hepatectomy: 14 mo Liver transplantation: 16 mo
Hart and White [43]	24/50 (48.0%)	24*		LTX: 4/16 Hx: 3/24 (12.5%)	Mean: 19.8 mo
This study	55/66 (83.3%)	51		Hx: 4/51 (7.8%)	Median: 3.1 yr
	Curative: 46	Curative: 45	19/46 (41.3%)	Curative: 3/46 (6.5%)	5-yr: 37.8%

Abbreviations: Hx, hepatectomy; LTX, liver transplantation.
*Central hepatic resection.
(Courtesy of Nimura Y, Hayakawa N, Kamiya J, et al: *World J Surg* 14:535–544, 1990.)

ing the drainage catheter with a 15-French catheter for superselective cholangiography and biopsy for definitive diagnosis of the histologic extent of the tumor and any variation of each segmental hepatic duct that joins the hepatic hilus. Curative resection was possible in 46 of the 66 patients, 45 of whom had various types of hepatic segmentectomy with caudate lobectomy; the morbidity rate was 41.3% and the operative mortality, 6.4%. Combined resection of the portal vein and hepatectomy was performed in 14 patients with advanced disease. Microscopic tumor involvement in the caudate branches was confirmed in 44 of 45 patients undergoing caudate lobe resection. The 43 patients surviving curative excision had a 3-year survival rate of 55.1% and a 5-year survival rate of 40.5%. All 11 patients with unresectable advanced disease died within 9 months (table; Figs 24–5 and 24–6).

Curative resection should be designed on the basis of preoperative findings of the extent of cancer in each segmental duct in patients with bile duct carcinoma of the hepatic hilus. Caudate lobe resection should be performed along with the smallest needed hepatic segmentectomy.

▶ This report chronicles a truly extraordinary operation. I had the opportunity of seeing a videotape of this demanding procedure, and the authors are to be complimented not only on the technical scene but on the results. Hadjis et al. (1) reported that 7 patients with cholangiocarcinoma had confluence of the ducts undergoing hepatic resection for cure. The overall median and mean survival times for patients who left the hospital were 25 months and 29 months, respectively. Twenty patients died later, and only 4 patients were alive after 48–54 months. These authors conclude that further progress is unlikely without significant advances in adjuvant therapy.—S.I. Schwartz, M.D.

Reference

1. Hadjis NS, et al: *Surgery* 107:597, 1990.

Carcinoma of the Main Hepatic Duct Junction: Indications, Operative Morbidity and Mortality, and Long-Term Survival
Tsuzuki T, Ueda M, Kuramochi S, Iida S, Takahashi S, Iri H (Keio Univ, Tokyo, Japan)
Surgery 108:495–501, 1990
24–12

In many cases carcinoma of the main hepatic duct junction spreads extensively along the hepatic ducts into the liver parenchyma. Extensive resection of the bile ducts and hepatic resection are therefore the treatments of choice for carcinoma of the main hepatic duct junction.

Between 1973 and 1989, 25 of 50 patients with carcinoma of the main hepatic duct junction underwent resection. Resection of the bilateral hepatic ducts, the common hepatic and bile ducts, and the gallbladder, along with hepatic lobectomy on the side of the longer extension of the cancer, was done. This was then followed by hepaticojejunostomy or hepatojejunostomy. Left medial segmentectomy was done when the cancer was located mainly in the common hepatic duct with extension to the main hepatic duct junction.

One patient died of staphylococcal sepsis 42 days after right trisegmentectomy and resection of the bile ducts. The hospital death rate was thus 4%. Among the 24 survivors discharged from the hospital, the 5-year actuarial survival rate was 19%. Four patients lived longer than 5 years postoperatively. The longest survival was 9 years after right trisegmentectomy and resection of the bile ducts.

Extensive resection of the bile ducts, combined with resection of the liver, is the procedure of choice for patients with carcinoma of the main hepatic duct junction. This procedure can be done with low operative mortality if jaundice is relieved preoperatively and if infection in the bile ducts is prevented.

▶ The Japanese have reported an increasingly aggressive surgical approach to manage carcinoma of the main hepatic duct junction. Ottow et al. (1) presented an excellent review of the subject, indicating that currently fewer than 10% of patients with malignancy of the biliary tract survive for 5 years. Iwasaki et al. (2) suggest that survival may be improved with intraoperative radiation therapy, but confirmed data substantiating this are not available.—S.I. Schwartz, M.D.

References

1. Ottow RT, et al: *Surgery* 97:251, 1985.
2. Iwasaki Y, et al: *World J Surg* 12:91, 1988.

Proximal Extrahepatic Bile Duct Tumors: Analysis of a Series of 52 Consecutive Patients Treated Over a Period of 13 Years

Fortner JG, Vitelli CE, Maclean BJ (Mem Sloan-Kettering Cancer Ctr, New York)
Arch Surg 124:1275–1279, 1989   24–13

Proximal extrahepatic bile duct tumors have a poor prognosis. Untreated, patients with a proximal bile duct tumor (PBDT) have a median survival of 1.2–4 months after diagnosis. Because of the relative rarity of these tumors, their management has been a matter of controversy. To evaluate factors affecting survival, data on 52 consecutive patients with a mean age of 59.8 years were reviewed.

Surgery was performed with either a palliative (group A) or curative (group B) intent. Group A (38) had a more advanced stage of disease and less favorable histologic features than group B (14). Adenocarcinoma was present in all of the tumor specimens.

The median survival for all patients in this series was 17.5 months. Group A had a median survival of 13.5 months, whereas group B had a median actuarial survival of 38 months (Fig 24–7). The choice of palliative procedure to relieve biliary obstruction did not significantly affect the length of survival. In-hospital mortality was 15.7% in group A; no hospital deaths occurred in group B.

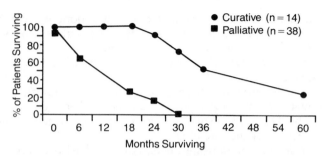

Fig 24–7.—Survival estimates. The median actuarial survival for patients undergoing curative procedures is 38 months. The median survival for patients undergoing palliative procedures is 13.5 months. (Courtesy of Fortner JG, Vitelli CE, Maclean BJ: *Arch Surg* 124:1275–1279, 1989.)

In group B, 6 patients (43%) had recurrence of tumor and 5 were dead within 12 months after the diagnosis of recurrence. Because 2 long-term survivors died of second primary tumors at 50 months and 80 months, respectively, after the original biliary procedure, careful follow-up of such patients is advised. In group B, length of survival was not affected by age, gender, grade of the lesion, extent of resection, or microscopic status of margins of resection.

Nontherapeutic laparotomies should not be performed in patients with a tentative diagnosis of PBTD because of the potential for locoregional neoplastic contamination that greatly reduces the chance for curative resection. Adjuvant radiotherapy offers more promising results than combination chemotherapy.

▶ With more refined surgical technique and a better appreciation of the potential for resection, including partial hepatic resection, more aggressive procedures have been carried out. Chen et al. (1) reported on 20 hepatic resections in patients with peripheral cholangiocarcinomas. The overall mean survival time was 20 months, and 1 patient was alive 5 years after the operation. Some of the most encouraging results have come from Cameron et al. (2). That group reported 96 patients managed surgically—53 resected, 39 curatively. Sixty-three patients also received postoperative radiotherapy. The 5-year survival was 5% and the 10-year survival, 2%. It was thought that the survival rate was better in the resected group than in those who were "stented." Radiotherapy appeared to extend survival in patients undergoing palliative stenting but not in those undergoing resection.—S.I. Schwartz, M.D.

References

1. Chen M, et al: *Cancer* 64:2226, 1989.
2. Cameron JL, et al: *Am J Surg* 159:91, 1990.

Significance of Tumor Spread in Adenocarcinoma of the Ampulla of Vater
Delcore R Jr, Connor CS, Thomas JH, Friesen SR, Hermreck AS (Univ of Kansas; Kansas City VA Med Ctr, Kansas City, Mo)
Am J Surg 158:593–597, 1989   24–14

Ampullary carcinoma is the most curable of all upper gastrointestinal tract malignancies, even in patients with lymph node metastases or invasion into adjacent organs. To determine the effect of pancreaticoduodenectomy on long-term survival, data on 28 patients with ampullary carcinoma who were treated in 1965–1988 were reviewed.

The patients had a mean age of 62 years; 18 (64%) were men. Common symptoms included jaundice (96%), abdominal pain (61%), and weight loss (43%). According to the Barton and Copeland staging system, 10 patients had stage III (extension to regional tissues or organs) and 11 had stage V (nodal metastases with regional extension) disease; 5 patients had disease localized to the ampulla and 1 had carcinoma in situ.

One patient died preoperatively of unrelated causes and a second patient refused surgery and died shortly thereafter. Palliative bypass procedures were performed in 3 patients. The remaining 23 patients underwent resection by either pancreaticoduodenectomy (22) or local resection (1).

The patient with stage I disease who underwent local excision only was alive and free of recurrence after 9 years. All patients in the bypass-only group died of progressive disease within 15 months of surgery; 1 patient died of a perioperative acute myocardial infarction, but the remaining 21 survived pancreaticoduodenectomy. The estimated 5-year survival rate for resected patients, 60%, was independently related to lymph node metastases and tumor size. The estimated 20-year survival was 42% for all resected patients.

Pancreaticoduodenectomy should be performed in all patients with ampullary carcinoma who have lymph node metastases or invasive tumors. Mortality and morbidity are low, and cures are achieved even when the disease has spread.

▶ A plea for an aggressive attitude in management of patients with ampullary carcinoma is in concert with our feelings. In our experience, 30% of patients who underwent pancreaticoduodenectomy and had positive nodes in the specimen have survived for 5 years. I feel a place remains for the use of ampullectomy for carcinoma in patients with small lesions who are regarded as poor risks for pancreaticoduodenectomy. Chiappetta et al. (1) reviewed 61 ampullectomies in which the mortality rate was 3% and the 5-year survival, 23%. I agree that the good-risk patient should receive the advantage of pancreaticoduodenectomy to more certainly effect cure.—S.I. Schwartz, M.D.

Reference

1. Chiappetta A, et al: *Am Surg* 52:603, 1986.

25 The Pancreas

Acute Pancreatitis and Normoamylasemia: Not an Uncommon Combination

Clavien P-A, Robert J, Meyer P, Borst F, Hauser H, Herrmann F, Dunand V, Rohner A (Univ Hosp, Geneva)

Ann Surg 210:614–620, 1989   25–1

To define the incidence of acute pancreatitis in patients with normal amylasemia on admission, 318 patients with 352 attacks of acute pancreatitis were examined by contrast-enhanced CT scans. The diagnosis was established by contrast-enhanced CT scan performed within the initial 36 hours of hospitalization in all but 4 patients. Amylase was measured spectrophotometrically in serum and peritoneal fluid. The clinical course was characterized as mild (62%), severe (29%), or necrotizing pancreatitis resulting in death (9%).

At admission, in 67 of 352 attacks of acute pancreatitis (19%) the serum amylase value was less than 160 IU/L; 50 of these attacks were in men and 17 in women. The hyperamylasemic group comprised 160 men and 125 women. The median duration of symptoms before admission was 2.4 days in the normoamylasemic group compared with 1.5 days in the hyperamylasemic group. Alcoholic pancreatitis was present in 39 of the 67 attacks of normoamylasemic acute pancreatitis. Biliary lithiasis prevailed slightly (38%) over alcohol (33%) as the cause in patients who had increased serum amylase levels. When graded by CT and Ranson's criteria, acute pancreatitis did not differ significantly whether or not amylase levels were increased. Normal serum amylase levels do not necessarily rule out acute pancreatitis. In some patients, amylase levels may have returned to normal by the time of admission. Serum lipase measurement increases the diagnostic sensitivity of amylase alone. Treatment should be the same regardless of serum amylase levels.

▶ The authors set out to attack a sacred cow, i.e., the concept that the diagnosis of acute pancreatitis should be questioned if the serum amylase value is normal (1). They used contrast-enhanced CT scanning as an admission study and then compared the results of the scan and the serum amylase value to Ranson's score and the clinical outcome. Computed tomography was found to be 99% accurate vs. 81% accuracy for serum amylase (as authenticated at operation or autopsy). Adding the serum lipase measurement raised the diagnostic accuracy from 81% with amylase alone to 94% for both enzymes.

Although the authors have demonstrated that pancreatitis exists in the face of normal amylase values, world-wide experience is firmly on the side of the value of the amylase measurement. Just think of how many cases of acute pancreatitis you have seen with normal amylase values. The patients I remember are those who come in nearly moribund with an infarcted pancreas. There certainly is no correlation between severity of disease and amylase levels, but as a screening diagnostic test, I am sure it will continue to be the most popular.—J.C. Thompson, M.D.

Reference

1. Moossa AR: *N Engl J Med* 311:639, 1984.

Acute Pancreatitis and Pancreatic Fistula Formation
Fielding GA, McLatchie GR, Wilson C, Imrie CW, Carter DC (Royal Infirmary, Glasgow)
Br J Surg 76:1126–1128, 1989   25–2

Pancreatic fistulas may occur as a complication of pancreatic disease or injury, or may follow surgical intervention. Fourteen men and 9 women (mean age, 40 years) had pancreatic fistulas that occurred after an attack of acute pancreatitis.

The pancreatitis resulted from gallstones in 12 cases and from a duodenal tumor in 1. Eight patients had alcohol-induced pancreatitis, and no precipitating cause was found in 2 patients. In 19 patients postoperative external fistulas were discharging through an abdominal wound or drain site. Four patients had 6 internal fistulas.

Patients with external fistulas underwent surgery when it was believed that the fistula would not close spontaneously with conservative treatment. Although internal fistulas that drained into the hollow viscera did not require surgical intervention, those that drained into peritoneal and pleural cavities were treated surgically after the patient was stabilized.

Four of the 19 patients with external fistulas died, 3 in the intensive care unit and 1 at 30 days after operation. Eleven of the 15 survivors, all of whom had low-output fistulas, experienced spontaneous closure at a mean of 12.3 weeks. The 4 remaining patients all had high-output fistulas and required some form of operative treatment. All 4 patients with an internal fistula underwent surgery. One, an alcoholic man aged 60 years with pancreatic ascites, died.

The mortality in this patient group (22%) reflects the severity of the underlying disease process. A successful outcome requires prompt recognition of the fistula; supportive therapy; active investigation by fistulography or endoscopic retrograde cholangiopancreatography, or both, as well as timely intervention.

▶ Bill Nealon in our department has shown communication with the main pancreatic duct in 44% of patients with pseudocysts (1), so we should not be surprised when a pancreatic fistula followed surgical operations in which a pseudocyst is opened and not drained into the gut. The 21% mortality in patients with external fistula is surprising and must reflect the septic condition of the patient. Most pancreatic fistulas are remarkably benign and will go away if everyone is patient. Rarely, if trypsinogen is activated to trypsin the fistula may digest the intra-abdominal wall, but for this to happen, the pancreatic juice usually must traverse the duodenum.—J.C. Thompson, M.D.

Reference

1. Nealon W, et al: *Ann Surg* 209:532, 1989.

On-Table Pancreatography: Importance in Planning Operative Strategy
Desa LA, Williamson RCN (Royal Postgrad Med School, London)
Br J Surg 77:1145–1150, 1990   25–3

Especially in patients with chronic pancreatitis, it is important to demonstrate the complete pancreatic ductal tree both for diagnosis and for planning operative treatment. There are several techniques for ductal imaging, but all may be inadequate, unsuccessful, or even misleading. On-table pancreatography (OTP) provides an alternative method.

Surgeons performed 124 OTPs on 112 patients undergoing 117 opera-

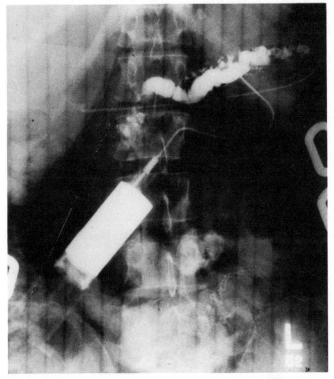

Fig 25–1.—Ambigrade pancreatogram in a patient with chronic pancreatitis. (The vertical striations in the background are caused by a water bed.) The need for operative pancreatography had not been anticipated in this patient in whom ERCP had indicated a complete ductal stricture in the neck of the pancreas. (Courtesy of Desa LA, Williamson RCN: *Br J Surg* 77:1145–1150, 1990.)

tive procedures. The median age of the 64 male and 44 female patients was 48 years. Preoperatively, 62 patients underwent ultrasonography, 71 CT, 30 visceral angiography, and 84 endoscopic retrograde cholangiopancreatography (ERCP). Five different techniques were used for OTP: retrograde, prograde, or ambigrade (Fig 25–1) ductography, cystography, and ascending loopography following pancreaticojejunostomy. Sixty-three patients had chronic pancreatitis; 6 had pseudocysts after acute pancreatitis, and 13 had recurrent acute pancreatitis. Of 14 patients with pancreas divisum, 9 had obscure abdominal pain and 5 had recurrent acute pancreatitis. Six of 8 patients with postcholecystectomy pain had positive results on an evocative morphine-prostigmine test.

There were 5 technical failures in 124 OTP attempts, but OTP provided important information about the main pancreatic duct in 23 patients with unsuccessful endoscopic visualization, in 17 with incomplete endoscopic visualization, and in 33 who did not have endoscopic visualization. In 35 patients, OTP provided either additional information or differing information from ERCP that led to changes in operative procedures. Nineteen extra procedures were scheduled, and 16 were altered as a result of information provided by OTP. Complete ductography was particularly helpful in the patients with chronic pancreatitis.

On-table pancreatography provides important information on ductal morphology in patients with pancreatic disease. There is a clear-cut role for this procedure for full operative evaluation, particularly of chronic pancreatitis and pancreas divisum.

▶ These folks seem to have greater facility with this than I do. I often find the papilla difficult to cannulate at operation and the duct, even when dilated, often a problem to locate. I feel much better if we can go into the operation with the pancreatic duct mapped out by ERCP. I know the authors would agree, and they are talking here about demonstrating the duct when the need had not been recognized preoperatively, or when preoperative attempts were unsuccessful. I do believe I could hit the duct shown in the illustration, but when they are smaller, we commonly have trouble.—J.C. Thompson, M.D.

The Natural History of Pancreatic Pseudocysts Documented by Computed Tomography

Yeo CJ, Bastidas JA, Lynch-Nyhan A, Fishman EK, Zinner MJ, Cameron JL (Johns Hopkins Med Insts)
Surg Gynecol Obstet 170:411–417, 1990   25–4

To determine whether a significant number of CT-documented pancreatic pseudocysts resolve without surgery, data on 75 such patients were reviewed. Patients without symptoms who were able to tolerate an oral intake were treated nonoperatively. Surgery was performed only for persistent abdominal pain or enlargement, or when the pseudocyst caused complications.

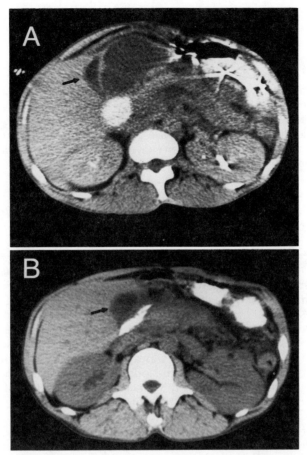

Fig 25–2.—**A,** a CT scan of a patient with alcohol-related pancreatitis and an 8-cm pseudocyst. The gallbladder *(arrow)* is compressed to the left (for the viewer) by the large pseudocyst. **B,** a CT scan of the same patient 1 month later. The patient was treated nonoperatively. The pseudocyst has completely resolved, and the gallbladder *(arrow)* is well visualized. (Courtesy of Yeo CJ, Bastidas JA, Lynch-Nyhan A, et al: *Surg Gynecol Obstet* 170:411–417, 1990.)

A total of 36 patients were treated nonoperatively. After a mean follow-up of 1 year, 60% of pseudocysts had totally resolved roentgenographically (Fig 25–2); the other pseudocysts had remained stable or decreased in size. Only 1 pseudocyst-related complication occurred in this group—a self-limited episode of intracyst hemorrhage that required transfusion.

Surgery was performed on 39 patients. Patients with pseudocysts greater than 6 cm in diameter more often required surgery. The most frequent operations were Roux-en-Y cystojejunostomy and cystogastrostomy. Five patients recovered slowly and 4 others required further surgery on the pancreas. A pseudocyst developed in 1 patient postoperatively. There were no deaths related to the pseudocyst. Many patients with pancreatic pseudocyst can be safely treated nonoperatively.

▶ We have gradually learned in the past 2 decades that many pancreatic pseudocysts simply go away. Because that is what we attempt to achieve when we operate, you can't ask for anything more. Cysts that are apt to go away are those that are small, those that have thin walls, and those that do not communicate with the pancreatic duct. The best plan is to operate on patients who are clearly symptomatic and have been so for 6 weeks or more and in whom the size of the cyst has been shown to be constant or enlarging. If the cyst is shrinking, don't operate, but follow it.—J.C. Thompson, M.D.

The Impact of Technology on the Management of Pancreatic Pseudocyst
Walt AJ, Bouwman DL, Weaver DW, Sachs RJ (Wayne State Univ, Detroit)
Arch Surg 125:759–763, 1990   25–5

The records of 299 patients who had 357 admissions for pancreatic pseudocyst in 1960–1989 were reviewed. Surgery had been performed in 233 patients. Of the patients, 82% were men; the median age at admission was 43 years. The median hospital stay was 30 days.

Alcoholism was the cause of pseudocyst formation in 70% of the patients. The next most frequent causes were biliary tract disease and blunt trauma. In only 35% of patients was a mass palpated at admission. Ascites was a feature at 17% of admissions. Pseudocysts were about equally frequent in the head and tail of the pancreas; they were less often present in the pancreatic body or at multiple sites.

Pancreatic pseudocysts now are recognized earlier, particularly through the use of endoscopic retrograde cholangiopancreatography. The data obtained have promoted nonoperative management but also more extensive operations. One fourth of the present patients who were operated on had partial resection of the pancreas along with the pseudocysts. Pseudocyst drainage by the percutaneous or transgastroduodenal route can avoid laparotomy in some patients. Nevertheless, major surgery will continue to be necessary in some patients with pancreatic pseudocysts.

▶ This study agrees with one from our department by Nealon et al. (1), which provided clear evidence that we could improve our operative results in patients with pseudocysts if we could delineate the relationship of the cyst to the pancreas and to the duct. Our study was undertaken, in part, in response to the demonstration of the usefulness of endoscopic retrograde cholangiopancreatography in categorizing ductal abnormality (2). The 3 studies taken together (that is, the 2 from Wayne State and the 1 from our institution) have given clear evidence that our previous efforts to treat pseudocysts surgically have often been misdirected and can be much better focused if we know the anatomy of the ductal system.—J.C. Thompson, M.D.

References

1. Nealon, W, et al: *Ann Surg* 209:532, 1989.
2. Sugawa C, Walt AJ: *Surgery* 86:639, 1979.

Endoscopic Retrograde Cholangiopancreatography in the Preoperative Diagnosis of Pancreatic Neoplasms Associated With Cysts

Pinson CW, Munson JL, Deveney CW (Oregon Health Sciences Univ, Portland; VA Med Ctr, Portland, Ore; Lahey Clinic Med Ctr, Burlington, Mass)
Am J Surg 159:510–513, 1990   25–6

Cystic neoplasms of the pancreas are relatively uncommon and difficult to diagnose. Because patients with true cystic neoplasms of the pancreas can be cured with prompt diagnosis and resection, accurate identification is important. The ability of endoscopic retrograde cholangiopancreatography (ERCP), CT, and ultrasonography to distinguish neoplastic from non-neoplastic pancreatic cysts was evaluated in 9 women and 2 men (mean age, 60 years). All complained of abdominal pain and had previously consulted a mean of 4 physicians. Other common symptoms were weight loss (73%), anorexia (55%), and an elevated serum level of amylase (27%). None was jaundiced.

Although CT revealed cysts in all 11 patients, 6 were mistakenly read

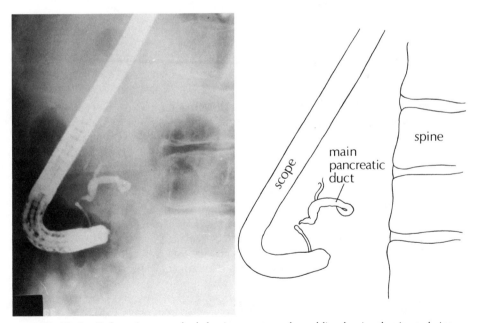

Fig 25–3.—Endoscopic retrograde cholangiopancreatography and line drawing showing occlusion of main pancreatic duct in same location as cyst in Figure 25–4. There were no findings of chronic pancreatitis. (Courtesy of Pinson CW, Munson JL, Deveney CW: *Am J Surg* 159:510–513, 1990.)

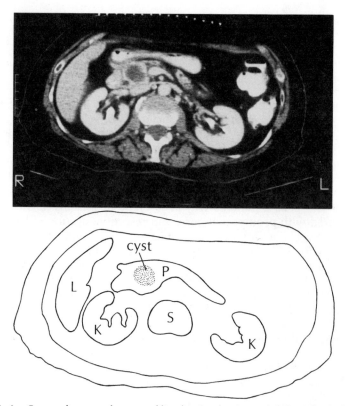

Fig 25–4.—Computed tomography scan and line drawing showing cystic lesion in head of pancreas. (Courtesy of Pinson CW, Munson JL, Deveney CW: *Am J Surg* 159:510–513, 1990.)

as pseudocysts. Findings at ultrasound, performed in 3 patients, were abnormal but not diagnostic. Findings on ERCP studies were abnormal and consistent with neoplasm in all 11 patients. None had the ductal changes seen in chronic pancreatitis. The pancreatic duct was occluded in 8 patients (Fig 25–3), narrowed in 2, and displaced in 1. Five patients with tumors in the pancreatic head (Fig 25–4) underwent pancreatoduodenectomy. Distal pancreatectomy was performed in 3 patients with tumors in the body or tail of the pancreas. The mean tumor size was 4.8 cm.

Cystic neoplasms of the pancreas occur most often in women with no history of alcoholism. When such patients present with abdominal pain, weight loss, and relatively normal laboratory findings, the possibility of a cystic neoplasm should be considered. The combination of CT scan and ERCP leads to the most accurate diagnosis.

▶ This is another demonstration of the value of preoperative ERCP. Hear and obey! This is a real finding. Whenever you have a patient upon whom you plan to operate who has a cystic lesion of the pancreas by ultrasound or by CT, ERCP is indicated. This is one of the many reasons that any surgeon planning a career working on patients with pancreatic or biliary disease must learn ERCP.—J.C. Thompson, M.D.

Papillary Cystic Neoplasm of the Pancreas: Radiological and Pathological Characteristics in 11 Cases
Yamaguchi K, Hirakata R, Kitamura K (Shinkokura Hosp, Kitayushu; Kyushu Univ, Fukuoka, Japan)
Br J Surg 77:1000–1003, 1990   25–7

Papillary cystic neoplasms of the pancreas (PCNP) are uncommon pancreatic tumors that usually affect the distal portion of the pancreas in

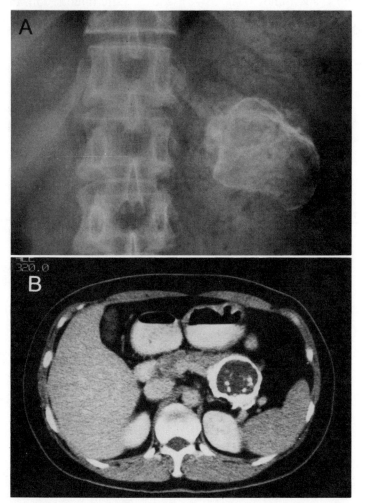

Fig 25–5.—Cystic type of papillary cystic neoplasm of the pancreas. **A,** a diffusely calcified mass in the *left upper quadrant* (abdominal radiograph). **B,** a calcified cystic mass (enhanced CT). (Courtesy of Yamaguchi K, Hirakata R, Kitamura K: *Br J Surg* 77:1000–1003, 1990.)

young women. A review was made of clinical charts, radiologic features, microscopic and macroscopic findings, and clinical follow-up data in 9 females and 2 males with PCNP. Patients ranged in age from 13 to 51 years (mean, 25 years). Eight patients with PCNP in the tail or body of the pancreas underwent distal pancreatectomy; 2 patients with PCNP in the head had complete resections of the tumor; and 1 with PCNP in the head underwent pancreaticoduodenectomy. In 1 patient familial adenomatosis coli, was diagnosed.

Tumors ranged in diameter from 2.5 to 14 cm (mean, 7.5 cm). Six tumors were found in the tail of the pancreas, 3 in the head, and 2 in the body. All but 1 patient complained of pain or of an abdominal mass. Findings on CT and/or ultrasonography showed 5 solid tumors, 4 mixed solid and cystic tumors (Fig 25–5), and 2 cystic tumors. On angiography, PCNP was shown to be either hypovascular or mildly hypervascular with displacement of the surrounding vessels. There was no vascular en-

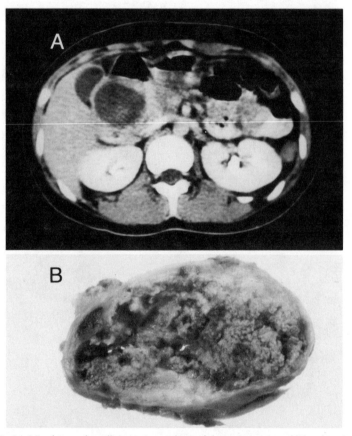

Fig 25–6.—Mixed type of papillary cystic neoplasm of the pancreas. **A**, a solid and cystic mass in the head of the pancreas seen on CT scan. **B**, a solid and cystic mass. (Courtesy of Yamaguchi K, Hirakata R, Kitamura K: *Br J Surg* 77:1000–1003, 1990.)

casement. Macroscopically, all 11 tumors were well-defined solid masses having degenerative changes of various widths. These changes included hemorrhage and necrosis or dystrophic calcification.

Radiologic findings showed a diffusely calcified mass in the upper abdomen in 2 patients (Fig 25–6) and amorphous calcification in 1 patient. Upper gastrointestinal radiography showed deformity of the stomach in 6 patients and enlarged duodenal loops in 2. Endoscopic retrograde pancreatography revealed displacement of the main pancreatic duct in 3 patients and disruption of the main pancreatic duct in 1. Survival was from 3 to 253 months after curative resection. There were no signs of local recurrence or distant metastases.

Patients with PCNP have an inherently good prognosis. Therefore, this tumor should be explored with aggressive surgical intent despite its large size.

▶ These tumors, found especially in young women, appear to be increasing in prevalence all over the world. We have seen 6 such patients in the past 18 months. The tumor has a variety of names (solid/cystic cystadenoma, microcystic cystadenoma, mucinous cystadenoma, or cystadenocarcinoma); some adenocarcinomas may also appear with cysts. There seems to be a slight predilection for the distal pancreas. Although many of them appear histologically benign, they are clinically malignant in that they recur and recur so that wide local excision is mandatory. Again, endoscopic retrograde cholangiopancreatography is reported in this study as being useful. These patients do have a good prognosis providing the tumor is widely excised.—J.C. Thompson, M.D.

Palliative Operations for Pancreatic Carcinoma
Potts JR III, Broughan TA, Hermann RE (Cleveland Clinic Florida, Ft Lauderdale; Cleveland Clinic Found, Ohio)
Am J Surg 159:72–78, 1990   25–8

Data on 142 patients were reviewed to determine which methods of biliary and enteric bypass provide the best palliation for pancreatic adenocarcinoma. The patients included 94 men and 48 women whose mean age was 62.2 years. Preoperative symptoms included weight loss in 121 patients, pain in 103, jaundice in 94, and vomiting in 34. Of 38 patients who were diabetic at surgery, 22 had become diabetic within the previous year. Surgery had been performed on 16 patients for pancreatic carcinoma and cholecystectomy had been performed on 26.

Biliary bypass was performed in 122 of the 142 patients; 74 patients had construction of some form of enteral bypass. Choledochoduodenostomy, performed in almost half of the patients, resulted in the lowest incidence of postoperative biliary sepsis and obstruction. These complications occurred most frequently with cholecystojejunostomy and least with direct choledochalenteric anastomosis. Loop gastrojejunostomy and Roux-Y gastrojejunostomy had similar complication rates and postoperative stays, but loop reconstruction was judged superior because it was less difficult to create.

These findings indicate that choledochoduodenostomy is the best method for relieving biliary obstruction caused by pancreatic adenocarcinoma. Gastric bypass, which may obviate the need for reoperation without increasing operative morbidity, should be liberally applied. Loop gastrojejunal reconstruction is the preferable method.

▶ The outcome of palliative operations for pancreatic cancer is so grim and the life expectancy so short that many physicians perform cholecystojejunostomy knowing that most patients will not live long enough to get into trouble. If the bile duct is greatly enlarged, anastomosis of the duct to the duodenum or to the jejunum is preferable. The ideal reconstruction would be a choledochal Roux-en-Y jejunostomy, so that any leak would be of bile only. The paper does not address the salient question in these patients, i.e., when to do a gastrojejunostomy. The authors say that the technique should be applied liberally, but what does that mean? Arguments have raged back and forth for years and have been well documented in these reviews in the past 5 years. We continue to reserve gastrojejunostomy for those patients whose tumor appears to press on the duodenum or the distal stomach. That will mean, inevitably, that some patients will live for a long time and will become obstructed and require another operation. The alternative is to do the procedure on everyone, and we find that hard to justify. The right answer is not yet available.—J.C. Thompson, M.D.

26 The Endocrine Glands

Lymph Node Metastasis from Papillary-Follicular Thyroid Carcinoma in Young Patients
Frankenthaler RA, Sellin RV, Cangir A, Goepfert H (Univ of Texas, Houston)
Am J Surg 160:341–343, 1990   26–1

Authorities disagree on the pathology, treatment, follow-up, and prognostic factors in pediatric thyroid cancer. Because of the controversies, data concerning a 39-year experience with thyroid carcinoma in young patients were reviewed to better define presentation, characteristics, relative frequency of occurrence by anatomical site, and mortality rate. In particular, the management of regional lymph node metastasis was investigated.

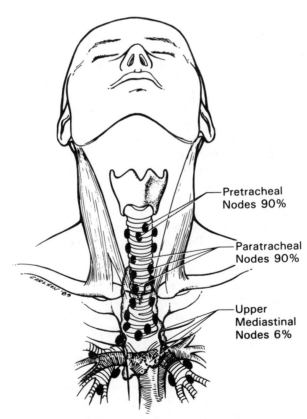

Pretracheal Nodes 90%

Paratracheal Nodes 90%

Upper Mediastinal Nodes 6%

Fig 26–1.—Anterior view of lymph node involvement in thyroid cancer diagnosed in young patients. (Courtesy of Frankenthaler RA, Sellin RV, Cangir A, et al: *Am J Surg* 160:341–343, 1990.)

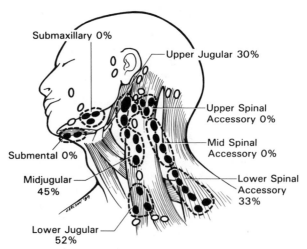

Fig 26–2.—Lateral view of lymph node involvement in thyroid cancer diagnosed in young patients. (Courtesy of Frankenthaler RA, Sellin RV, Cangir A, et al: *Am J Surg* 160:341–343, 1990.)

The series included 117 patients whose mean age at presentation was 16 years. The ratio of female to male patients was 2.9:1. Patients had thyroid cancer of papillary and/or follicular histologic type. Three percent had family histories of thyroid cancer, and 20% had received irradiation for chronic adenoiditis (57%), thymic hyperplasia (30%), and acne (13%). A mean of 11 years elapsed between previous irradiation and the diagnosis of thyroid cancer. A solitary, painless cervical mass was the most common presenting symptom. The mass was in the thyroid in 40% of patients; it represented regional lymph node metastasis in 60%. Few patients had either hoarseness or dysphagia, and none had signs of thyroid dysfunction. The duration of symptoms ranged from 1 month to 10 years (mean, 14.5 months).

In the 39-year study period the trend in treatment has been toward surgery plus postoperative irradiation with iodine-131. All patients also received postoperative hormone suppression therapy. In 79% of patients the cancer was papillary-follicular, with 12% being pure papillary and 9% pure follicular. Twenty-seven percent of patients had soft tissue invasion at the primary site, 6% had strap muscle invasion, and 5% had extracapsular spread from lymph nodes. Pathologic examination revealed lymph node involvement in 26% of cases that were clinically N_0 (Figs 26–1 and 26–2). Overall, the recurrence rate was 29%. The most frequent site of recurrence was the neck. Relapse was rare at both primary and distant sites. All distant metastases were pulmonary. For all sites the average time to recurrence was 3.5 years. No patients died of thyroid cancer during an overall follow-up of 14.5 years.

Surgery and postoperative irradiation with iodine-131 for initial control of local and regional thyroid cancer should lower the rate of neck recurrences and decrease morbidity. Near-total or total thyroidectomy with modified neck dissection followed by iodine-131 treatment is recommended. The prognosis is excellent in these patients if initial treatment is aggressive, there is vigilant surveillance for recurrence, and early treatment when recurrent disease is discovered.

▶ There is a message here if we were only smart enough to receive it. What is going on in young people with thyroid cancer? When a cancer is sufficiently virulent to invade the strap muscle, you would certainly suspect a significant incidence of fatality. What do young people, especially young women, have that protects them? Many older surgeons have the experience of following healthy patients for 40 or more years, operating occasionally to remove a local recurrence. What is it that keeps the disease from becoming systemic, and why is it that even patients with spread to the lungs seem to survive for extraordinary lengths of time? If we could answer this, we would have the key to other important locks.—J.C. Thompson, M.D.

Anaplastic Carcinoma of the Thyroid: A Clinicopathologic Study of 121 Cases
Venkatesh YSS, Ordonez NG, Schultz PN, Hickey RC, Goepfert H, Samaan NA (Univ of Texas, Houston)
Cancer 66:321–330, 1990   26–2

Up to 14% of primary thyroid carcinomas are anaplastic. Anaplastic carcinoma is extremely aggressive, with a 5-year survival rate of only 7.1% and a mean survival period of 6.2 months. Data were reviewed on 121 cases of anaplastic carcinoma of the thyroid.

The tumors were classified as either initial anaplastic or transformed anaplastic. In the latter category, the patients had received a diagnosis of well-differentiated thyroid carcinoma at presentation but anaplastic carcinoma developed subsequently. The stage of disease was categorized as "gland only," "gland and nodes," "gland, nodes, and neck," or "distant disese." Survival data were calculated from the time of tissue diagnosis. Immunohistochemical studies were performed on 30 tumors.

Patients ranged in age from 24 to 91 years (mean, 61.3 years); only 4 patients were younger than 40 years. There were 54 men and 67 women. The most common presentation was a rapidly enlarging neck mass, with or without previous goiter. In addition to anaplastic carcinoma, 35% of the patients had areas of well-differentiated thyroid carcinoma elsewhere and 53% had metastases. Of the metastases, 88% were to the lung and 15% to the bones. Tumors that consisted primarily of spindle cells contained cells having a sarcomatoid appearance; these were often arranged in fascicles similar to fibrosarcoma (Fig 26–3). Some tumors consisted primarily of large anaplastic cells containing single or multiple hyperpyknotic nuclei and eosinophilic cytoplasm that sometimes had a rhabdoid-like appearance (Fig 26–4). Of the 30 tumors analyzed, 84% stained for keratin, 93.3% stained for vimentin, and 33% stained for epithelial

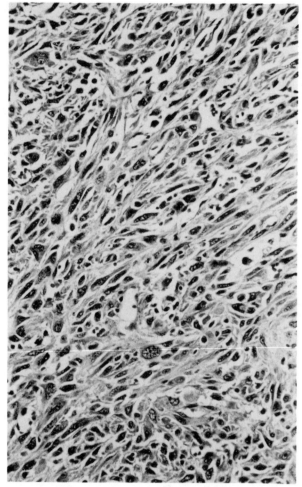

Fig 26–3.—Spindle cell growth pattern mimicking soft tissue sarcoma hematoxylin-eosin; original magnification, ×200. (Courtesy of Venkatesh YSS, Ordonez NG, Schultz PN, et al: *Cancer* 66:321–330, 1990.)

membrane antigen. Men and women had similar durations of survival. The mean survival of patients was 7.2 months, but younger patients lived longer than older patients, and those whose disease was in an earlier stage at presentation responded better to treatment than those with metastatic disease. The duration of survival was not increased significantly by radical surgery vs. less radical surgery. Ten of 12 long-term survivors received combined radiotherapy and chemotherapy postoperatively.

Anaplastic carcinoma has a bleak prognosis, but combined multimodality therapy may offer the possibility of long-term survival. The outcome is most hopeful in younger patients with less disease at the time of diagnosis.

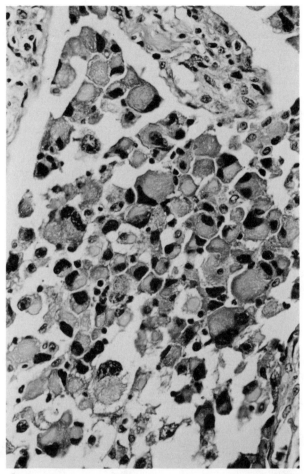

Fig 26–4.—Giant cell pattern. The cells have abundant eosinophilic cytoplasm and eccentric nuclei. Hematoxylin-eosin; original magnification, ×300. (Courtesy of Venkatesh YSS, Ordonez NG, Schultz PN, et al: *Cancer* 66:321–330, 1990.)

▶ We tell residents: Some day you are going to be called to the emergency room to see a patient with a huge mass in the neck who is severely dyspneic, nigh unto death, and someone will be standing there with a tracheostomy set urging you to provide a transtracheal airway. We say: Don't do it. These huge tumors are highly vascular, and many patients have bled to death while someone is attempting to establish a tracheostomy. These patients should be intubated and subjected to irradiation of the neck mass in hopes of shrinking the tumor sufficiently so as to allow removal of the endotracheal tube. As far as I know, surgery is never helpful, and recurrence is so rapid you can almost watch the tumor grow. Aggressive young surgeons often fail to heed admonitions of caution and proceed to operation, almost always making the patient worse.—J.C. Thompson, M.D.

Primary Hyperparathyroidism Associated With Two Enlarged Parathyroid Glands

Roses DF, Karp NS, Sudarsky LA, Valensi QJ, Rosen RJ, Blum M (New York Univ)

Arch Surg 124:1261–1265, 1989   26–3

A major issue in the surgical management of primary hyperparathyroidism is the extent to which all parathyroid glands should be identified and removed. Although most patients have an adenoma of a single parathyroid gland, others have involvement of more than 1 gland. Accurate assessment of abnormal glands may be difficult at surgery. Experience with 9 patients having 2 enlarged parathyroid glands was reviewed to assess criteria that might be used in managing such cases.

Five patients remained normocalcemic after both enlarged glands were excised at the initial operation, but 4 patients required a second operation. In 3 patients the second abnormal gland was not removed initially because it was only slightly enlarged. Hyperparathyroidism recurred in 2 patients after a period of normocalcemia following the first operation. Another patient had hypercalcemia immediately after the initial operation and was returned to surgery on the third postoperative day. The fourth patient underwent neck exploration and biopsy of 3 normal-appearing parathyroid glands. These glands were confirmed as normal, but levels of calcium remained elevated. A selective angiogram of the left internal mammary artery revealed a mass in the superior mediastinum (Fig 26–5), which was found to be an additional parathyroid gland. Removal of this gland resulted in an immediate return to normal serum levels of calcium.

Hyperplasia or neoplasia may affect parathyroid glands unevenly.

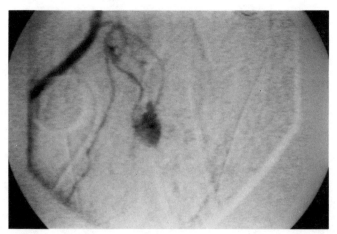

Fig 26–5.—Selective angiogram of left internal mammary artery (lateral view). Hypervascular mass within mediastinum supplied by a branch of left internal mammary artery is consistent with presence of parathyroid adenoma. (Courtesy of Roses DF, Karp NS, Sudarsky LA, et al: Arch Surg 124:1261–1265, 1989.)

Thus a leading cause of failure after surgery for primary hyperparathyroidism is the failure to detect and remove all affected glands. Even a slight enlargement of a parathyroid gland may be significant.

▶ The formerly clear lines of distinction between hyperplasia and adenomas of the parathyroid are becoming blurred. Most surgeons with interests of hyperparathyroidism have had the occasional experience of serially removing multiple enlarged parathyroid glands, each of which is labeled as an adenoma. The present series reports 9 patients with 2 enlarged glands, 5 of which were recognized at the initial procedure, but 4 of whom required second operation. Anyone operating for hyperparathyroidism should be aware of the need to identify all parathyroid glands. It is never safe to stop after identifying 1 large gland.— J.C. Thompson, M.D.

Clinical Characteristics and Surgical Treatment of Sporadic Primary Hyperparathyroidism With Emphasis on Chief Cell Hyperplasia
Wallfelt C, Ljunghall S, Bergström R, Rastad J, Åkerström G (Univ of Uppsala, Sweden)
Surgery 107:13–19, 1990   26–4

The number of operations for primary hyperparathyroidism (HPT) has increased. There is agreement on the liberal use of parathyroid surgery, but opinions vary on the optimal extent of parathyroid resection in patients with chief cell hyperplasia. The clinical characteristics and results of surgery in patients with sporadic primary HPT were investigated.

In a 28-year period, 437 female and 133 male patients underwent primary parathyroid exploration. The mean age was 59.3 years. Renal stone formation was more prevalent in men (58%) than in women (28%). Women were more likely than men to have neuromuscular and psychiatric symptoms (27% vs. 11%) and to have apparently asymptomatic HPT (31% vs. 11%). Younger (<50 years) patients had considerably more renal stone formation (75% vs. 25%) than older patients but fewer neuromuscular and psychiatric symptoms (14% vs. 29%).

Adenoma was diagnosed in most (78%) of the patients. Ninety-eight patients had chief cell hyperplasia, and 2 had parathyroid carcinoma. No histopathologic diagnosis was found in 24 patients. The serum calcium concentration was positively correlated to the glandular weight of both adenomas and hyperplasias. Renal stone disease was more common among patients with chief cell hyperplasia (47%) than among those with adenoma (32%).

After surgery, 91% of patients with adenoma and 80% of those with hyperplasia who were available for follow-up became normocalcemic. Failure in patients with adenoma resulted from difficulties in visualizing the parathyroid glands, whereas persistent and recurrent hypercalcemia seemed to increase with serum calcium values in patients with hyperplasia.

It appears sufficient to remove only the enlarged glands in hyperplasia with asymmetric and more markedly enlarged glands. In patients with more symmetrically or less enlarged hyperplastic glands, a subtotal 3- to 3.5-gland resection is recommended.

▶ This large series is interesting because of the high incidence of symptomatic hyperparathyroidism (69% of women and 89% of men were symptomatic). In the past 2 decades, most patients in the United States are operated on for asymptomatic hypercalcemia found incidentally on chemical screening. Ordinarily, parathyroid cancer is said to be responsible for 1% of hyperparathyroidism; if that is true, the incidence is low in this series (2/570). What is the significance of the finding that nephrolithiasis is more common in patients whose hyperparathyroidism is caused by chief cell hyperplasia rather than by adenoma? I find that hard to understand but difficult to dismiss in such a large series of patients.—J.C. Thompson, M.D.

Arteriographic Ablation of Cervical Parathyroid Adenomas
Pallotta JA, Sacks BA, Moller DE, Eisenberg H (Beth Israel Hosp, Boston; Harvard Med School)
J Clin Endocrinol Metab 69:1249–1255, 1989   26–5

An alternative to surgery may be needed in some patients with primary hyperparathyroidism, especially when neck exploration has been unsuccessful. The acute and chronic metabolic effects of angiographic destruction by angiographic contrast infusion of solitary parathyroid adenomas were studied in 18 patients with symptomatic disease. Fourteen had previously had unsuccessful surgery, and 4 were extremely high surgical risks. Seventeen patients had cervical adenomas and 1 had a mediastinal adenoma.

Selective parathyroid venous catheterization was done in 16 cases, which facilitated subsequent arteriographic localization. In all patients selective arteriographic localization and attempted ablation were done with standard contrast, renografin-60.

In all patients the serum level of calcium dropped to normal or subnormal within 48 hours of attempted ablation. A mean follow-up of 35 months showed that ablation was curative in 12 patients and partially effective in 1. Overall, the serum level of calcium dropped from 3.14 mmol/L at presentation to 2.42 mmol/L at the end of follow-up. Hypercalcemia recurred within 2 weeks in 4 of 5 failed cases. All 5 patients had curative surgery, which was aided by accurate localization during the angiographic procedure. There were several transient complications and in 1 case hypoparathyroidism was permanent.

Angiographic ablation of cervical parathyroid adenomas is a possible alternative to medical treatment or reoperation in patients in whom initial neck exploration has failed or who are extremely high surgical risks. However, the radiologic techniques are difficult, may produce serious complications, and should be attempted only by experienced angiographers at specialized centers. The consequences of failed ablation are negligible, and patients may go on to definitive surgery with the lesion well localized and displayed.

▶ The problem with this interesting technique is that it is only a matter of time (and that statement may be redundant) until aggressive angiographers convince someone that it should be tried primarily. In the setting described, i.e., in patients with unsuccessful previous operations or patients who are poor surgical risks, the procedure was helpful. The authors warning that the method may produce serious complications warrants careful attention. Attempts at ablation of tumors in other areas by injection of high concentrations of contrast material have often resulted in wide necrosis, with later massive hemorrhage.—J.C. Thompson, M.D.

Clinical Features of Adrenocortical Carcinoma, Prognostic Factors, and the Effect of Mitotane Therapy
Luton J-P, Cerdas S, Billaud L, Thomas G, Guilhaume B, Bertagna X, Laudat M-H, Louvel A, Chapuis Y, Blondeau P, Bonnin A, Bricaire H (Hôp Cochin; Hôp Fernand Widal; Hôp Broussais, Paris)
N Engl J Med 322:1195–1201, 1990   26–6

Data were reviewed on 105 patients referred to a single center with adrenocortical carcinoma in 1963–1987. A single group of physicians followed 88 patients for a mean time of 25 months; 80 of these patients were operated on, 57 curatively. Second operations were performed on 11 patients for locally recurrent disease; 59 surgically treated patients also received mitotane therapy.

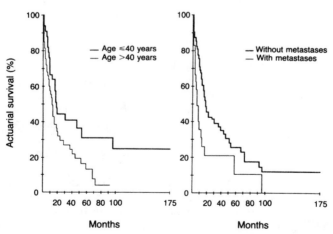

Fig 26–6.—Actuarial survival rates from the time of diagnosis in 88 patients with adrenocortical carcinoma, according to age and initial staging. For the comparison of the younger and older groups, $P = .035$ and the Tarone-Ware statistic = 4.467. For the comparison of patients with and without metastases, $P = .007$ and the Tarone-Ware statistic = 7.245. (Courtesy of Luton J-P, Cerdas S, Billaud L, et al: *N Engl J Med* 322:1195–1201, 1990.)

Patients were symptomatic for 9 months on average before diagnosis. Two thirds had endocrine symptoms at the time of diagnosis, and hormonal studies indicated that 79% of the tumors were functional. Distant metastases were noted at the time of presentation in 30% of patients.

The median disease-free interval after curative surgery was 1 year. More than 80% of the 67 deaths were caused by metastatic disease. Patients older than 40 years and those with distant metastases at diagnosis had significantly reduced survival (Fig 26–6). Disease regressed transiently in 8 of 37 evaluable patients given mitotane for 2 months or longer. Treatment did not significantly influence survival. Major side effects occurred in 12 patients as a result of mitotane therapy.

Mitotane should be used after aggressive surgery for adrenocortical carcinoma. It also is an appropriate reference treatment for use in controlled trials of other drugs. Although mitotane may control endocrine symptoms, the prognosis remains poor.

▶ This is an extraordinary series—an average of more than 4 patients per year for 24 years. As far as I know, this is the largest series reported and confirms the dismal outlook of the disease. The drug under test appeared to cause transient regression of tumor in some patients but did not effect cure in any. Preserved endocrine function supposedly indicates relative differentiation of the tumor, but 4 of every 5 of these tumors were functional, and the median survival was 14.5 months.—J.C. Thompson, M.D.

Gastrinoma Excision for Cure: A Prospective Analysis
Howard TJ, Zinner MJ, Stabile BE, Passaro E Jr (UCLA Ctr for the Health Sciences; West Los Angeles VA Hosp; San Diego VA Hosp)
Ann Surg 211:9–14, 1990   26–7

To determine the surgical cure rate for gastrinoma, 15 consecutive patients (mean age, 49 years), treated in a 6-year period, were studied prospectively. Criteria for surgery were sporadic gastrinoma without associated multiple endocrine neoplasia type I (MEN I) syndrome, no preoperative evidence of hepatic metastases, and an acceptable surgical risk. Because of MEN I syndrome or hepatic metastases, 4 patients were excluded from the study.

Long-term follow-up data were available for 8 of 11 surgical patients and an external historic control group of 11 patients. All patients in the control group had laparotomies, and tumor resection was attempted. The mean tumor size, incidence of multiple tumors, and occurrence of tumors in extrapancreatic/extraintestinal sites and within lymph nodes were similar in the 2 groups. All 24 tumors found were within the anatomical boundaries of the gastrinoma triangle (Fig 26–7).

The surgical cure rate was significantly greater in patients in the study group (82%) than in controls (27%). In contrast to the control group, all peptic ulcer complications in the study group occurred after the diagnosis of gastrinoma had been made. From a technical standpoint, the major

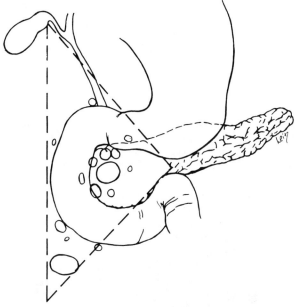

Fig 26–7.—Intra-abdominal location of 16 tumors found in 10 patients in the study group. (Courtesy of Howard TJ, Zinner MJ, Stabile BE, et al: *Ann Surg* 211:9–14, 1990.)

differences between the 2 groups were the thorough dissection and extensive tissue sampling performed in patients in the study group. Morbidity was acceptable (10%) in the study group, and no surgical deaths occurred. In selected patients, abdominal exploration and surgical excision for cure is the optimal treatment for gastrinoma.

▶ The Los Angeles group headed by Dr. Passaro has the highest incidence of gastrinoma excision for cure in the world. This prospective study provides the most optimistic outlook I have seen. The differences in the results of the 2 groups (study and control) is difficult to understand. Exactly what changes in technique led to the astounding differences in results? The authors have confirmed the high incidence of tumors in the so-called gastrinoma triangle. For "high incidence" in this study, read "exclusive appearance," because all of the tumors found were within the magic zone.

The high incidence of peptic ulcer complications seen in Zollinger-Ellison patients receiving long-term H$_2$-receptor antagonist therapy was confirmed (6 of 11 patients). It will be of great interest to follow those patients who have had resections that are apparently curative. Will they stayed cured?—J.C. Thompson, M.D.

Endogenous Peptide YY Is Dependent on Jejunal Exposure to Gastrointestinal Contents

Rudnicki M, McFadden DW, Liwnicz BH, Balasubramaniam A, Nussbaum MS, Dayal R, Fischer JE (Univ of Cincinnati College of Medicine; Cincinnati Dept of Veterans Affairs Med Ctr)

J Surg Res 48:485–490, 1990
26–8

Peptide YY (PYY), a polypeptide hormone sharing substantial sequence homology with pancreatic polypeptide, is released after colonic mucosal stimulation by bile and fatty acids. The roles of the proximal jejunum and biliary system in regulating and circulating PYY were examined in rats, and the distribution of PYY-containing cells was studied in the rat intestine.

Groups of rats underwent proximal jejunal bypass, Roux-en-Y cholangiojejunostomy, and sham surgery. Feeding studies were performed using mixed and pure fat meals 3 months postoperatively in unanesthetized animals. Plasma PYY was estimated by radioimmunoassay.

A mixed meal produced a significant increase in plasma PYY in control animals only. The fat meal had a similar effect in control rats. In bile-diverted animals with a Roux-en-Y anastomosis, the fat meal produced a significant but delayed increase in plasma PYY. The PYY-containing cells increased distally along the bowel. Both experimental groups had fewer such cells in the proximal/bypassed jejunum than were present in comparable areas of the bowel in sham-operated rats.

Release of PYY may depend in part on stimulatory neural or endocrine signals emanating from the proximal jejunum. Bile may modulate its release but does not seem to be a primary factor.

▶ Peptide YY appears to be important in feedback suppression of gastric and pancreatic secretion. The impressive early release of PYY after a meal is something of an enigma because major PYY stores are located in the distal small bowel and proximal colon. Clearly, some signal—we believe it to be endocrine—is released from the proximal bowel on eating. Peptide YY and neurotensin, and probably enteroglucagon (whatever that is), qualify the colon as an endocrine organ.—J.C. Thompson, M.D.

Combined Computerized Tomography and Angiography in the Diagnosis of Insulinoma

Merine DS, Fishman EK, Siegelman SS (Johns Hopkins Med Insts)

South Med J 83:595–596, 1990
26–9

Computed tomography, angiography, and transhepatic venous sampling have all been used for preoperative assessment of insulinoma. The best reported sensitivity for CT has been 66% and that for angiography, 80%. Combined CT and angiography (CTA) were used to show the presence and extent of pancreatic insulinoma.

Woman, 43, had a 10-month history of hypoglycemic symptoms. Fasting hypoglycemia was diagnosed on the basis of simultaneous insulin and glucose assays. Abdominal CT scan with contrast showed a normal pancreatic contour and no evidence of a mass. Celiac arteriography was suboptimal, but there was suggestion of a hypervascular mass in the body of the pancreas. Visualization with CTA showed a 1.5-cm hypervascular mass arising at the junction of the head and body of the pancreas. No other lesions were visible, and there was no evidence of metastatic disease. A 1.5-cm mass was palpated in the body of the pancreas at laparotomy. The patient underwent distal pancreatectomy and splenectomy. Pathologic examination of the resected specimen revealed a well-circumscribed 1.5-cm nodule in the pancreas. Histopathologic evaluation was consistent with insulinoma. The postoperative course was uneventful, and the patient has had no recurrence of hypoglycemia.

In this case, pancreatic insulinoma was diagnosed by combined CT and angiography. In selected cases, CTA is preferable to dynamic enhanced CT in the detection of small pancreatic islet cell tumors.

► By and large, results with CT (plain or enhanced) have not been favorable because of the small size of most lesions. Endocrine surgeons have waited anxiously for some tests that would provide clear localization of insulinomas. Because 10% of insulinomas are multiple, how do we know that a small tumor is not present that will later develop autonomous function? We don't know, and we never do whenever we take out an insulinoma. We must always search for multiple foci.—J.C. Thompson, M.D.

Effects of Hemipancreatectomy on Insulin Secretion and Glucose Tolerance in Healthy Humans
Kendall DM, Sutherland DER, Najarian JS, Goetz FC, Robertson RP (Univ of Minnesota)
N Engl J Med 322:898–903, 1990   26–10

Since 1977, tissue taken from healthy donors by hemipancreatectomy has been transplanted into recipients having type I diabetes. The metabolic consequences were examined in 28 donors a year after hemipancreatectomy using the oral glucose tolerance test and 24-hour monitoring of the serum glucose and urinary C-peptide levels. All donors were adults and at least 10 years above the age at which diabetes developed in the recipient. The 20 women and 8 men had a mean age of 34 at the time of hemipancreatectomy.

The mean fasting serum level of glucose was significantly higher a year after hemipancreatectomy (5.4 mM/L vs. 4.9 mM/L), as was the serum glucose level 2 hours after oral administration of glucose (Fig 26–8). Fasting serum insulin levels were lower than at baseline, as was the case for the area under the insulin curve during oral glucose tolerance testing. Urinary C-peptide excretion was lower after hemipancreatectomy. Seven subjects had abnormal glucose tolerance, but none had a fasting serum

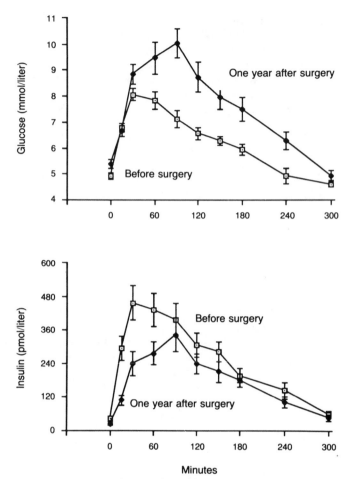

Fig 26–8.—Mean (± SE) serum glucose and serum insulin levels, measured before and 1 year after hemipancreatectomy, during 5-hour oral glucose-tolerance tests in 28 transplant donors. (Courtesy of Kendall DM, Sutherland DER, Najarian JS, et al: *N Engl J Med* 322:898–903, 1990.)

glucose level above 7.8 mM/L. All subjects had a normal mean 24-hour plasma glucose level. Hemipancreatectomy diminishes glucose tolerance, but it is not clear whether clinical diabetes is an inherent risk of the procedure.

▶ I am sure that everyone who read about these pancreatic donors wondered how they would fare. This careful study shows that they have, indeed, sustained significant loss of endocrine function. Because diabetes is relatively common, one must face what appears to be the inevitable consequence—giving up half of your pancreas may convert later subclinical diabetes to a major problem. This all must be viewed in perspective: We are almost certainly currently going through a phase before development of effective techniques for isolation of human pancreatic islets. The ultimate treatment of diabetes will almost certainly depend on selective transplantation of islet tissue alone. Everyone would hope that this will relieve the necessity of living-related donor procedures.—J.C. Thompson, M.D.

Subject Index

A

Abdomen (*see* Intraabdominal)
Acid
  aspiration-induced organ injury
    mediated by TNF-α, 21
Acoustic
  properties of skin and wound and tissue
    constituents, 141
Adenocarcinoma
  of ampulla of Vater, spread of, 379
  appendix, primary, 323
  lung, K-*ras* oncogene in, 137
Adenoma
  colorectal, dysplasia in, patient and
    polyp characteristics, 327
  parathyroid, cervical, arteriographic
    ablation of, 400
Adrenal
  cortex carcinoma, mitotane in, 401
Aerodigestive tract
  upper, synchronous and
    metasynchronous cancer, 168
Aged
  burn care in, 84
  trauma, outcome, 33
Aging
  duodenal bicarbonate secretion and,
    304
Air
  embolism, arterial, in penetrating lung
    injury, 180
  transport, critical care, in severe injury,
    survival, 27
Albumin
  in prime for cardiopulmonary bypass,
    outcome, 233
Alcoholic cirrhosis (*see* Cirrhosis,
  alcoholic)
Allograft (*see* Transplantation)
Alopecia
  burn, tissue expansion in, 85
Amino acids
  branched-chain vs. standard, in
    parenteral nutrition, 8
Ampulla of Vater
  adenocarcinoma spread, 379
Amputation
  in peripheral vascular disease, wound
    healing in, 57
Anastomosis
  colorectal, stapling in, 334
  end-to-end, for coarctation of aorta
    correction in infant, 197
  of intestine, small, duodenojejunostomy
    as alternative to, 311

Aneurysm
  aortic, small abdominal, expansion rate
    and outcome, 264
  ascending aorta and transverse aortic
    arch, surgery of, 253
  false, after prosthesis for aortoiliac
    obstruction, 266
Angiography
  with CT of insulinoma, 404
Angioplasty, coronary
  failure, myocardial salvage after, 225
  percutaneous transluminal
    failure, coronary artery bypass in,
      outcome, 226
    practice patterns, 224
Angioscopy
  intraoperative, and completion
    arteriography in femorodistal
    bypass, 275
Anomalies
  bronchopulmonary, congenital, 190
Anorectal
  melanoma, characteristics and surgery
    results, 336
Antibacterial
  drug delivery into fibrotic cavities, 73
Antibiotic(s)
  intraperitoneal, by liposomal carrier, 74
  prophylaxis
    perioperative, for herniorrhaphy and
      breast surgery, 4
    in trauma, underdosing, 32
Antibody(ies)
  -dependent cellular cytotoxicity in
    kidney transplant, 94
  to interleukin-2 receptor, 123
  monoclonal (*See* Monoclonal antibody)
  -*Pseudomonas* exotoxin A in marrow
    elimination from breast cancer, 126
Anti-CD3
  in combination immunotherapy, 122
Anti-CD4
  monoclonal antibody in kidney
    transplant (in monkey), 107
Antigen(s)
  carcinoembryonic, monitoring in colon
    cancer, 135
  Epstein-Barr virus-associated, in B cell
    disorders after immunosuppression,
    114
  HLA-DR, in trauma outcome, 54
  major histocompatibility complex, in
    thyroid transplant, 97
  papilloma virus, in colon cancer, 134
  xero antigen-matched cyclosporine-
    treated kidney transplant, survival,
    89

Author Index